Heg PocketGuide to Treatment in Speech-Language Pathology

Second Edition

M. N. Hegde, Ph.D.

Department of Communicative Sciences and Disorders
California State University-Fresno

SINGULAR

™

THOMSON LEARNING

Hegde's PocketGuide to Treatment in Speech-Language Pathology, Second Edition
by M. N. Hegde, Ph.D.

Business Unit Director:
William Brottmiller

Acquisitions Editor:
Marie Linvill

Development Editor:
Kristin Banach

Executive Marketing Manager:
Dawn Gerrain

Channel Manager:
Tara Carter

Production Manager:
Barbara Bullock

Production Editor:
Sandy Doyle

Library of Congress Cataloging-in-Publication Data

Hegde, M. N. (Mahabalagiri N.), 1941–
   Hegde's pocketGuide to assessment in speech-language pathology / by M. N. Hegde.—2nd ed.
     p. ; cm.
   Rev. ed. of: PocketGuide to assessment in speech-language pathology. c1996.
   Includes bibliographical references.
   ISBN 0-7693-0158-4 (softcover : alk. paper)
   1. Speech disorders— Diagnosis—Handbooks, manuals, etc. I. Title: PocketGuide to assessment in speech-language pathology. II. Hegde, M. N. (Mahabalagiri N.) 1941–
   PocketGuide to assessment in speech-language pathology. III. Title.
   [DNLM: 1. Speech Disorders—diagnosis— Handbooks. 2. Language Disorders—diagnosis— Handbooks. WL 39 H462h 2001]
   RC423 .H38286 2001
   616.85'5075—dc21
                              00-049225

ABBREVIATED CONTENTS: ENTRIES BY DISORDERS

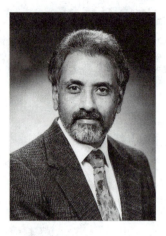

M. N. (Giri) Hegde is Professor of Communicative Sciences and Disorders at California State University-Fresno. He holds a master's degree in Experimental Psychology from the University of Mysore, India, a post-master's diploma in Medical (Clinical) Psychology from Bangalore University, India, and a doctoral degree in Speech-Language Pathology from Southern Illinois University at Carbondale.

A specialist in fluency disorders, language disorders, research designs, and treatment procedures in communicative disorders, Dr. Hegde has made numerous scientific and professional presentations to national and international audiences. He has extensive clinical and research experience and has published research articles on a wide range of subjects, including fluency and language, their disorders, and treatment. Dr. Hegde has authored or co-authored several highly regarded and widely used scientific and professional books, including *Clinical Research in Communicative Disorders, Introduction to Communicative Disorders, Treatment Procedures in Communicative Disorders, Treatment Protocols in Communicative Disorders, A Coursebook on Scientific and Professional Writing in Speech-Language Pathology, Clinical Methods and Practicum in Speech-Language Pathology, A Pocket-Guide to Assessment in Speech-Language-Pathology, A Singular Manual of Textbook Preparation, A Coursebook on Language Disorders in Children, An Advanced Review of Speech-Language Pathology,* and *Assessment and Treatment of Articulation and Phonological Disorders in Children.* He is the Editor of the Singular Textbook Series and has served on the editorial boards of several scientific and professional journals. Dr. Hegde has received many honors and awards, including the Distinguished Alumnus Award from Southern Illinois University Department of Communication Sciences and Disorders, Outstanding Professor Award from California State University-Fresno, Outstanding Professional Achievement Award from District Five of California Speech-Language-Hearing Association, and Fellowship in the American Speech-Language-Hearing Association.

Preface

The second edition of this PocketGuide to treatment procedures in speech-language pathology has been updated and expanded by more than 100 pages. Information on ethnocultural variables that affect treatment has been added under each disorder and the steps involved in administering certain treatment procedures are described in more detail in the second edition. Simultaneous revision of the companion volume, *Hegde's PocketGuide to Assessment in Speech-Language Pathology* has also helped to streamline the information in the two books.

This PocketGuide to treatment procedures in speech-language pathology has been designed for clinical practitioners and students in communicative disorders. The PocketGuide combines the most desirable features of a specialized dictionary of terms, clinical resource book, and textbooks and manuals on treatment. It is meant to be a quick reference book like a dictionary because the entries are alphabetized; but it offers more than a dictionary because it specifies treatment procedures in a "do this" format. The PocketGuide is like a resource book in that it avoids theoretical and conceptual aspects of procedures presented; but it offers more than a resource book by clearly specifying the steps involved in treating clients. The PocketGuide is like standard textbooks that describe treatment procedures; but it organizes the information in a manner conducive to more ready use. By avoiding theoretical background and controversies, the PocketGuide gives the essence of treatment in a step-by-step format that promotes easy understanding and ready reference just before beginning treatment. The PocketGuide does not suggest that theoretical and research issues are not important in treating clients; it just assumes that the user is familiar with them.

How the PocketGuide is Organized
Each main entry is printed in bold and burgundy color. Each cross-referenced entry is underlined in burgundy. Each main

disorder of communication is entered in its alphabetical order. Subcategories or types of a given disorder are described under the main entry (e.g., *Broca's Aphasia* under *Aphasia*).

Specific techniques, most of them with general applicability across disorders (e.g., *Modeling, Biofeedback,* or *Turn Taking*) also are alphabetized. Such specific techniques generally are described at their main alphabetical entry (e.g., *Modeling* under M). When appropriate, the reader also is referred to the disorders for which the techniques are especially appropriate.

For most disorders, a general and composite treatment procedure is described first. For example, there is a general treatment program described for *Stuttering, Treatment* or *Language Disorders in Children.* Following this description of a generic treatment procedure, specific techniques or treatment programs are described (e.g., treating auditory comprehension problems in aphasia, pragmatic problems in language disorders in children, or rate reduction in stuttering; and such treatment programs as *Helm Elicited Program for Syntax Stimulation* or the *Monterey Fluency Program*). Organization of entries varies somewhat for different disorders, but an example of a general organization used in the guide follows:

Articulation and Phonological Disorders. (Definition)
  A General Articulation Treatment Procedure
  Treatment of Articulation and Phonological Disorders: Specific
    Techniques or Programs
    Behavioral Approaches
    Contrast Approach
    Cycles Approach
    Distinctive Feature Approach
    Multiple Phoneme Approach
    Paired Stimuli Approach
    Phonological Knowledge Approach
    Phonological Process Approach
    Sensory Motor Approach
    Traditional Approach

Preface

Many treatment concepts and procedures are cross-referenced. All cross-referenced entries are underlined in burgundy. Therefore, the reader who comes across an underlined term can look up that term in a different place or context.

How to Use This PocketGuide

There are two methods for the clinician to use this guide. In the **first method**, the clinician looks up treatment procedures by disorders in their alphabetical order; an **Abbreviated Contents: Entries by Disorders** on page v will quickly refer the reader to specific communication disorders described in the guide. Treatment procedures of the following major disorders are described in their alphabetical order:

> Aphasia
> Apraxia of Speech
> Articulation and Phonological Disorders
> Cerebral Palsy
> Cleft Palate
> Cluttering
> Dementia
> Dysarthria
> Dysphagia
> Hearing Impairment
> Language Disorders in Children
> Laryngectomy
> Right Hemisphere Syndrome
> Stuttering
> Traumatic Brain Injury
> Voice Disorders

Under each of the main entries for major disorders, the clinician may look up subentries or specific types of disorders. For example, under **Dysarthria**, the clinician will find the following alphabetized subentries and their treatment procedures:

Ataxic Dysarthria
Flaccid Dysarthria
Hyperkinetic Dysarthria
Hypokinetic Dysarthria
Mixed Dysarthria
Spastic Dysarthria
Unilateral Upper Motor Neuron Dysarthria

In the **second method**, the clinician looks up treatment procedures by **their name**. For example, the clinician can look up such specific treatment techniques as the following in their alphabetic order:

Activity-Based Language Intervention
Airflow Management in Stuttering
Augmentative Communication
Behavioral Momentum
Child-Centered Approaches to Language
Intervention
Collaborative Model
Conversational Repair
Delayed Auditory Feedback
Differential Reinforcement of Alternative Behaviors
(DRA)
Environmental Language Intervention Strategy
Event Structure
Functional Equivalence Training
Joint-Action Routines
Incidental Teaching Method
Isolated Therapy Model
Mand-Model
Melodic Intonation Therapy
Narrative Skills Training
Prolonged Speech

Preface

Rate Reduction in Treating Dysarthria

Whole Language Approach

and so forth.

If appropriate, the reader who finds a specific treatment technique in the general alphabetized order is referred to the specific disorder for which the technique is relevant.

A Caveat

Serious attempts have been made to include most treatment techniques described in the literature. However, the author is aware that not all techniques have been included. Some have been excluded because of their transparent lack of logic, appropriateness, or even an expectation of desirable effects. A few are defined because they are popular or being advocated. However, they are not described fully because of the presence of strong negative evidence. Most important, in any task such as this that requires encyclopedic review of literature, omission of a procedure that deserves inclusion is an acknowledged and unintended limitation. The reader may be more often correct in assuming that a technique was omitted inadvertently than to assume that it was considered and rejected.

The author did not set for himself the impossible goal of including all treatment techniques. The practical goal was shaped more by such descriptors or qualifiers of treatment techniques as the *most,* the *major,* the *generally effective,* the *most widely* practiced, and so forth. Such qualifiers necessarily involve judgment, with which clinicians will disagree. If some techniques included do not meet these qualifiers, that is fine; the author would rather err in that direction. Conversely, errors of omission are correctable through future revisions of this book. Therefore, the author is open to suggestions from clinicians and researchers.

Although most treatment techniques in communicative disorder are in need of treatment effectiveness or efficacy data, those that are especially deficient are noted in their description or definition. Those treatment techniques that have especially strong supportive evidence also are noted. In most cases, unfortunately, information on effects and efficacy is unavailable or ambiguous. This guide is not a means of evaluating treatment techniques; such evaluation is solely the responsibility of the clinician who selects treatment techniques. To help the clinician make such evaluations, procedures and experimental designs that are used in treatment efficacy research are included in this guide. Also included are suggested *Treatment Selection Criteria.*

Abbreviation Used Throughout the Book
PGASLP: Hegde's PocketGuide to Assessment in Speech-Language Pathology (2nd ed.) by M. N. Hegde (2001). San Diego, CA: Singular Thomson Learning.

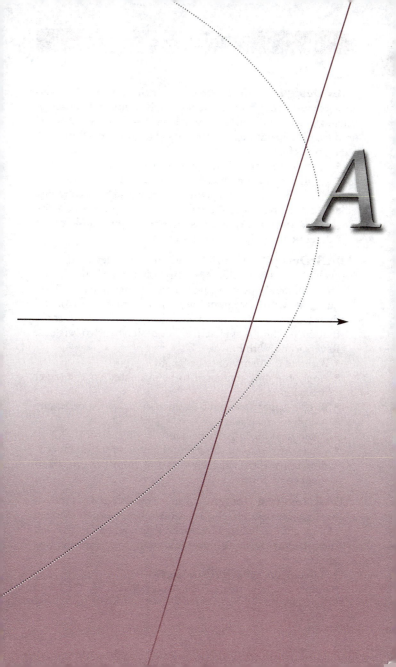

A

ABA Design. A single-subject research design used to evaluate treatment effects; a target behavior is first baserated (A), taught with the procedure to be evaluated (B), and then reduced (A) by withdrawing treatment to show that the teaching was effective.

- Baserate the target behavior to be taught
- Apply the new treatment to be evaluated
- When the target behavior increases, withdraw treatment
- Chart the results to show that the results for the baserate and withdrawal conditions were similar but those for the treatment condition were different.

ABAB Design. A single-subject research design used to evaluate treatment efficacy; a target behavior is first baserated (A), taught by applying the treatment program (B), reduced by withdrawing or reversing the treatment (A), and then taught again by reapplying the treatment (B) to show that the teaching was effective. The design has two versions: Reversal and Withdrawal.

- Baserate the behavior to be taught
- Apply the new treatment to be evaluated for the target behavior
- Briefly, apply treatment to another behavior or simply withdraw treatment
- Again treat the target behavior
- Chart the results to show that the two no treatment conditions were convincingly different from the two treatment conditions.

ABAB Reversal Design. A single-subject design for evaluating treatment effects; a desirable behavior is baserated (A), taught (B), reduced by teaching its counterpart (A), and then taught again (B) to show that the teaching was effective.

- Baserate the behavior to be taught
- Apply the new treatment to be evaluated for the target behavior

- Briefly, apply treatment to an incompatible behavior
- Again treat the target behavior
- Chart the results to show that the behavior varied according to the treatment and reversal operations

ABAB Withdrawal Design.   A single-subject research design for evaluating treatment effects; a desirable behavior is baserated (A), taught (B), reduced by withdrawing the treatment (A), and then taught again (B) to show that teaching was effective.

- Baserate the target behavior to be taught
- Apply the new treatment to be evaluated
- When the behavior increases, withdraw treatment
- Reapply treatment to the target behavior
- Chart the results to show that the behavior varied according to the treatment and withdrawal operations

Hegde, M. N. (1994). *Clinical research in communicative disorders: Principles and strategies* (2nd ed.). Austin, TX: Pro-Ed.

Abduction.   Separation of the vocal folds.

Adduction.   Approximation of the vocal folds.

Agraphia.   Loss or impairment of writing skills associated with cerebral pathology or injury; may be associated with reading problems (Alexia); not the same as writing problems found in children; often found in patients with aphasia; for treatment procedures, see Treatment of Aphasia: Writing Problems; see *PGASLP* for description of different types and assessment procedures.

Airflow Management.   A stuttering treatment target; includes inhalation of air, slight exhalation before initiating phonation, and sustained air flow throughout an utterance; for procedures see Stuttering, Treatment; Treatment of Stuttering: Specific Techniques or Programs.

Alaryngeal Speech.   Speech without a biological larynx; a mode of communication for persons whose larynges have been surgically removed; may be electronically assisted, pneumatically assisted, or esophageal; for treatment procedures, see Laryngectomy.

Alerting Stimuli. Various means of drawing the client's attention to the imminent treatment stimuli; include such statements as "Get ready! Here comes the picture!" or "Look at me, I am about to show you how," or such nonverbal cues as touching the client's hand just before presenting a stimulus.

Alexia. Reading problems in children and adults; in children, often due to inadequate instruction or learning disabilities; in adults, often due to neurological problems and is associated with aphasia, dementia, and related disorders; some use the term dyslexia synonymous with alexia; others apply the term dyslexia to reading problems in children whose instruction is adequate; may be associated with writing problems (Agraphia) in some, isolated in others; for treatment of alexia in patients with neurological communication disorders, see Treatment of Aphasia: Reading Problems; see *PGASLP* for description of different types of alexia and their assessment.

Alphabet Board. A communication board with the alphabet printed on it; may also contain a few words and sentences; the client simultaneously speaks and points to the first letter of each spoken word printed and displayed on the board; helps slow down the rate of speech in clients whose speech rate is excessive (e.g., clients with hypokinetic dysarthria).

Alphabet Board Supplementation. A technique used in reducing the speech rate and thus improving intelligibility in clients with dysarthria; to reduce rate, the method requires clients to point to the first letter of each word on an alphabet board.

- Arrange an alphabet board with large capital letters
- Ask the client to point to the first letter of each word to be spoken on the board

Yorkston, K. M., Beukelman, D. R., Strand, E. A., & Bell, K. R. (1999). *Management of motor speech disorders in children and adults.* Austin, TX: Pro-Ed.

Alternating Motion Rates (AMR). A measure of the speed with which certain syllables (e.g., "puh, puh, puh") are repeated when asked to; the same as the diadochokinetic rate; used in the assessment of dysarthria or articulation disorders in children; see *PGASLP* for assessment procedures.

Alternative Communication. Methods of nonoral, nonvocal communication that serve as alternatives to oral speech and language; only in a few extreme cases are the methods totally alternative; most nonoral, nonvocal means of communication augment oral and vocal communication; treatment techniques described under Augmentative Communication, a term some prefer.

Alzheimer's Disease. A degenerative neurological disorder caused by Neurofibrillary Tangles, Neuritic Plaques, Granulovacuolar Degeneration, and neurochemical changes; characterized by deterioration in behavior, cognition, memory, language, communication, and personality; most common of the irreversible dementias; consider the following suggestions and see Dementia for management details:

Management of Patients With Alzheimer's Disease: General Guidelines

- A thorough assessment of not only the patient, but also of the family resources and needs is necessary before rehabilitation can be started; see the cited sources and the *PGASLP*
- Management of symptoms and behaviors of the patient for as long as possible is a practical clinical goal of rehabilitation
- Counseling and supporting the family and teaching them the skills to cope with the disease are important elements of rehabilitation

- Finding resources and services for disadvantaged families and ethnoculturally diverse families is a part of rehabilitation
- Putting the family in touch with local support groups and national information centers on dementia and Alzheimer's disease is useful to the families
- Some patients with Alzheimer's disease may have a slow progression with several years of relatively stable behavior patterns; rehabilitation efforts with such patients and their families may be especially productive
- Family members and caregivers should not automatically assume that a patient with Alzheimer's disease is incapable of making decisions in the early and middle stages of the disease

Working With Caregivers and Family Members

Ask caregivers and family members to:

- Use good lighting when communicating with the patient, especially if the patient has a visual-perceptual deficit
- Initiate interaction in a helpful manner
  - approach the patient within his or her visual field; do not surprise the patient
  - establish eye contact before speaking
  - always identify yourself before you start saying something; remind the patient about your earlier encounters, activities done together, and so forth
  - speak slowly to the patient
- Keep communication at a simple level but not overly simplified
  - keep your instructions simple and direct
  - use gestures, smile, and posture to enhance your verbal communication
  - ask the patient to do one thing at a time; avoid multiple and sequentially given commands
  - speak clearly

- be redundant, restate important information
- keep topic familiar and observable
- speak in simple, short sentences
- repeat instructions every time you ask a patient to do something
- have all caregiving staff use similar expressions, directions, and instructions
- always say "good-bye" or give other departing signals
- Be consistent with standard expressions
  - use the same spoken phrases to inform the client about routine tasks (e.g., say, "Let's go out" when it is time to go out and say "Your food is ready" when it is time to eat)
  - use the same greetings every morning
  - use the same phrase at night (e.g., "Good night" or "Let's go to bed")
- Make sure the patient understood what you just said before saying more
  - ask questions about what you just said
  - let the patient restate what you said
  - ask questions about actions you asked the patient to perform
- Keep the patient's day structured
  - reduce variability in daily activities
  - schedule activities at the same times every day (e.g., serve meals at the same time every day; have specific times for bathing; wake up the patient the same time every morning; schedule recreational activities for the same time every day)
- Simplify the patient's living environment
  - remove unnecessary items or objects the patient does not use from the bedroom
  - remove unnecessary clothing items from the closet and the chest of drawers

- keep only the shoes he or she uses
- reduce desktop, coffee table, and countertop clutter
- Provide printed prompts for actions
  - print the patient's daily schedule on a poster board
  - post it in more than one, conspicuous place
  - teach the patient to consult the schedule frequently (note that just posting notices may not do any good to the patient who may not consult them)
  - print only the essential information; keep displays simple
- Help support the patient's continued orientation to time, place, persons, and events
  - help support the patient's familiar activities, interests, and hobbies (let the patient watch his or her familiar TV shows, listen to music, engage in recreational activities)
  - make recent pictures of family members, family cars, home, and so forth and show them frequently to the patient to help keep orientation
  - frequently ask orientation questions (e.g., "Where are you?" "What day is it today?" "What time is it?"); reinforce the patient's correct answers; model and have the client imitate correct answers if the responses are incorrect
  - ask multiple choice questions about orientation (e.g., "Is this Friday or Saturday?" "Are you at home or in a hospital?")
  - post printed signs about the place, date, month, and year in clear view of the patient and in multiple settings; teach the patient to use them frequently
  - frequently remind the patient about the day, date, time, month, and so forth
  - post a larger calendar the patient can see often and mark the current day with a color border or some such device

- keep up the patient's habit of looking at the clocks and reading the time; reinforce the client for correctly reading the time
- keep a map of frequently visited places (e.g., homes of relatives and friends, shops, restaurants)
- when prompting the patient to perform an action or attend an event, remind him or her of the day and time as well (e.g., "It's 3 o'clock on Tuesday; time to watch the ------ show on TV.")
- note that orientation problems are confounded with memory impairments; therefore, help sustain memory skills to the extent possible
- Minimize stimulation and reduce the frequency of events that disrupt the patient's behaviors
  - reduce noise and loud music
  - have only a few people visit at any one time
  - reduce or eliminate loud and big parties
  - eliminate any chaotic situation
  - teach grandchildren to play more quietly around the patient
- Reduce or eliminate products and situations that pose danger to the patient
  - lower the thermostat on the hot water heater to reduce the danger of burning while taking a shower
  - keep all chemical cleaners, medications, manual and power tools (e.g., hammers, all kinds of saws, lawn mowers, grass edgers, sledgehammers and such other tools in the garage) out of the patient's reach and preferably under lock and key
  - remove stove knobs or install special devices to turn them on
  - keep the family car keys in a secured place

Direct Management of Communication and Memory Skills

- Teach superordinate category names (e.g., *tools* and *furniture*) instead of basic level names (e.g., *socket*

wrench and *footstool*) because superordinate category names appear to be relatively unaffected
- Teach compensatory strategies for lost functions
- Teach gestures as a means of communicating
- Use intensive auditory stimulation
- Provide new information that is an extension of the familiar
- Develop a theme for each treatment session
- Use praise that is appropriate for an adult
- Speak slowly during direct treatment sessions
- Wait for a sign that the client has understood before progressing to the next topic
- Manage the memory skills
  - teach the client to use a Memory Log
  - use techniques described under Memory Impairments
- See Dementia for additional suggestions

Brookshire, R. H. (1997). *Introduction to neurogenic communication disorders* (5th ed.). St. Louis, MO: Mosby.

Hegde, M. N. (1998). *A coursebook on aphasia and other neurogenic language disorders* (2nd ed.). San Diego: Singular Publishing Group.

American Indian Hand Talk (AMER-IND). A system of nonverbal communication used by Native Americans to communicate with members of other tribes with different languages; a manual interlanguage; the signs represent ideas and many are pictographic; gestures may be produced in series to express more complex ideas, called agglutination; many signs are one-handed; used in teaching Augmentative Communication, Gestural (Unaided).

American Sign Language (ASL or AMESLAN). A highly developed manual (gestural) language used mostly by deaf persons in the United States; a communication target for certain nonverbal or minimally verbal persons; each sign or gesture may represent a letter of the English alphabet, a word, or a phrase; signs provide phonemic, morphologic, and syntactic information; used in teaching <u>Augmentative Communication, Gestural (Unaided)</u>.

Amyotrophic Lateral Sclerosis (ASL).   A progressive neurological disease in which the upper and lower motor neurons degenerate; initial symptoms vary depending on the neurons involved, but in the final stages all levels of motor neurons are involved; symptoms of the final stage include severe impairment of movement; one of the several causes of dysarthria.

Analogies.   Logical inferences that are based on the assumption that if two things are similar in certain aspects, then they must be alike in other aspects.

Anomia.   Difficulty in naming people, places, or things; a major symptom of <u>Aphasia</u>.

Antecedents.   Events that occur before responses; stimuli or events the clinician presents in treatment. Antecedents may be:
- Objects
- Pictures
- Re-created or enacted events
- Instructions, demonstrations, modeling, prompting, manual guidance, and other special stimuli

Aphasia.   A language disorder caused by recent brain injury in which (a) all aspects of language comprehension and production are impaired to varying degrees (a nontypological definition); (b) one or more aspects of language comprehension and language production may be affected (a typological definition).

Treatment of Aphasia: General Guidelines
- Conduct a detailed assessment; see the cited sources and *PGASLP*
- Reduce the effects of the residual deficits on the personal, emotional, social, family, and occupational aspects of the client's life

- Teach compensatory strategies (e.g., signing, gestures)
- Counsel family members to help them cope with the residual deficits
- Give a realistic prognosis that modifies the clients' and the family members' expectations
- Structure the treatment and let the client repeatedly practice the target behaviors
- Develop a variety of client-specific treatment procedures
- Exploit the client's strengths (e.g., use the stronger visual mode to supplement the weaker auditory mode)
- Judge when it is not useful or ethical to continue the treatment
- Observe the client carefully
- Choose client-specific target behaviors that enhance functional communication rather than grammatical correctness
- Sequence target behaviors in treatment
- Move from simple to complex tasks
- Use such extra stimuli as instructions, prompts, modeling, pictures, and objects in initial stages of treatment
- Fade extra stimuli used in treatment
- Use only natural stimuli (e.g., only a question, not a prompt) to evoke speech in later stages of treatment
- Program natural consequences for functional communication targets (e.g., smile and approval to reinforce verbal expressions; real objects to reinforce requests for objects)
- Provide immediate, response-contingent feedback
- Encourage the client to self-monitor
- Train family members to evoke, prompt, reinforce, and maintain communicative behaviors

Treatment of Aphasia: Ethnocultural Guidelines

Consider the ethnocultural, linguistic, and economic background of the client in planning treatment. There is little or no controlled experimental research on the effectiveness of different treatment approaches when applied to different ethnocultural clients with aphasia. However, the clinician should:

- Gain an understanding of the client's family and its economic resources to pay for extended treatment, afford regular transportation, ability and willingness to keep regular appointments
- Help find public and private resources that support a client's continued treatment and rehabilitation
- Assess the family members' educational level, emphasis on communication skills, and their willingness and time available for helping the client
- Understand the client's family constellation and communication patterns (e.g., living in an extended family; the client's role in educating and raising grandchildren)
- Evaluate client's linguistic background and especially if the client speaks a different dialect or form of standard English (e.g., African American English or Spanish-influenced English); premorbid literacy level and the current need for literacy skills (e.g., Does the client need treatment for reading and writing or will functional communication suffice?)
- Assess communication needs of a bilingual client in both languages or, at the least, in the dominant language
- Select treatment targets that are functional and effective in the client's natural environment and are appropriate for the communicative needs of the client and the family
- Select treatment stimuli that are available in the client's home, and, if appropriate, work environment
- Carefully describe the treatment procedures and note the effects they produce or fail to produce; modify the treatment procedure in light of the client's performance and ethnocultural background

Payne, J. C. (1997). *Adult neurogenic language disorders: Assessment and treatment.* San Diego: Singular Publishing Group.

Treatment of Aphasia: Auditory Comprehension

In planning auditory comprehension treatment, consider the following **factors that promote better comprehension** in an aphasic patient:

- More frequently used words
- Nouns rather than verbs, adjectives, and adverbs
- Picturable verbs and other words
- Unambiguous pictures
- Shorter sentences
- Syntactically simpler sentences
- Active sentences
- Personally relevant information
- Slower speech with frequent pauses
- Slower rate with additional stress on key terms
- Speech in quieter environment
- Redundant messages
- Repeated verbal messages
- Connected speech rather than isolated words or sentences
- Limited response choices
- Accompanied auditory stimuli with appropriate visual stimuli
- Visibility of the speaker's face
- <u>Alerting Stimuli</u> presented before the evoking stimulus is presented (e.g., "Look at my face." "Here comes the picture.").
  In treating auditory comprehension, avoid the following that are known to be detrimental to improved auditory comprehension:
- Louder speech, which is generally ineffective
- Telephone presentations, which may have a negative effect in some clients
- Audio- or videotaped presentations, which are ineffective

Sequence of Auditory Comprehension Treatment
Comprehension of Single Words
  Ask the client to point to:
  - Body parts
  - Objects
  - Pictures of objects
  - Clothing items
  - Food items
  - Actions in pictures

Comprehension of *Spoken Sentences*

Accept an appropriate verbal or nonverbal (gestural) response that suggests comprehension. Treat comprehension of:

- Simpler sentences before more complex sentences
- More redundant sentences before less redundant sentences
- Sentences with familiar information before those with unfamiliar information

Comprehension of *Spoken Questions*

Ask questions of the following kind and accept a correct verbal or nonverbal response of any length or complexity:

- Concrete yes/no questions ("Are you sitting in the wheelchair?")
- Abstract yes/no questions ("Is a plant bigger than a tree?")
- Simpler open-ended questions ("What pet do you have?")
- More complex open-ended questions ("How many states are in the United States?")

Comprehension of *Spoken Directions*

- Start with pointing to, and manipulation of, objects:
  - point to single objects (nouns) or actions in pictures (single verbs)
  - point to objects in sequence ("Point to the pen and then the paper.")
  - manipulate stimuli in sequence ("Point to the pen and then lift up the paper.")
  - manipulate objects according to directions ("Put the ball in the box.")
- Use Manual Guidance if the client cannot point to the pictures (e.g., take the client's hand and make it touch the requested objects)

Comprehension of *Discourse*

Target such skills as:

- Understanding narratives (e.g., tell or read a short story aloud and ask questions to test comprehension of details and the main story idea)
- Understanding questions in a conversational format (asking questions about personal interests and hobbies while engaging the client in conversational speech)

Treatment of Aphasia: Verbal Expression

Treatment of Naming: Designing Problem-Specific Strategies

Design treatment to suit the kind of anomia present:

- *Word production anomia:* Anomia due mainly to motor problems; often does not need direct treatment; provide such simple cues as the first sound of target words.
- *Word selection anomia:* Clients can describe, gesture, write, and draw to suggest a word they cannot say or can correctly recognize the name when given; cueing, including gestures, descriptions, and drawing is not very effective.
- *Semantic anomia:* Patients do not recognize the words they cannot produce; train word recognition.
- *Limited anomia:* Disconnection anomias; such category-specific problems as difficulty naming animals or vegetables; pair unimpaired skills with impaired naming.
- *Delayed response:* Presumably due to the slow activation of the naming process; shape progressively faster reaction time.
- *Self-corrected errors:* Prompting might be effective; reinforce self-correction.
- *Perseveration:* Persisting errors; reduce their frequency.
- *Unrelated words:* Irrelevant responses; reduce their frequency.
  Paraphasias: Unintended word or sound substitutions; reduce their frequency by increasing the production of target words.

Treatment of Naming: General Considerations

Use stimuli or strategies that facilitate correct naming:

- High frequency words
- Names of manipulable objects
- Names of objects rather than pictures
- Realistic drawings rather than line or abstract drawings
- Phonemic cues
- Client-regulation of stimulus presentation
- Extra time to respond
- Longer (30 seconds or more) stimulus exposure time
- Simultaneous visual and auditory stimulus presentation

Treatment of Naming: Targets and Techniques

Confrontation Naming: Treatment Procedure. Confrontation naming is naming an object when asked "What is this?"

- Start with more familiar objects and move on to less familiar objects
- Place a picture or an objects in front of the client
- Ask "What is this?"
- Prompt the correct response
- Reinforce the correct response

Naming in General: Treatment Procedure

- Use cueing hierarchies (Response evoking stimuli arranged in hierarchies)
- Find a stimulus (cue) that evokes the response
- Use a stronger cue only when weaker cues do not evoke the response
- Start with a few cues and add more only when necessary
- Use different types of cues
- Fade the cue so that natural stimuli come to evoke the response

Types of Cues
Modeling

- Ask a question ("What is this?")

- Immediately model the response ("Say, *a book*.")
- Let the client imitate
- Reinforce the client for correct imitation

Sentence completion tasks as cues: Give parts of sentences as cues.

Clinician (CN): "You write with a _____ ."

Client (CT): "Pen."

CN: " You write with a ball-point _____ ."

CT: "Pen."

Initial sound of words as cues: Give initial sounds as cues.

CN: "You write with a (pause); the word starts with a p _____ ."

CT: "Pen."

Syllables as cues: Give syllables of words as cues when the sound cue is not effective.

CN: "This is a spoo___."

CT: "Spoon."

Silent phonetic gestures as cues: Give articulatory postures without vocalizations as cues.

CN: "This is a ___." (silent articulatory posture for *p*).

CT: "Pen."

Functional descriptions as cues: Give a description of the use of an object as its cues.

CN: "This is a round object that you roll or kick. What do you call it?"

CT: "Ball."

Description and demonstration of an action as cues: Request the target name, describe its use, and demonstrate an action as cues.

CN: "What is this? You use this to write" (demonstrate writing).

CT: "Pen."

Client description as cues: Ask a client to first say what an object is used for and then name it.

CN: "Tell me what you use this for and then tell me its name."

CT: "I use it to write. It is a pen."

Patient's demonstration of functions as cues: Ask the client to first demonstrate the function of an object and then name it.

CN: "Show me how you use this and then tell me the name."

CT: Demonstrates the action of drinking and then says "cup."

Objects or pictures with their printed names as cues: Present an object or a picture with its printed name and ask the client to name it.

CN: Presents a book (or a picture of a book), the printed word book, and then asks the client, "What is this?"

CT: "Book."

Patient's oral spelling as cues: Ask the client to spell a word orally and then say the word (name).

Patient's spelling and writing as cues: Ask the client to spell a word, write it, and then say it.

An associated sound as a cue: Present a sound associated with an object and then ask the client to name it.

An associated smell as a cue: Present an object and let the client smell the fragrance typically associated with it and then ask the client to name it.

A synonym as a cue: Say "dwelling" to evoke the word "house" from the patient.

An antonym as a cue: Say "woman" to evoke the word "man."

A typically associated word as a cue. Say, "plate" to evoke the word "cup."

A superordinate as a cue: Say "It is something you eat" to evoke "cake."

A rhyming word as a cue: Say "It rhymes with *hog*" to evoke "dog."

Deblocking: Direct and Indirect. Treating naming or word-finding problems in clients with aphasia by presenting a variety of stimuli to which the person can respond and then presenting the target stimulus for the client to respond to.

Direct deblocking: Present several unrelated words along with the target word (e.g., say several words along with "cup"; then ask the client to name the picture of a cup)

Indirect deblocking: Present a word typically associated with a target word and then ask the client to produce it; do not present the target word (e.g., say "woman" to evoke the word "wife").

Fade the special cues: Gradually reduce the amount and extent of cues and ask typical questions to evoke naming; reinstate previously successful cues when necessary; again, try to fade them out.

Teach self-cueing: Teach the client to first produce an antonym, a synonym, or an associated word that may lead to the target word; teach the client to first spell the word, describe the use, demonstrate the use that may lead to the target word; teach the client to self-generate effective cues in natural settings.

Treatment of Aphasia: Expansion of Verbal Expressions. Expand words into phrases, phrases into sentences, and sentences into narratives and conversational speech. For expansion, select verbal expressions that are:

- Most useful to the client and his or her caregivers
- Most effective in expressing personal experiences, basic needs, emotions, and thoughts
- Most meaningful in social contexts to sustain conversation

Teach Verbal Expressions

- While asking the client to describe scenes in a picture, model simple sentences for the client to imitate
- Fade the model and ask a question to evoke the sentence the client imitated
- Ask questions about the client's daily activities
- Ask the client to describe actions in a picture
- Supply functional words and ask the client to make sentences with those words
- Tell a story and ask the client to retell it
- Tell a story and ask questions about the details
- Show sequenced pictures and ask the client to construct a story
- Give such cues as "say more'" or "elaborate on that" to have the client expand limited expressions
- Ask the client to describe such familiar tasks as making an omelet, planting flowers, or changing flat tires
- Engage the client in more naturalistic conversation
- Have family members engage the client in conversation in and out of the treatment setting
- Reinforce the client for correct or functionally appropriate productions

A

- Give corrective feedback ("That is not correct"; "That was a wrong word"; or "How about this _____ ?")
- Repeat successful trials several times to strengthen the responses

Treatment of Aphasia: Functional Communication and Maintenance

Functional communication skills are those that are useful in social situations; final targets of aphasia treatment; in addition to the following generic treatment procedure, consider using one of several special programs described later in this section under Treatment of Aphasia: Specific Techniques or Programs; integrate compatible procedures.

- Target communication as opposed to linguistic accuracy
- Select words, phrases, and sentences that are most useful:
  - for the client and his or her caregivers
  - in expressing the client's personal experiences, bodily needs, emotions, and thoughts
  - in simple, everyday social situations and conversational contexts
- Design client-specific treatment programs in which you shape progressively longer utterances
- Start with what the client can say, perhaps a few words or even syllables
- Add other syllables to create words, or words to create phrases
- Add additional words to create sentences
- Evoke a variety of sentence structures
  - noun and verb combinations
  - active declarative sentences
  - requests, commands, demands
  - wh-questions
  - structures with adjectives
  - structures with comparatives
  - yes/no questions

- structures with prepositions, pronouns, present progressives, and so forth
- Use special stimuli that are necessary (pictures, modeling, prompting, and so forth)
- Fade the special stimuli out, and fade in the naturalistic stimuli
- Reinforce the client productions
- Move to conversational speech
  - engage the client in meaningful, functional conversation
  - ask the client to describe personal experiences, hobbies, professional experiences, family-related events, favorite foods, entertainment, books read, vacations taken, and so forth
  - narrate a story and ask the client to retell it
  - role play Turn Taking
  - reinforce the client for staying on a topic; extend the duration of Topic Maintenance
- Implement a maintenance program
  - train the client to generate his or her own cues for better speech
    → teach the client to self-monitor
    → implement treatment in naturalistic settings
    → use natural response consequences
  - conduct group sessions in which the clients learn to monitor and reinforce each other's verbal or nonverbal expressions
  - train health care professionals to support and socially reinforce the communicative behaviors
  - train family members to
    → evoke and reinforce speech
    → reduce demands when it is appropriate
    → pay attention to the client's strengths
    → express emotional support for the client
    → include the client in communicative and other social activities

Treatment of Aphasia: Reading Problems

Treatment of reading problems may or may not be a major part of aphasia rehabilitation. When it is, use the following guidelines:

- Assess whether reading skills are important for the client
- Consider the level of premorbid reading skills and the current need to read
- Depending on the need, teach functional reading skills to persons who have mild or moderate aphasia
- Target comprehension of silently read material rather than oral reading
- Select client-specific, basic, and functional (survival) reading skills for treatment
- Target newspaper- and book-reading skills only when functional and basic reading skills are intact
- Teach comprehension of printed words in the beginning
  - Have the client read aloud selected printed words
  - Model and prompt the responses
  - Repeat successful trials for each word
  - Have the client read the words silently and state their meaning
  - Provide positive reinforcement and corrective feedback
- Construct phrases and sentences with words already comprehended
- Have the client read those phrases and sentences aloud with the help of modeling and prompting
- Have the client read them silently and state their meanings
- Present progressively complex reading material and assess comprehension at each level of complexity

Treatment of Aphasia: Writing Problems

Treatment of writing problems may or may not be a major part of aphasia rehabilitation. When it is, use the following guidelines:

- Assess whether writing skills are important for the client
- Consider the level of premorbid writing skills and the current need to write
- Depending on the need, teach functional writing skills to persons who have mild or moderate aphasia
- Consider the preferred hand and whether it is free from neuromuscular disorders
- Consult with the client, family members, and other care-givers to select words, phrases, and sentences that are important to the client and are useful in his or her daily living (e.g., names of family members, address and phone numbers, grocery lists, short letters, filling-out forms, writing down appointments)
- Target correct spelling of words and grammatical accuracy of sentences
- Name a target alphabet and have the client point to its printed form
- Name a target word and have the client point to its printed form
- Have the client trace printed letters and words
- Have the client copy letters and words
- Have the client write letters and words to dictation
- Have the client copy sentences
- Have the client spontaneously write sentences
- Have the client write paragraphs, short letters, lists, and so forth
- Give writing homework the client completes
- Train family members to help sustain the writing skills at home

Treatment of Aphasia: Apraxic Speech in Persons With Aphasia

Persons with aphasia are likely to exhibit verbal apraxia or Apraxia of Speech, especially those who have Broca's aphasia. Prognosis for severe apraxia beyond 4 weeks postonset is thought to be poor. In treating apraxic speech in patients with aphasia, use the following guidelines:

- Make a thorough assessment of apraxia and its severity as treatment procedures vary somewhat, depending on the severity
- Note that clients with aphasia and apraxia do not necessarily have sound discrimination problems
- Auditory discrimination training to improve apraxic symptoms are unnecessary and unproductive
- An early suggestion that persons with aphasia and apraxia are deficient in oral sensation and oral form recognition has not been sustained
- Treatment procedures described under <u>Apraxia of Speech</u> are appropriate for patients who have both aphasia and apraxia of speech

Brookshire, R. H. (1997). *Introduction to neurogenic communication disorders* (5th ed.). St. Louis: Mosby.

Chapey, R. (1994) (Ed.). *Language intervention strategies in adult aphasia.* Baltimore, MD: Williams & Wilkins.

Davis, G. A. (2000). *Aphasiology.* Boston: Allyn & Bacon.

Haskins, S. (1976). A treatment procedure for writing disorders. In R. H. Brookshire (Ed.), *Clinical aphasiology conference proceedings* (pp. 192–199). Minneapolis, MN: BRK.

Hegde, M. N. (1998). *A coursebook on neurogenic language disorders* (2nd ed.). San Diego: Singular Publishing Group.

LaPointe, L. L. (Ed.) (1997). *Aphasia and related neurogenic language disorders* (2nd ed.). New York: Thieme.

Rosenbek, J. C., LaPointe, L. L., & Wertz, R. T. (1989). *Aphasia: A clinical approach.* Austin, TX: Pro-Ed.

Treatment of Aphasia: Specific Types of Aphasia

Treatment suggestions offered for specific types of aphasia are based on the symptom complex and expert opinion. Substantive, experimentally validated treatment procedures that are specific to certain types of aphasia are limited. Treatment techniques with experimentally documented effects for such types as transcortical sensory aphasia and conduction aphasia are lacking. Clinicians generally design behavioral procedures to teach and strengthen skills that are impaired and are judged appropriate for remediation in a given client.

Broca's Aphasia. A type of aphasia characterized by nonfluent, effortful speech with missing grammatical elements; marked difficulty in naming; slow rate of speech and limited word output; limited syntax; better auditory comprehension; may have associated dysarthria and apraxia of speech; usually associated with lesions in the third frontal convolution of the left or dominant hemisphere.

- Use procedures described under Aphasia; Treatment of Aphasia: Verbal Expression; specifically:
  - Increase length of utterances in gradual steps
  - Increase complexity of responses in gradual steps
  - Decrease grammatical errors
  - Treat naming difficulties
  - Decrease stereotypic utterances by giving corrective feedback
  - Use modeling
  - Model progressively longer utterances and ask the client to imitate
  - Teach nouns and verbs on successive trials
  - Provide immediate, positive feedback
  - Ask questions to evoke responses
  - Encourage pointing, gestures, drawing, writing, and reading to improve verbal expression
  - Teach a sign language system (e.g., AMER-IND) if necessary
- In addition, consider the following:
  - Combine gestures with verbal expressions as this combination is known to facilitate naming and other verbal expressions
  - Teach self-cueing strategies
  - Find out the compensatory strategies a client uses (e.g., singing, gesturing, or writing key words to

effectively communicate) and incorporate them into training; reinforce their use in and out of the clinic
- Reinforce even telegraphic productions and then model more complete productions using the client's telegraphic productions
- Reinforce the client's imitation of more complete productions
- Select one of the special programs described under Aphasia; Treatment of Aphasia: Special Programs (e.g., A Program of Changing Criteria, the Helm Elicited Language Program for Syntax Stimulation, or Promoting Aphasics' Communicative Effectiveness or Response Elaboration Training)

Global Aphasia. A type of aphasia characterized by severe deficits in comprehension and production of language; all sensory modalities may be affected; caused by widespread damage to language areas of the brain.

- Note that traditional aphasia therapy for some very severely globally aphasic patients may not be effective or appropriate; in such cases, train the health care staff and family members to:
  - be alert to the patient's communicative efforts of any kind including eye contact, head nodding, facial expressions, postures, simple gestures, and so forth
  - not to expect linguistic accuracy and expansions
  - eliminate distractions while talking to the client
  - face the client while talking to him or her
  - draw the client's attention before each attempt at communication
  - speak slowly
  - pause at syntactic junctures and between stimulus presentations
  - use appropriate stress and intonation
  - use short, simple sentences; simplify all messages
  - pause between sentences

- use nonverbal cues to improve communication
- allow extra time for the client to respond
- be unhurried
- verbally state the guessed response from the client so he or she can confirm it
- let the client know if there is difficulty in understanding him or her (e.g., "I am sorry, I do not understand.")

To implement a more formal treatment program:

- Establish realistic goals for the client
- Use procedures to improve auditory comprehension of simple commands and requests
- Select basic, simple, functional words and phrases for initial treatment
- Teach *yes/no* responses to basic questions
- Teach a few unequivocal gestures to express basic needs
- Teach simple line drawing to express basic needs
- Select words and phrases that express basic needs
- Accept any mode of response: verbal, gestural, or signed
- Provide both auditory and visual stimulation; combine verbal responses with gestures
- Provide multiple stimuli (modeling, pictures, written stimuli, objects, gestures)
- Begin treatment with modeling and require immediate imitation
- Ask for delayed imitation later; give the client time to respond
- Fade modeling and other additional stimuli
- Shape the response to achieve more complex forms if found appropriate
- Provide manual guidance in shaping gestures, nodding the head, and pointing to objects
- Give prompt, natural, and social reinforcement
- Teach responses to simple questions

- Teach simple requests
- Teach simple descriptions
- Move to basic conversational skills training if judged appropriate
- Improve writing skills if found necessary and appropriate
- Teach an organized gestural system and consider techniques described under Augmentative Communication (including AMER-IND, Communication Boards, and Blissymbolics).
- Consider one of the special programs (Aphasia; Treatment of Aphasia: Special Programs, including Visual Action Therapy and Gestural Reorganization)
- Counsel the family about the effects of stroke, the communication problems and prospects of treatment, home strategies to enhance communication, and so forth

Collins, M. (1991). *Diagnosis and treatment of global aphasia.* San Diego: Singular Publishing Group.

Transcortical Motor Aphasia. A type of nonfluent aphasia characterized by agrammatic, paraphasic, and telegraphic speech; distinguishing feature is intact repetition; lesion is typically outside Broca's area, found often in the deep portions of the left frontal lobe or below or above Broca's area.

Use imitation and naming to improve speaking

- Select pictures as stimuli
  - ask the client to say or write nouns and verbs that the pictures suggest
  - if the client fails, point out dominant aspects of the stimulus or prompt nouns and verbs
  - obtain from the client or supply three or more words for each picture
- Ask the client to form sentences with one of the words produced or supplied

- Ask the client to expand the sentence with other words
- Reinforce all attempts in the right direction

Use relatively intact reading skills to prime or promote speaking

  - Begin treatment sessions with client reading general printed materials aloud to deblock speaking
  - Begin controlled conversational treatment after an extended period of reading
  - Relate conversation to the reading if necessary, or unrelated if possible
  - Have the client read selected utterances (prepared for the client) and then say them if general reading does not deblock speaking
  - Have the client read more complex materials and answer questions about them
  - Model if necessary
  - Use story books with pictures, ask the client to first read the story, and then describe the pictures in the same book

    Rosenbek, J. C., LaPointe, L. L., & Wertz, R. T. (1989). *Aphasia: A clinical approach.* Austin, TX: Pro-Ed.

Wernicke's Aphasia. A type of fluent aphasia characterized by good or even excessive fluency of speech, rapid rate, normal articulation and prosody, good grammatical structures, paraphasia, neologism, jargon, and generally meaningless speech; poor auditory comprehension is a major distinguishing feature; the lesion is in Wernicke's area.

- Reduce the impulsive and incessant talking:
  - structure the treatment sessions and reduce distracting stimuli
  - ask the client to listen
  - use gestures and manual guidance to stop the client from talking (touch your lips with your index

finger to suggest "be quiet," touch the client's hand to make him or her stop talking)
- ask yes/no questions and accept only such answers, not elaborate utterances
- Expand utterances in a controlled manner
- Train the client to listen carefully, instead of rushing to speak
- Reduce the rate of speech directed toward the client as this helps improve comprehension
- Train the client to reduce his or her rate of speech and self-monitor the rate
- Treat auditory comprehension deficits; use relevant procedures described under Treatment of Aphasia; Auditory Comprehension
- Use one of the special programs described under Aphasia; Treatment of Aphasia: Special Techniques or Programs, including Treatment for Wernicke's Aphasia (TWA)

Graham-Keegan, L., & Caspari, I. (1997). Wernicke's aphasia. In L. L. LaPointe (Ed.), *Aphasia and related neurogenic language disorders* (2nd ed.) (pp. 42–61). New York: Thieme.

Treatment of Aphasia: Specific Techniques or Programs

Gestural Reorganization. A method of teaching verbal expression by first pairing them with gestures and then fading the gestures; described by J. Rosenbek, L. LaPointe, and R. Wertz.
- Select phrases or sentences for training
- Select gestures that mean the same as those target expressions
  - use gestures from American Indian Hand Talk (AMER-IND) or other systems
  - invent gestures that are appropriate for the expressions
  - explain the gestures and the treatment approach to the client

- Teach the gestures to the client
  - ask the client to match your gesture
  - ask the client to match pictures of gestures
  - teach functional and spontaneous use of gestures
- Combine the learned gestures with speaking (verbal expression)
  - model the gesture and the verbal expression
  - model only one of them
  - use Manual Guidance if necessary (manually help form the gesture)
  - have the client practice the two separately, only if necessary; combine them
- Fade the gestures and continue to evoke and reinforce the verbal expressions

Rosenbek, J. C., LaPointe, L. L., & Wertz, R. T. (1989). *Aphasia: A clinical approach.* Austin, TX: Pro-Ed.

Helm Elicited Program for Syntax Stimulation. An aphasia treatment program designed to increase the production of syntactically correct utterances in agrammatic clients with moderate to well-preserved auditory comprehension and some speech production; developed by N. Helm-Estabrooks; uses pictures and a story completion method to evoke the following 11 sentence types at two levels (Level A and Level B):

1. Imperative Intransitive ("Lie down.")
2. Imperative Transitive ("Wash the dishes.")
3. Wh-interrogative ("What are you doing?")
4. Declarative Transitive ("She cleans teeth.")
5. Declarative Intransitive ("She skates.")
6. Comparative ("They're funnier.")
7. Passive ("The suitcases were lost.")
8. Yes/No Questions ("Did you buy the paper?")
9. Direct and Indirect Object ("They give Pat a cake.")
10. Embedded Sentences ("She wanted him to be healthy.")
11. Future ("He will hike.")

Background and Preparation
- Obtain the entire treatment program or prepare your own questions, stories, and pictures
- Baserate the responses

Level A
- Select sentence type 1.
- Read a story containing a target sentence; ask the client to produce the target sentence:

  Clinician (CN): "My friend feels dizzy, so I tell him, 'lie down.' What do I tell him?"

  Client (CT): "Lie down."
- Upon reaching a 90% accuracy criterion, move to Level B.

Level B
- Read a short story again, but without the target sentence; ask the client to produce the target sentence:

  CN: "My friend feels dizzy, so I tell him what?"

  CT: "Lie down."
- Upon reaching 90% accuracy criterion for sentence type 1 at Level B, select sentence type 2 for training; use the same procedure as for sentence type 1.
- Complete training on all 11 sentence types

Helm-Estabrooks, N. (1981). *Helm elicited program for syntax stimulation.* Austin, TX: Pro-Ed.

Helm-Estabrooks, N., & Albert, M. L. (1991). *Manual of aphasia therapy.* Austin, TX: Pro-Ed.

Melodic Intonation Therapy (MIT). An aphasia treatment program for clients with severe nonfluent aphasia with good auditory comprehension; developed by M. Albert, R. Sparks, and N. Helm; uses musical intonation, continuous voicing, and rhythmic tapping to teach verbal expression; hierarchically structured; contraindicated for clients with Wernicke's, transcortical motor or sensory, and global aphasia; has three levels.

General Procedures
- Select high probability words, phrases, and sentences
- Use pictures or environmental cues for each target utterance
- Intone each word, phrase, or sentence slowly and with constant voicing
- Maintain pitch and stress variations of normal speech
- Tap the client's left hand once for each intoned syllable
- Signal with your left hand when to listen and when to intone
- Generally, move to the earlier step when the client fails at a step

Level I
- Humming: Show a picture, hum the target item, and tap; no response required
- Unison singing: Intone in unison with the client and tap
- Unison with fading: Intone, tap, and fade halfway through the phrase
- Immediate repetition: Ask the client to listen to you as you intone the phrase and tap; let the client imitate
- Response to a probe question: Following a correct imitation, intone a probe question (e.g., "What did you say?")

Level II
- Introduction of item: Intone the phrase twice and tap; no response required
- Unison with fading: Intone, tap, and fade halfway through the phrase
- Delayed repetition: Intone and tap, and after 6 seconds of delay, let the client tap with assistance; ask the client to intone without help

- Response to a probe question: Six seconds following the client's response, intone the probe question; do not hand tap; let the client intone the phrase

Level III

- Delayed repetition: Tap and intone and let the client intone the phrase after 6 seconds and give tapping assistance
- Introducing *sprechgesang* (speech song): Present the target phrase twice slowly, without singing, but with exaggerated rhythm and stress; no tapping and no response required
- Delayed spoken repetition: Present the phrase in normal prosody, without hand tapping and let the client imitate after 6 seconds in normal prosody
- Response to a probe question: Ask a probe question with normal prosody after a 6-second delay; let the client respond with normal prosody

Albert, M., Sparks, R., & Helm, N. (1973). Melodic intonation therapy for aphasia. *Archives of Neurology, 29,* 130–131.

Helm-Estabrooks, N., Nicholas, M., & Morgan, A. (1989). *Melodic intonation therapy program.* San Antonio, TX: Special Press. *See this source for a complete description of steps, scoring procedure, and stimulus materials.*

Program of Changing Criteria. An aphasia treatment program described by J. Rosenbek, L. LaPointe, and R. Wertz to increase the length and quality of language; uses systematic shaping and progressively higher response criteria requiring longer utterances; uses differential reinforcement and extensive practice.

- Select realistic human action pictures to evoke responses
- Write about 10 questions, some of which you will use with each picture (e.g., "How many people do you see?" "What are they doing?" "What is the person wearing?")

- Begin at Criterion I. Require a one- or two-word response
  - give directions, present a picture, and ask a question
  - if no or incorrect response, use the <u>Cloze Procedure</u>
  - if the client fails, model the response
  - if the client fails, use any other procedure to evoke the response
  - if the client fails, use another program
  - reinforce and give repeated practice on correct responses
- Move to Criterion II. Require a three- to five-word response
  - give cloze-like cues when the response is incorrect
  - if the client fails, model the correct response
  - if no imitation, use any other method to evoke the response
  - if still no success, return to Criterion I or shift to another program
  - reinforce and give repeated practice on correct responses
- Move to Criterion III. Require six- to eight-word responses; use the same procedures as under Criterion II.
- Move to Criterion IV. Require spontaneous description of pictures with sentences containing nine or more words; but be flexible about this to promote natural productions.

Rosenbek, J. C., LaPointe, L. L., & Wertz, R. T. (1989). *Aphasia: A clinical approach.* Austin, TX: Pro-Ed.

Promoting Aphasics' Communicative Effectiveness (PACE). An aphasia treatment program designed to promote face-to-face conversation; developed by G. A. Davis and J. Wilcox; emphasis on exchange of new information, functional communication (as against linguistic precision) with turn taking, free choice for the client to communicate in any modality; and natural feedback.

- Use a large number of stimulus cards that contain pictured objects, actions, and stories; stack the cards face down on the table
- Take turns drawing cards from the stack; communicate information about the stimulus
- Encourage any mode of expression (words, gestures, drawings, writing, pointing, or a combination of these)
- Add new stimulus cards to promote the exchange of new information
- Provide natural consequences (e.g., "What did you say?" "Do you mean _____ ?" "I am not sure . . .")
- Acknowledge the client's message while suggesting the correct word or words (e.g., "I understand. You mean *book,* right?")
- Make variations and adaptations
- Exchange the roles of speaker and listener with the client

Davis, G. A. (1993). *A survey of adult aphasia* (2nd ed.). Englewood Cliffs, NJ: Prentice-Hall.

Davis, G. A. (2000). *Aphasiology.* Boston: Allyn & Bacon.

Response Elaboration Training. A treatment approach that uses a loose training format; designed to expand utterances of aphasic clients; emphasis is on shaping and chaining client- rather than clinician-initiated utterances; allows a wide variety of responses as against a predetermined correct response; developed and researched by K. Kearns and his associates.

- Select line drawings to stimulate speech
- Show a stimulus card and evoke an initial response, any response (e.g., the client may say "Man . . . sweeping" to a line drawing of a person with a broom)
- Reinforce the client; also, shape and model the client's response (e.g., say, "Great. The man is sweeping.")

- Ask a wh-question to evoke an elaboration of the initial utterance (e.g., ask "Why is he sweeping?")
- Reinforce the client's elaboration and shape and model the initial response combined with the subsequent elaboration (e.g., the client may answer by saying "wife . . . mad" and you say, "Way to go! The man is sweeping the floor because his wife is mad.")
- Model the longer response a second time and ask the client to "Try and say the whole thing after me. Say. . . ."
- Ask the client to imitate after a delay if the client is successful at the previous step
- Continue until the client fails to elaborate any more
- Introduce another picture for a similar sequence or initiate a different initial response for the same picture

Kearns, K. P., & Scher, G. P. (1989). The generalization of response elaboration training effects. In T. E. Prescott (Ed.), *Clinical aphasiology* (Vol. 18, pp. 223–245). Austin, TX: Pro-Ed.

Schuell's Auditory Stimulation Approach for Aphasia.
The method concentrates on intensive auditory stimulation or auditory bombardment; developed by H. Schuell; the method needs more clinical efficacy data.

- Find varied and abundant stimulus materials
- Design a sequence of auditory stimulation
- Work systematically and intensively
- Begin with easy and familiar tasks and increase their complexity; ask the client to:
  - point to objects named, described, spelled, and so forth
  - follow directions (simpler to more complex)
  - answer yes/no questions
  - respond to alternate items (switch responses) (e.g., "Show me the horse/Tell me your name.")

- repeat words, phrases, and sentences
- complete your sentences
- answer different kinds of questions
- form simple sentences
- retell stories
- describe pictures and events
- engage in conversation
- copy and write words
- Provide intensive auditory stimulation
- Combine auditory stimulation with visual stimulation
- Elicit responses to each stimulation, but do not force them
- Elicit many and varied responses
- Do not correct responses; instead repeat stimulation
- Give such feedback as visual charting of progress made in treatment sessions
- Introduce new materials that contain or extend old materials

Duffy, J. R. (1994). Schuell's stimulation approach to rehabilitation. In R. Chapey (Ed.), *Language intervention strategies in adult aphasia* (3rd ed., pp. 146–174). Baltimore, MD: Williams & Wilkins.

Treatment for Wernicke's Aphasia (TWA). A method of aphasia treatment developed by N. Helm-Estabrooks and P. Fitzpatrick to treat auditory comprehension problems; appropriate for clients with severe Wernicke's aphasia who can read and understand single picturable words:

- Select a corpus of words printed in lowercase that the client can read aloud and point to pictured stimuli
- Provide a printed word that the client can read, but cannot point to when named
- Ask the client to match the printed word to the picture depicting the word

- Ask the client to read the word aloud
- Ask the client to repeat the word "chair" as you say it without showing the picture
- Ask the client to point to the picture of a chair placed among other pictures
- Introduce new words as the client shows progress
- If new words cannot be introduced by about the fifth session, reevaluate the procedure; select another procedure
- Chart correct and incorrect responses on a recording sheet

Helm-Estabrooks, N., & Albert, M. L. (1991). *A manual of aphasia therapy.* Austin, TX: Pro-Ed.

Visual Action Therapy (VAT). A nonvocal, visual/gestural communication approach to the rehabilitation of globally aphasic clients; developed by N. Helm-Estabrooks and her associates; neither the clinician nor the client talk during treatment; a client who cannot match an object with the tracing of that object is not a good candidate for VAT; more treatment efficacy data are needed.

- Select seven real objects, shaded line drawings of the objects, and seven action pictures involving the objects
- Select some contextual props (e.g., a screw in a block of wood to use a screwdriver)

Level I

1. Matching pictures and objects
   - Placing objects on pictures. Place all 7 line drawings of the objects on the table; give each object to the client and gesture to place it on the correct drawing
   - Placing pictures on objects. Arrange objects on table, and ask the client to place the picture on the object

- Pointing to objects. Rearrange objects on table, show a picture one at a time, and gesture the client to point to the object the picture represents
- Pointing to the pictures. Rearrange pictures, show one object at a time, and gesture the client to point to the correct picture

2. Object use training
   - Pick up each object separately
   - Use props; demonstrate its use
   - Place it back on the table
   - Ask the client to pick it up and demonstrate its use

3. Action picture demonstration
   - Place an object and its corresponding action picture in front of the client
   - Point to the picture
   - Pick up the object and demonstrates its use

4. Following action picture commands
   - Place all objects and props on the table
   - Hold up an action picture
   - Gesture the client to manipulate the corresponding object

5. Pantomimed gesture demonstration
   - Place each object on the table
   - Demonstrate a gesture that represents the object; do not use props from this step on

6. Pantomimed gesture recognition
   - Produce a pantomimed gesture to represent one of the objects on the table
   - Gesture the client to point to the corresponding object

7. Pantomimed gesture production
   - Show one object at a time
   - Gesture the client to produce a gesture that suggests the object

8. Representation of hidden objects demonstration
   • Demonstrate a gesture each for two objects
   • Hide the objects in a box
   • Take one object out and gesture the hidden object.
9. Production of gestures for hidden objects
   • Have the client gesture for two objects
   • Hide them
   • Take one object out and suggest that the client gesture for the hidden object.

Level II
• Do not use objects; replace objects with action pictures beginning with Step 5 of Level I

Level III
• Use only the drawings; begin with Step 5.

Helm-Estabrooks, N., & Albert, M. L. (1991). *A manual of aphasia therapy.* Austin, TX: Pro-Ed.

Aphonia.   Loss of voice; a voice disorder.

Apraxia.   Disordered volitional movement in the absence of muscle weakness, paralysis, or fatigue; disorder of movement needed to execute learned actions; involuntarily, the same movements may be executed normally; often due to damage to the premotor cortex.

Apraxia of Speech (AOS) in Adults.   A neurogenic speech disorder with documented neuropathology in the left cerebral hemisphere including such areas as Broca's and supplementary motor; also known as verbal apraxia; primarily an articulatory (phonologic) disorder characterized by sensorimotor problems in positioning and sequentially moving muscles for the volitional production of speech; associated with prosodic problems; not caused by muscle weakness or neuromuscular slowness; presumed to be a disorder of motor programming for speech; rare as an isolated disorder; typically associated with Broca's aphasia.

Treatment of Apraxia of Speech: General Guidelines

- Make a thorough assessment of apraxia of speech; see the cited sources and *PGASLP* for details
- Assess associated aphasia, dysarthria, or both
- Note that treatment of AOS is essentially behavioral, highly structured, focused on speech production, repetitive, and intensive
- Do not recommend prosthetic and medical management for AOS as their effects are limited, indirect, and temporary
- Do not use delayed auditory feedback in treating AOS as data contraindicate it
- Do not spend time on oral sensation and form recognition exercises in treatment as they are unlikely to result in improved speech production
- Consider client preference of certain techniques (e.g., some may not like melodic speech or clinician's manipulation of articulators)
- Drop techniques that do not produce results or modify them to increase their effectiveness
- Defer treatment for AOS until treatment for a severe aphasia produces some language production
- Counsel the client and the family on the nature of apraxia of speech and expected treatment efforts and potential outcomes
- Start management early
- Hold frequent treatment sessions
- Organize sessions to move from easy to difficult tasks
- End sessions with success
- Emphasize communicative efficiency and naturalness as you would with most clients in communicative disorders
- Emphasize articulatory accuracy
- Select treatment target words that are functional for the client, medical caregivers, and the family

AOS: General Procedures

- Carefully sequence the speech tasks; train:
  - automatic speech before spontaneous speech
  - frequently occurring sounds before less frequently occurring sounds
  - stimulable sounds before nonstimulable sounds
  - sounds in word-initial positions before those in other positions
  - visible before nonvisible sounds
  - oral-nasal distinctions before voicing distinctions
  - voicing distinctions before manner distinctions
  - manner distinctions before place distinctions
  - bilabial and lingua-alveolar sounds before others
  - singletons before clusters
  - high-frequency words before low-frequency words
  - meaningful words
  - single-syllable words before multisyllable words
  - single words before phrases or sentences
- Teach the client self-monitoring skills

Treatment of Apraxia of Speech: General Procedures

- Provide counseling and support for the client and family
- Use consistent and variable practice
- Model sound productions frequently for the patient to imitate
- Provide systematic practice in producing the target speech sounds (drill)
- Reduce speech rate initially
- Increase speech rate as articulatory accuracy improves and stabilizes
- Use shaping to promote natural prosody
- Use phonetic placement and Phonetic Derivation
- Use a variety of sounds and sound combinations
- Practice sound productions with meaningful material
- Provide instruction on and demonstration of speech production
- Provide immediate, specific feedback

- Use instrumental feedback or biofeedback, when appropriate
- Focus treatment activities on speech tasks
- Use contrastive stress tasks
- Use the Key Word technique
- Use cueing techniques
- Use phonetic contrasts
- Use automatic speech tasks initially to evoke speech
- Use carrier phrases
- Use singing
- Push on abdomen to achieve vocal fold closure and phonation for the speechless client
- Employ an artificial larynx for the speechless patient
- Emphasize total communication (combined use of verbal expressions, gestures, writing, augmentative devices)
- Teach Self-Control (Self-Monitoring) skills
- Use techniques of treating Articulation and Phonological Disorders

Brookshire, R. H. (1997). *An introduction to neurogenic communication disorders* (5th ed.). St. Louis, MO: Mosby Year Book.

Duffy, J. R. (1995). *Motor speech disorders: Substrates, differential diagnosis, and management.* St. Louis, MO: C. V. Mosby.

Freed, D. (2000). *Motor speech disorders: Diagnosis and treatment.* San Diego: Singular Publishing Group.

Halpern, H. (2000). *Language and motor speech disorders in adults* (2nd ed.). Austin, TX: Pro-Ed.

Johns, D. F. (Ed.), *Clinical management of neurogenic communicative disorders* (2nd ed.). Boston: Little, Brown

Wertz, R. T., LaPointe, L. L., & Rosenbek, J. C. (1991). *Apraxia of speech.* San Diego: Singular Publishing Group.

Treatment of Mild Apraxia of Speech

- Note that persons with mild AOS are:
  - good candidates for massed-trial treatment of articulatory accuracy
  - likely to learn to communicate well in social and occupational situations

- • not likely to exhibit severe forms of aphsaia
- Counsel the patient and the family; tell them about the good prospects of recovered or vastly improved communication
- Keep the focus on articulatory accuracy, good prosody, and appropriate rate of speech
- Select meaningful and personally relevant words for treating sound productions
- Model sound productions in words initially
- Fade modeling in gradual steps
- Move to modeled and evoked productions of phrases and sentences in graduated steps
- Use visible and simple utterances in the beginning
- Give visual feedback of movement of articulators (e.g., "See how I produce the sound and do the same.")
- Encourage the client to listen to his or her own sound productions to judge their adequacy
- Require immediate imitation of modeled productions because it is easier than delayed imitation
- Reduce the client's rate of speech
- Extend treatment to utterances that are more complex and sound productions that are less visible in carefully graded steps
- Use the Phonetic Placement Method
- Use Contrastive Stress Drills to promote articulatory proficiency and prosodic features of speech; in constructing contrastive drill materials:
  - • use a single sound target initially in any phrase or sentence
  - • use simpler and more familiar sounds initially
  - • use shorter phrases or sentences initially
  - • use longer words and sentences subsequently
  - • add more sound targets to each utterance
  - • use infrequently occurring words later
  - • increase rate of speech gradually

- Use the Eight-Step Continuum Treatment, described under Treatment of Apraxia of Speech: Specific Techniques or Programs following this section
- Use the Darley, Aronson, and Brown Procedure for AOS, described under Treatment of Apraxia of Speech: Specific Techniques or Programs following the end of these sections
- Encourage the patient to create original sentences
- Ask open-ended questions
- Encourage the patient to ask questions to practice normal rhythm
- Encourage the patient to read aloud and self-correct mistakes
- Improve ability to talk under stress or interference
- Encourage self-correction
- Increase speed of response (reduced reaction time)

Brookshire, R. H. (1997). *An introduction to neurogenic communication disorders* (5th ed.). St. Louis, MO: Mosby Year Book.

Freed, D. (2000). *Motor speech disorders: Diagnosis and treatment.* San Diego: Singular Publishing Group.

Halpern, H. (2000). *Language and motor speech disorders in adults* (2nd ed.). Austin, TX: Pro-Ed.

Wertz, R. T., LaPointe, L. L., & Rosenbek, J. C. (1991). *Apraxia of speech in adults: The disorder and its management.* San Diego: Singular Publishing Group.

Treatment of Moderate Apraxia of Speech

- Note that persons with moderate AOS are likely to be:
  - hemiparetic or hemiplegic
  - mildly or moderately aphasic
  - apraxic in other respects (e.g., limb apraxia, buccofacila apraxia)
- Counsel the patient and the family about:
  - variability in symptoms
  - faster recovery of speech during the earlier weeks and slower recovery later
  - prospects for improved communication

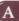

- potential need for long-term speech treatment
- need to work hard in treatment
- coping strategies
- Encourage the patient to make decisions about the future (returning to work, changing assignments at work, driving, and so forth)
- Use modeling to promote imitation of carefully selected speech sound contrasts
  - provide patients with auditory and visual cues
  - ask the patient to imitate a model
  - place a single target in varied linguistic contexts (e.g., for the target /t/, a typical list of stimuli might be *tea, tie, toe,* and *two*)
  - ask the patient to contrast the target with other sounds
  - replace single-syllable words with polysyllabic ones
  - construct phrases and sentences out of practiced words for more practice
  - make contrasts harder
  - use slow rate initially with difficult targets
  - use varying rhythm and stress (e.g., begin with equal and even stress and progress toward normal)
  - use multiple contrasts
  - encourage greater independence
- Use Contrastive Stress Drills
- Use Melodic Intonation Therapy (MIT)
- Use imitation initially
- Use a question-and-answer dialogue

Use Reading in Treatment
- Ask the client to read aloud
- Fade the printed stimuli by having the client:
  - look at the text and talk about it
  - look at the text and wait before talking about it
- Teach the client to Self-Monitor rate, rhythm, stress, and errors

AOS: Treatment of Moderate Forms

Use Gestural Reorganization to Improve Communication

- Explain the need and usefulness of Gestural Reorganization (described under Aphasia; Treatment of Aphasia: Special Techniques or Programs) to the client
- Begin with frequently used and simpler gestures (tapping with a finger, drumming with one or more fingers, squeezing the thumb and the index finger, tapping with the foot)
- Model the gesture that works for the client and ask the client to imitate
- Give Manual Guidance (e.g., physical assistance in tapping) if the client needs it
- Tap on the client's hand if this helps
- Give verbal modeling and other cues as well
- Stabilize the gesture
- Model gestures with speech and ask the patient to imitate both
- Pair gestures with words or phrases initially and pair longer utterances subsequently
- Fade your tapping first
- Fade your verbal modeling
- Use gestures with Contrastive Stress Drills
- Move on to more spontaneous conversational speech
- Fade the client's gestures if they persist as the client becomes verbally more proficient
- Use a Pacing Board

Brookshire, R. H. (1997). *An introduction to neurogenic communication disorders* (5th ed.). St. Louis, MO: Mosby Year Book.

Freed, D. (2000). *Motor speech disorders: Diagnosis and treatment.* San Diego: Singular Publishing Group.

Halpern, H. (2000). *Language and motor speech disorders in adults* (2nd ed.). Austin, TX: Pro-Ed.

Wertz, R. T., LaPointe, L. L., & Rosenbek, J. C. (1991). *Apraxia of speech in adults: The disorder and its management.* San Diego: Singular Publishing Group.

Treatment of Severe Apraxia of Speech
- Note that persons with severe AOS:
  - may not have volitional speech at all
  - may have other kinds of apraxia (often limb and buccofacila)
  - may be moderately aphasic
  - may be hemiparetic or hemiplegic
- Counsel the family members and the patient
  - give the family a reasonable statement of prognosis
  - discuss the severity of accompanying aphasia and how it might complicate apraxia treatment
  - ask the family members and health care workers to speak slowly, use shorter sentences, reduce background noise, talk only when the client is focused, and use Total Communication
  - teach family members and health care staff to use various prompts (cues) including the use of the Cloze Procedure, suggesting the first letter of the word, the first syllable of a word, paraphrasing what the client may have said for the client to indicate *yes* or *no,* and so forth.
  - ask the family and the patient to allow for some failures
  - ask the family to observe treatment and learn from it
  - tell the client what the family members are asked to do and what he or she can expect from treatment and with what efforts
- Educate the other members of the team about the client's communication problems, strengths, and the treatment program
- Begin direct treatment with modeling and ask the client to imitate; be aware that it may not work very well with severely apraxic clients who tend to perseverate
- Use the Phonetic Placement Method to help improve articulatory accuracy; encourage the client to
  - use manner distinctions (especially plosive and fricative)
  - use simultaneous manner and place distinctions

- make voicing distinctions (evoke any kind of sound including humming or grunting and then shape it)
- make oral-nasal distinctions
- Use <u>Phonetic Derivation</u> (<u>shaping</u> or progressive approximation) if other techniques fail
- Combine modeling, phonetic placement, and shaping (phonetic derivation) techniques
- Use rhythm to evoke speech sounds, syllables, and words; use aspects of <u>Melodic Intonation Therapy</u> described under <u>Aphasia; Treatment of Aphasia: Specific Techniques or Programs</u>
- Use the <u>Key Word</u> technique to have the client practice correct articulation
- For the most severely apraxic, consider using <u>Augmentative Communication</u> techniques

Brookshire, R. H. (1997). *An introduction to neurogenic communication disorders* (5th ed.). St. Louis, MO: Mosby Year Book.

Freed, D. (2000). *Motor speech disorders: Diagnosis and treatment.* San Diego: Singular Publishing Group.

Halpern, H. (2000). *Language and motor speech disorders in adults* (2nd ed.). Austin, TX: Pro-Ed.

Wertz, R. T., LaPointe, L. L., & Rosenbek, J. C. (1991). *Apraxia of speech in adults: The disorder and its management.* San Diego: Singular Publishing Group.

Treatment of Apraxia of Speech: Specific Techniques or Programs

Darley, Aronson, and Brown's Procedure for AOS. A procedure for treating AOS by systematic shaping of articulatory productions and capitalizing on automatic productions. It includes intensive trails for phoneme productions (phonemic drills).

- Shape vowels, consonants, and consonant-vowel (CV) syllables:
  - identify a vocal response the client can make (perhaps an "ah"; if not, a voluntary cough or a hum that can be shaped into a vocal response)

- have the client repeat the "ah" or any other phonated sound several times, varying its duration and intensity
- shape different vowel sounds from the phonated and repeated sound productions (e.g., "ee," "oh," "oo")
- move to consonants; model /m/ for the client to imitate; give repeated trials
- shape syllables out of /m/ (e.g., *me, moe, moo*)
- have the client produce other combinations of consonants and vowels
- Move to automatic responses; have the client:
  - count to 10
  - recite days of the week and months of the year
  - produce such routine expressions as "Hello," "How are you?" "Fine," "Good morning," "Thank you," and so forth
  - sing songs
- Move to intensive practice of phoneme productions ("phonemic drills")
  - produce or hum /m/ and ask the client to imitate it
  - model CV combinations with initial /m/ and ask the client to imitate them (e.g., *my, moe, maw, moo, may, me*)
  - model doubled CV combinations and ask the client to imitate each at least 20 times (e.g., *my-my*)
  - model consonant-vowel-consonant (CVC) combinations and ask the client to imitate them (e.g., *mom, moom, meem*); when successful, evoke CVC combinations without modeling
  - model simple words with initial /m/ and have the client imitate each 10 to 20 times (e.g., *man, mine, moon, more*); when successful, evoke the words
  - model two-word phrases, both the words with initial /m/, and have the client imitate them multiple

times (e.g., *my mom, miss me, much more*); when successful, evoke the phrases

- model two-word phrases, both the words ending in /m/, and have the client imitate them multiple times (e.g., *come home, name him*); when successful, evoke the phrases
- model two-word phrases with /m/ in the initial position of the first word and in the final position of the second and have the client imitate them (e.g., *my home, meet them*); when successful, evoke the phrases
- model longer phrases containing multisyllabic words (e.g., *moment by moment, Monday morning*)
- introduce other sounds and sound combinations; use essentially the same procedure to create syllables, words, and phrases
- introduce sentences containing practiced words and phrases

Darley, F. L., Aronson, A. E., & Brown, J. R. (1975). *Motor speech disorders*. Philadelphia: W. B. Saunders.

Eight-Step Continuum Treatment for AOS. A procedure for treating AOS developed by J. C. Rosenbek and associates. The main feature of this technique is the systematic shaping of words with the use of cues that are faded out.

- Select the sounds and words for training
  - select words for initial training that contain easier sounds in them (vowels, nasals, and stops as against fricatives and affricates)
  - select words that contain sounds produced with closer articulatory contacts for initial training (e.g., words with only bilabial sounds) and increase the distance between the articulatory contact gradually (e.g., words with bilabial and lingua-alveolars moving on to velar sounds)

- select short, simple, and frequently used words for initial training and increase the length of words gradually
- Apply a sequenced treatment
  - say "Watch me" and "Listen to me" and then model a target word
  - ask the client to say the word along with you; this is unison production
  - say "Watch me" and "Listen to me" and then say the word; ask the client to produce the word aloud as you silently mouth the word
  - say "Watch me" and "Listen to me" and then say the word; ask the client to produce the word without any cues
  - say "Watch me" and "Listen to me" and then say the word; ask the client to produce the word several times without any cues
  - present the target word printed on a card and ask the client to produce it
  - show the printed target word briefly, remove it, and then ask the client to produce it
  - ask a question to evoke the target word and let the client respond with it
  - arrange role-playing conversational situations in which the client has opportunities to produce target words; get family members and others involved in this role-playing

Rosenbek, J. C., and associates (1973). A treatment for apraxia of speech in adults. *Journal of Speech and Hearing Disorders, 38,* 462–472.

Prompts for Restructuring Oral Muscular Targets (PROMPTS). A procedure for treating AOS in children and adults that emphasizes the use of tactile-kinesthetic cues in teaching correct production of phonemes; uses manual guidance to position articulators or suggest their appropriate movement; developed by P. Square-Store and D. Hayden.

- Note that kinesthetic and tactile cues may be effective only in the context of speech production; by themselves, such cues may be ineffective
- Learn the cues that are described in the cited source; note that cues are given for articulatory positions, voicing, extent of jaw opening, syllable timing, manner of articulation, coarticulation, and so forth
- Learn the many contact positions on the face, neck, jaw, and so forth
- Provide cues by touching the client's face, neck, jaw, and other structures
- Manually guide the articulators to correct positions
- Model target words for the client to imitate
- Give cues if the imitative production was incorrect
- Manually guide the articulators to correct positions
- Ask the client to produce the sound as the articulators are being moved to correct positions
- Give other cues to suggest articulatory movements that cannot be manually guided

Square-Store, P., & Hayden, D. (1989). PROMPT treatment. In P. Square-Store (Ed.), *Acquired apraxia of speech in aphasic adults* (pp. 165–189). London: Taylor and Francis.

Voluntary Control of Involuntary Utterances. A procedure for treating AOS, although it was originally developed for clients with severe aphasia with little voluntary speech; based on the assumption that most severely aphasic and apraxic individuals can produce a few words involuntarily and that from such involuntary productions, it is possible to shape voluntary productions; developed by N. Helm and B. Baresi.

- Write down all utterances the client produces during the initial interview and testing situations
- Select words from the client's involuntary or spontaneous productions

- Write down each word the client produced on a separate sheet of paper
- Present the words one at a time, in the printed format
- Present some emotionally laden and personally relevant words to see if the client would read them correctly; if so, write them down on separate cards to be used in therapy
- Discard a word if the client struggles with it or produces neologistic utterance
- Select a word the client substitutes, but produces correctly, for a word presented (e.g., select the word *mother* if the client read the printed word *father* as "mother")
- Give the selected words, each printed on a separate index card, to the client and ask him or her to practice reading them aloud at home
- Introduce the selected and printed words, one at a time, during the treatment session; withdraw a word on which struggle appears; reintroduce it later
- Draw a picture to represent the word on the other side of the card (e.g., a line drawing of a heart to prompt *love*)
- Use the picture to evoke confrontation naming by asking "What is this?"
- Turn the card over and show the printed word if the response is incorrect or the client struggles with it
- Continue to add new words to the target word list as you observe new word productions
- Construct phrases and sentences from practiced words and present them to read
- Ask questions that would evoke responses in which practiced words, phrases, and sentences are likely to be used
- Use other techniques to expand utterances and correct production of phonemes when a core set of

words that were involuntarily or spontaneously produced initially begin to be used in conversational speech or oral reading

Helm, N., & Baresi, B. (1980). Voluntary control of involuntary utterances: A treatment approach for severe aphasia. In R. Brookshire (Ed.), *Clinical aphasiology conference proceedings* (pp. 308–315). Minneapolis, MN: BRK Publishers.

Articulation and Phonological Disorders. Disorders of speech characterized by difficulty in producing speech sounds correctly; sounds may be omitted, distorted, or substituted; difficulty in producing a few sounds with no pattern or derivable rule is often described as an articulation disorder; multiple errors that can be grouped on some principle or characteristics and thus form patterns are typically described as <u>Phonological Disorders</u>.

- Make a thorough assessment of articulation and phonological disorders; consult the sources cited and the *PGASLP*

Treatment of Articulation and Phonological Disorders: General Guidelines

Consider the issues and approaches in treating articulation and phonological disorders:

- *Phonetic or phonemic approach?* Note that some experts recommend that the clinician decide whether the child needs a motor (phonetic) approach in which single sounds are trained at different levels or a phonemic approach in which errors are grouped and a phonological process (linguistic) approach is used; note also that even in the phonemic approaches, single phonemes must be trained.

- *What are the treatment targets?* Note that treatment targets may be defined either as the correct production of phonemes in error or the remediation or elimination of phonological process; note also, that either way, individual sounds need to be taught; correct production of all phonemes in conversational speech produced in natural settings is the final treatment target

- *How are the targets sounds sequenced?* Although all sounds need to be taught, multiple sounds misarticulated cannot be taught all at once; consider selecting certain sounds for initial training, certain others for subsequent training, and the remaining sounds for training during the final stages of therapy:

  - select sounds that are *functional* for the child for immediate training; sounds that are important from the standpoint of social and academic performance (e.g., even though /r/ may not be an initial target for all 4-year-old children who misarticulate that sound, it may be for a child named Robert Roberson who refers to himself as "Wobert Woberson"; in this case, /r/ is *functional* for the child)

  - select for immediate training sounds that are *stimulable*; sounds the child misarticulates in spontaneous speech but imitates correctly when modeled may be more easily taught; hence, select sounds that are imitated correctly for initial training; select sounds not imitated correctly for training in later stages; note that some children may learn equally fast the sounds that are not easily imitated, but shaped in therapy

  - select for immediate training sounds that are typically misarticulated but *correctly produced in some words;* use these words as key words to teach correct production of the sounds in other words by using the Paired-Stimuli Approach described later in this section

  - select for immediate training sounds that are *more visible*; visible sounds provide visual feedback when the clinician models them and this might facilitate initial success; select nonvisible sounds for later training

  - select *high frequency* sounds for immediate training; teaching correct production of sounds that are more frequently used in speech will improve intelligibility faster and more noticeably than correcting sounds that occur less frequently; see <u>Frequency of Occurrence of English Consonants</u>

- select sounds that are normally *acquired earlier* before selecting those that are acquired later; this recommendation is based on the normative logic that behaviors acquired earlier are easier to teach than those that are acquired later; may not hold true for all sounds that need to be taught

- select sounds that the child *does not produced at all* for immediate training; this recommendation is contrary to the one that suggests inconsistently produced sounds for immediate training; this is based on the assumption that sounds that are totally missing contribute the most to unintelligibility of speech and that teaching them will improve intelligibility the most

- select for immediate training sounds whose training may results in *generalized production* of some untrained sounds; this means that training time and effort can be saved for some sounds; for instance, consider training voiced sounds when voiced and voiceless cognates are both misarticulated to see if unvoiced, untrained sounds will begin to be produced because of generalization; always probe untrained sounds to confirm generalized productions; note that all phonological process approaches *assume* that some sounds trained within a process is sufficient to have other sounds within it produced without training; note that this may or may not happen

- *How is the Response Topography Sequenced?* Use the following guidelines in sequencing response topography (levels of response complexity at which the sounds are trained); consider <u>Specific Techniques or Programs</u> described in a later section for somewhat varied recommendations:

- teach the target sounds at the highest level of response complexity that the client can initially handle with success
- do not begin teaching at a lower level if the client can handle training at a higher level (e.g., do not train at the syllable level if in the initial treatment trials the client can learn to imitate the modeled productions at the word level)
- begin training a sound minimally at the word level; if practical at the phrase level; or even at the sentence level; expect in most cases to begin training at the word level
- drop to syllable level only if a the child fails to imitate the modeled production of sounds in words on several trials
- drop to the isolated phoneme level only if the child fails to imitate the modeled production of sounds in syllables on several trials
- to begin with, experiment with a higher level; you can always drop to a lower level if necessary
- move up to a higher level of complexity when training is completed at a lower level (e.g., move on to training the sound in phrases when it has been trained in words)
- end training at the level of conversational speech level produced in more naturalistic settings

Ethnocultural Considerations in Treating Articulation and Phonological Disorders

- Note that variables related to ethnic, cultural, and linguistic background of clients significantly affect the assessment, diagnosis, and treatment of articulation disorders; see *PGASLP* for assessment guidelines of clients with varied ethnocultural background
- Do not recommend treatment for a client who speaks a different dialect of English as all dialects of a language

are its accepted forms with its own cultural heritage; note that this is the official position of the American Speech-Language-Hearing Association on social dialects

- Note that African American English (AAE) is an accepted form of English; see <u>Treatment of Articulation and Phonological Disorders in African American Children</u> in this section
- Note that English spoken by a bilingual child is influenced by his or her primary language; thus, there is Spanish-influenced English or Chinese-influenced English; see <u>Treatment of Articulation and Phonological Disorders in Bilingual Children</u> in this section
- Recommend treatment only if there is an articulation disorder within the dialectal framework of a client's speech
- Offer treatment to teach the sound patterns of standard English only if the client's errors are not due to the influence of a primary language, an accepted social dialect, or African American English
- Offer treatment to change someone's otherwise acceptable dialect (such as African American English or Spanish-influenced English) only if the client, the family, or both seek it

A Comprehensive Treatment Program for Articulation and Phonological Disorders

- Assess the client's articulation and phonological skills; determine any patterns that may exist (based on distinctive features or phonological processes); consult the cited sources and *PGASLP*
- Select the target speech sounds for modification;
  - use previously described criteria for selecting treatment targets (functional targets, sounds that greatly improve intelligibility, sounds that are acquired earlier, sounds that are produced inconsistently, or, alternatively, sounds that are not produced at all)

- sequence the target sounds for training them in the early, middle, and final treatment phases using the previously described guidelines
- group the target sounds—especially in the case of multiple misarticulations—according to distinctive features or phonological processes (e.g., establishing voiced/voiceless contrasts or elimination of the final consonant deletion process)
- Write measurable objectives for each target sound; include in each objective statement:
  - the response to be taught (e.g., "The production of /s/ . . .")
  - the complexity level at which the response will be taught initially (e.g., "The production of /s/ *in words . . .*")
  - the position of the target sound in words (e.g., "The production of /s/ in word-*initial positions . . .*"; and similar statements for other word positions)
  - the performance criterion to judge success (e.g., "The production of /s/ in word-initial positions *at 90% accuracy in a set of 10 training words . . .*")
  - the response setting (e.g., "The production of /s/ in word-initial positions *at 90% accuracy in a set of 10 training words . . .*"); note that for initial training, only one setting—the clinical setting—may be specified and as training advances, new objectives may be written to include additional settings
  - the number of speech samples or sessions in which the production of sounds is measured (e.g., "The production of /s/ in word-initial positions at 90% accuracy in a set of 10 training words *measured across three consecutive speech samples or treatment sessions.*")
- Write different measurable target objectives for different levels of response complexity
  - at the word level (e.g., "The production of /l/ in word-final positions at 90% accuracy in a set of *10 training*

words measured across three consecutive speech samples recorded in the clinic.")

- at the phrase level (e.g., "The production of /t/ in word-medial positions at 90% accuracy in a set of *10 two-word training phrases* measured across three consecutive speech samples recorded in the clinic.")

- at the sentence level (e.g., "The production of /d/ in word-initial positions at 90% accuracy in a set of *10 training sentences* measured across three consecutive speech samples recorded in the clinic.")

- at the conversational speech level (e.g., "The production of /k/ in word-medial positions at 90% accuracy in three consecutive, spontaneous conversational speech samples recorded in the clinic.")

- Write different measurable target objectives for different settings

  - for the clinical setting (e.g., "The production of /k/ in word-medial positions at 90% accuracy in three consecutive, spontaneous conversational speech samples produced in the clinic."); write similar objectives for other word positions and for phrases and words

  - for the setting just outside the clinic, but within the clinic premises (e.g., "The production of /z/ in 10 training phrases at 90% accuracy produced outside the clinic but within the general clinical setting."); write similar objectives for other word positions and for words and sentences

  - for the client's home setting (e.g., "The production of /k/ in conversational speech at 90% accuracy in three consecutive samples evoked by parents in their home setting."); write similar objectives for other sound targets; note that when the parents do the home training and measurement, the response mode is typically conversational speech; parents are rarely asked to pay attention to position of sounds in words although they can monitor sound productions in words

- for the client's classroom (e.g., "The production of /t/ in conversational speech at 90% accuracy in three consecutive samples evoked by the teacher in the child's classroom setting."); write similar objectives for other sound targets; note that when the teachers monitor production of target speech sounds, the response mode is typically conversational speech; teachers are rarely asked to pay attention to position of sounds in words although they can monitor sound production in words
- for the client's school setting other than the classroom (e.g., "The production of /t/ in conversational speech at 90% accuracy in three consecutive samples evoked by the teacher in the school's dining hall."); write similar objectives for all target phonemes to be monitored in all academic settings (e.g., library, playground)
- for the client's varied settings (e.g., "The production of /b/ in conversational speech at 90% accuracy in three consecutive samples evoked by family members or others in such natural settings as restaurants and shopping centers."); write similar objectives for all target sounds; note that when the production of a target sound is monitored in natural contexts and settings, the response mode is usually conversational speech

- Prepare stimulus materials to be used in therapy sessions
  - prepare 20 words, phrases, and sentences for each target sound in each word position (i.e., 20 words *each* for initial, medial, and final word positions; 60 target words for each sound to be trained); select picturable words to the extent possible
  - select pictures, drawings, objects, or a combination of these to evoke each target word, phrase, or sentence; preferably, select colorful and realistic pictures from popular magazines

- test the stimulus materials with the child to make sure that the child is familiar with them; show the materials to parents to get their feedback; replace any ethnoculturally inappropriate stimulus material (including picture, objects, words, and phrases) with those that are appropriate, familiar to the child, and approved by the parents

- Design a treatment response recording sheet of the following kind; modify as necessary with the required features of space available to list the target behaviors and score the child's responses as correct, incorrect, or absent (no response):

Name:	Treatment target:
Clinician:	Date: Session #:
Target Behavior: Correct production of /s/ in word-initial positions	Responses (+ = correct; − = incorrect; 0 = no response; m = modeled; e = evoked)
1. soup	+ m
2. sun	− m
3. soap	+ m
4. seed	0 m
. . . 20.	

Note that in the beginning, all trials will be modeled; subsequently, when modeling is dropped, evoked trials are administered.

- Write training and probe criteria that help make clinical decisions throughout training:
  - *Imitative accuracy criterion:* When the child gives five consecutively correct imitated responses, modeling will be discontinued
  - *Modeling reinstatement criterion:* When the child gives three incorrect responses on evoked (without

modeling) trials, modeling will be reinstated and then withdrawn after five correct imitated response as before; reinstated and withdrawn in this manner

- *Shaping criterion:* When the child fails to correctly imitate the target sound in the first word selected for training on 10 consecutive trials, a different word will be selected for training; if the child fails to imitate the sound in the second word in 10 trials, the training of the sound will be initiated in syllables or at the level of isolated sounds; when the child gives five correct responses at the phoneme level, the training will shift to syllable level; five correct responses at the syllable level will move training to the word level.
- *Training criterion:* A 90% accurate production of a sound at each level of response complexity (i.e., 90% accuracy in sound production at the word, phrase, and sentence levels evoked on a block of 10 trials; and 90% accuracy in conversational speech with at least 20 productions of the target sound)
- *Probe criterion:* A 90% accuracy in the production of sounds in untrained words presented on a series of Probe trials with at least 10 untrained words
- *Probe timing and frequency criterion:* A probe will be administered when a child meets the training criterion on four to five stimulus items or exemplars (e.g., when the child's correct response rate on four words— soup, soap, sun, and seed—reaches 90% accuracy on a block of 10 evoked training trials, a probe will be conducted with at least 10 untrained words interspersed with trained words; the same criterion for all word positions, phrases, and sentences)
- *Reinstatement of training criterion:* Treatment on the same sound in the same word position will be reinstated if the probe criterion is not met (similar criterion for phrases and sentences); after training the sound in four new words, a probe will be conducted

again; training and probes will be alternated until the probe criterion of 90% accuracy in untrained words is achieved

- Establish <u>Baselines</u> of target sounds in words, phrases, sentences, and conversational speech
  - measure the correct production of target sounds in conversational speech; use the initial sample recorded during assessment; repeat the procedure to obtain another sample in the first intervention session; if the initial assessment sample and the first intervention-session sample show different percentage of errors for the same sound, repeat the sample
  - measure the production of target sounds in words with the discrete trial procedure; administer one set of trials with modeling and one without:
    1. place a picture or an object in front of the child
    2. ask a relevant question (e.g., "What is this?")
    3. model the correct response (e.g., "Say *soup*."); emphasize the target sound
    4. wait a few seconds for the child to imitate
    5. move the picture toward you and record the sound production as correct, incorrect, or no response
    6. present the same picture; ask the same question; but do not model the response; record the response as before
    7. administer all target words once with modeling (modeled trial) and once without (evoked trial)
    8. calculate percent correct imitated and evoked response rate for each sound and each word-position
- Teach **sound production** in words, phrases, and sentences using the discrete trial procedure; initially, train the target sound at the word (or syllable) level with <u>Modeling</u>:
  1. describe the target sound and how it is produced; demonstrate its production; and point out its <u>Pho-</u>

netic Placement; if necessary, use Manual Guidance to move articulators to their correct production; see Sound-Evoking Techniques for English Consonants that describe specific instructions and manipulations that facilitate the production of specific sounds

2. place a picture or an object in front of the child

3. ask a relevant question (e.g., "What is this?")

4. model the correct response (e.g., "Say *sun*."); emphasize the target sound

5. wait a few seconds for the child to imitate

6. positively reinforce the child by verbal praise, a token, or a primary reinforcer as soon as he or she correctly imitates the sound

7. give corrective feedback if the child does not imitate correctly (say "That is not correct; you said _____; I want you to say _____."); use Time-out or Response Cost to control incorrect sound productions and uncooperative or interfering behaviors

8. move the picture toward you and record the sound production as correct, incorrect, or no response

9. represent the same picture; repeat the instructions on correct production; show the phonetic placement for its production; ask the same question; model the response; record the response as before

10. continue this training with modeling until the child gives five consecutively correct imitated responses; discontinue modeling

11. if the child fails to imitate the sound in a word in 10 trials, use Shaping by dropping to the syllable or isolated phoneme production level; when the child correctly imitates the phoneme on 5 trials, move up to the syllable level; with 5 correct imitative responses at the syllable level, move up to the word level; with 5 correct imitations at the word level, discontinue modeling

- Administer evoked trials
  1. present the same picture, ask the same question, but do not model
  2. reinforce the correct responses or give corrective feedback for incorrect responses; repeat instructions, demonstrations of phonetic placement if necessary
  3. continue this training without modeling until the child gives 9 correct responses in a block of 10 trials; when this happens, consider the particular word tentatively trained
  4. select another word with the same target sound and begin training with modeling; discontinue and reinstate modeling as before; drop to phoneme or syllable level if necessary; move up to the word level; when the child gives 9 correct evoked responses in a word in a block of 10 trials, consider this word tentatively trained; follow this procedure until the child is trained on at least 4 words, perhaps up to 6 words
- Probe for generalized production of the trained sound
  - note that a probe is done to assess generalized production of trained sounds in untrained contexts
  - initially, conduct an <u>Intermixed Probe</u> with at least 10 untrained words intermixed with trained words; alternate trained and untrained words; reuse trained words; note that untrained words are also called the probe words; correct production of the sound in probe words indicates that the child will produce the sound in new and untrained words
  - prepare an <u>Intermixed Probe Recording Sheet</u> as shown here and record the probe responses
  - note that all probe trials are evoked only; do not model correct productions
  - reinforce or provide corrective feedback for sound productions only in already trained words; do not reinforce or provide corrective feedback for correct or

incorrect productions in untrained (probe) words; see also Probe Procedure

Intermixed Probe Response Recording Sheet	
Name:	Treatment target:
Clinician:	Date: Session #:
Target Behavior: Correct production of /s/ in word-initial positions	Responses (+ = correct; − = incorrect; 0 = no response
1. soup (trained)	
2. superman (untrained)	
3. sun (trained)	
4. sunflower (untrained)	
5. soap (trained)	
6. soda (untrained)	
7. seed (trained)	
8. seal (untrained)	

Note: Repeat the trained words until at least 10 probe words are administered.

5. calculate the percent correct probe response rate based only on the number of probe words, ignoring the trained words in this calculation (e.g., If the child's production of the target sound was correct in 5 of the 10 probe words, the correct probe response rate is 50%.)

- Alternate between probe and training
  - if the child's probe response rate is below 90%, provide additional training with new training words; after training four or six more words, administer another intermixed probe; if the probe criterion is not met, train more words and probe again until the child meets the probe criterion

- when the intermixed probe criterion is met, administer a <u>Pure Probe</u> in which only untrained words are presented; calculate the percent correct pure probe response rate; if it is below 90% correct, provide a few additional training trials on all the trained words until the pure probe criterion is met
- switch training to another target sound or the same sound in a different word position; follow the same procedure as outlined to complete training the sound at the word initial, medial, and final positions; train other sounds at the word level with the same procedure

- Shift training to higher levels of response complexity
  - when a sound meets either the intermixed or pure probe criterion for a given word-position (e.g., the initial position), construct two- or three-word phrases that contain a word in which the sound is produced correctly
  - administer the phrases the same way as the words; model initially; withdraw modeling when at least five correct imitations are produced; reinstate modeling if incorrect responses return; withdraw modeling again
  - after training four to six phrases to the same training criterion as 90% correct on a block of 10 trials, administer an intermixed probe; provide additional training on new phrases if the intermixed probe criterion is not met; when the intermixed probe criterion is met, administer a probe; when the pure probe criterion is met, shift training to sentence levels in which the word with correct production of the target sound is included
  - train sentences in the same manner as words and phrases; after presenting the stimulus item, ask a question that would evoke a sentence (e.g., ask "What is the boy doing?" to evoke "He is having some *soup.*"); initially, model the sentences and withdraw

modeling: probe generalized production of sounds in conversation in the same way as described for words and phrases

- when the pure probe criterion is met for sentences, shift training to conversational speech level; with the help of pictures and other stimulus materials, engage the child in conversational speech and positively reinforce correct productions on an Intermittent <u>Reinforcement Schedule</u>; prompt the correct productions; give corrective feedback

- periodically, conduct pure conversational probes in which you engage the child in conversation without reinforcement or corrective feedback; continue training until the child meets the 90% correct production of all target sounds in conversational speech with little or no prompting and reinforcement

• Note that within the framework of this comprehensive treatment program, you can use components of various programs of articulation treatment described under <u>Treatment of Articulation and Phonological Disorders: Specific Techniques or Programs</u>; for instance:

- use aspects of the <u>Contrast Approach</u>; in using the <u>Minimal Pair Contrast Method</u>, write minimal pair contrast words for training each sound; for instance, in teaching a child to produce final consonants (elimination of final consonantal deletion), write such word pairs as *bow-boat, bee-beet, toe-toad, pie-pine*; to teach the correct production of a single phoneme such as /b/ for which the child substitutes /p/, write such pairs as *bye-pie, bat-pat, beat-peat, bike-pike*; instead of placing a single stimulus item as previously described, place a pair of stimulus items in front of the child; model both the words and ask the child to imitate; withdraw modeling and prove evoked trials; move through response complexity levels as described earlier

- use aspects of the Paired-Stimuli Approach; instead of presenting only the target word in which the child misarticulates the sound (as described earlier), present both the target word and a Key Word in which the sound is correctly produced; ask the child to produce the key word first and then the target word; see Paired-Stimuli Approach for details; when the client meets the training criterion for words, move on to probes and then to training the words in sentences
- use aspects of the Multiple Phoneme Approach if the child exhibits multiple errors; instead of training one sound at a time as described, train multiple phonemes; see the description of the procedure for details
- use aspects of the Phonological Process Approach if the client exhibits multiple misarticulations with identified patterns; note that the phonological process approach does not have a unique treatment *procedure*; to eliminate a process, individual phonemes still need to be taught; this teaching involves instructions, modeling, phonetic placement, manual guidance, positive reinforcement, corrective feedback, and so forth; in using the phonological process approach, identify patterns or processes in misarticulations; select processes for elimination; teach the phonemes as described in the comprehensive program; when you teach a few phonemes within a process, probe the other phonemes within the process to see if they are now produced on the basis of generalization; if they are, move on to the other processes or to higher levels of response complexity; if they are not produced, train additional sounds within the process
- Implement a maintenance program
  - Always train the correct production of sounds in sentences and in naturalistic conversational speech during the final stages of treatment

- Conduct informal training sessions in Extraclinical Settings; monitor the child's correct speech sound production outside the therapy room but within the clinic, outside the clinic but in the surround areas, and in such natural settings as the classroom, the shool dining hall, and the library
- Train family members, teachers, and peers in reinforcing the correct production of sounds in Natural Settings; ask the parents or other caregivers to observe your treatment session; educate them about the correct production of target sounds; ask them to pay attention to the correct method of providing positive reinforcement and corrective feedback; train them to prompt and promptly reinforce the correct productions at home; train them to hold brief training sessions at home; ask parents to tape-record the session and review the tape to give them feedback
- Teach the client Self-Control (Self-Monitoring) techniques to self-manage the correct and incorrect productions; in the treatment sessions, ask the child to judge the accuracy of his or her productions; give feedback on this judgment; ask the child to mark on a sheet his or her own responses as either correct or incorrect; teach the child to pause briefly as soon as an error is produced and then try to produce it correctly
- Follow up the child periodically and assess the correct production of phonemes in conversational speech; provide booster treatment when the correct production in conversational speech falls below 90% accuracy

Peña-Brooks, A., & Hegde, M. N. (2000). *Assessment and treatment of articulation and phonological disorders in children.* Austin, TX: Pro-Ed.

Hegde, M. N. (1998a). *Treatment procedures in communicative disorders* (3rd ed.). Austin, TX: Pro-Ed.

Hegde, M. N. (1998b). *Treatment protocols in communicative disorders: Targets and strategies.* Austin, TX: Pro-Ed.

Treatment of Articulation and Phonological Disorders in African American Children

African American English is a product of unique historical and cultural forces; it is a recognized form of English; therefore, note that:

- African American English (AAE) has its own phonologic, syntactic, semantic, and pragmatic rules and conventions
- The phoneme inventory of children speaking AAE will consist of the same phonemes as in Standard American English (SAE); only some phonemes will be used differently, substituted for other phonemes, or omitted in certain contexts
- A majority of phonemes are used in the same way in both AAE and SAE
- The clinician needs to know which AAE phonemic usages that differ from those of SAE are indeed characteristics of AAE; the following phonological patterns are accepted in AAE and hence are not to be treated as disorders:
  - /l/ lessening or omission (e.g., *too'* for *tool; a'ways* for *always*)
  - /r/ lessening or omission (e.g., *doah* for *door; mudah* for *mother*)
  - /θ/ substitution for /f/ in word final or medial positions (e. g., *teef* for *teeth, nofin'* for *nothing*)
  - /t/ substitution for /θ/ in word initial positions (e.g., *tink* for *think*)
  - /d/ substitution for /ð/ in word initial and medial positions (e.g., *dis* for *this* and *broder* for *brother*)
  - /v/ substitution for /ð/ at word final positions (e.g., *smoov* for *smooth*)
  - omission of consonants in clusters in word initial and final positions (e.g., *thow* for *throw* and *des'* for *desk*)

- consonant substitutions within clusters (e.g., *skrike* for *strike*)
- unique syllable stress patterns (e.g., ***gui** tar* for *guitar* and ***Ju** ly* for *July*)
- modification of verbs ending in /k/ (e.g., *li-id* for *liked* and *wah-tid* for *walked*)
- metathetic productions (e.g., *aks* for *ask*)
- devoicing of final voiced consonants (e.g., *bet* for *bed* and *ruk* for *rug*)
- deletion of final consonants (*ba'* for *bad* and *goo'* for *good*)
- /i/ substitution for /e/ (e.g., *pin* for *pen* and *tin* for *ten*)
- /b/ substitution for /v/ (e.g., *balentine* for *valentine* and *bes'* for *vest*)
- diphthong reduction or ungliding (e.g., *fahnd* for *find* and *ol* for *oil*)
- /n/ substitution for /g/ (e.g., *walkin'* for *walking* and *thin'* for *thing*)
- unstressed syllable deletion (*bout* for *about* and *member* for *remember*)
- A treatable articulation disorder for a child who speaks AAE is a disorder in the context of AAE, not in the context of SAE
- Note that not all African Americans speak AAE; hence, it should not be stereotypically assumed that AAE articulatory patterns are automatically targets for African American children; family communication patterns and the parents' preferences will dictate the target phonological patterns
- Plan an articulation and phonological treatment program for an African American child, with the following guidelines:
  - select the speech patterns of AAE (even if they vary from those of standard English) as treatment goals for a speaker of AAE

- accept and reinforce sound patterns that are accepted in AAE (e.g., a child's production of *baftub* for *bathtub* is acceptable and reinforceable in treatment)
- treat first the phoneme usages that are the same in AAE and SAE (many actually are)
- treat next the unique phoneme usages of AAE that the child does not use correctly; the goal is to teach what is acceptable in AAE, even if it deviates from SAE
- change AAE dialectal patterns to SAE patterns only if the client, the family, or both demand it; in this case, treatment of SAE sound patterns is *elective*

- As with all children, select functional speech sounds, child-specific sounds, and sounds that when treated will rapidly improve the child's speech intelligibility

- Select stimulus items for treatment from the child's home environment; consult with parents about pictures, objects, toys, and other materials for their appropriateness and child familiarity

- Consult the family members about appropriate reinforcers for the child; ask the child about his or her preferences; but as always, determine that a consequence is a reinforcer only after data show that correct productions have increased during treatment

- Unless data show otherwise, assume that standard treatment procedures (e.g., modeling, phonetic placement, positive reinforcement involving especially verbal praise, and a token system backed up with a variety of culturally appropriate reinforcers) will be effective with African American children; in all treatment sessions, record the response rates systematically to support or correct this assumption

Peña-Brooks, A., & Hegde, M. N. (2000). *Assessment and treatment of articulation and phonological disorders in children.* Austin, TX: Pro-Ed.

Roseberry-McKibbin, C. (1995). *Multicultural students with special needs.* Oceanside, CA: Academic Communication Associates.

Stockman, I. (1996). Phonological development and disorders in African American children. In A. G. Kamhi, K. E. Pollock, & J. L. Harris (Eds.), *Communication development and disorders in African American children* (pp. 117–153). Baltimore: Paul H. Brookes.

Treatment of Articulation and Phonological Disorders in Bilingual Children

Bilingual children are a large and varied group. In the United States, children whose primary language is Spanish constitute a large and growing group. Other groups include children whose primary language is an Asian language or a Native American language. Because of the variety of primary languages that influence the secondary English spoken in the United States, it is not possible to list the characteristics of all the various primary languages that influence American English. Follow the guidelines specified below to develop appropriate articulation and phonological treatment programs for bilingual children:

- Make a thorough assessment of articulation and phonological skills in children who are bilingual; assess in primary language as well as in the secondary Standard American English (SAE); consult the cited sources and the *PGASLP*
- Analyze errors in the primary language; select these as the treatment targets; note that such treatment requires the working knowledge of the child's primary language; in the absence of such knowledge, refer the child to a speech-language pathologist (SLP) who has the knowledge
- Analyze errors in SAE that are *not* due to the influence of the primary language; these errors, too, may be treatment targets; note that a monolingual English-speaking SLP can offer this treatment, assuming that an assessment was made with the help of a bilingual clinician
- Analyze English sound productions that vary from those in SAE but are due to the influence of the child's

primary language; these are not normally the targets of articulation treatment

- Treat SAE articulatory variations in English only if the client or the family request such treatment because of the advantage SAE offers in educational, social, and occupational settings
- Treat errors in phonemes that are common to the child's primary language and the secondary SAE on a priority basis
- As with all children, select functional speech sounds, child-specific sounds, and sounds that when treated will rapidly improve the child's speech intelligibility
- Select stimulus items for treatment from the child's home environment; consult with parents about pictures, objects, toys, and other materials for their appropriateness and child familiarity
- Consult the family members about appropriate reinforcers for the child; ask the child about his or her preferences; but, as always, determine that a consequence is a reinforcer only after data show that correct productions have increased during treatment
- Unless data show otherwise, assume that standard treatment procedures (e.g., modeling, phonetic placement, positive reinforcement involving especially verbal praise, and a token system backed up with a variety of culturally appropriate reinforcers) will be effective with bilingual children; in all treatment sessions, record the response rates systematically to support or correct this assumption
- Modify treatment techniques to suit the individual child; keep good records of such modifications to evaluate whether they were needed because of individual differences or ethnocultural variations
- Refer the child to a bilingual clinician who knows the child's primary language

- Use the following characteristics of **Spanish-influenced English** in treating articulation and phonological disorders in a child whose primary language is Spanish:
  - Spanish has only 5 vowels (as against 15 in English)
  - the English consonants /v/, /θ/, /ð/, /z/, and /ʒ/ are not in Spanish; while speaking English, some of these may be produced as allophonic variations of phonemes present in Spanish
  - some Spanish consonants, though similar to certain consonants in English, may be produced differently
  - Spanish has only a few consonants in word final positions (only /s/, /n/, /r/, /l/, and /d/)
  - Spanish consonantal clusters are fewer and simpler; the /s/ cluster, most common in English, does not occur in Spanish; final clusters are rare in Spanish
  - English /t/, /d/, and /n/ tend to be dentalized
  - final consonants may be devoiced (e.g, *dose* for *doze*)
  - /b/ may be substituted for /v/ (e.g., *bery* for *very*)
  - weak or deaspirated stops, giving the impression of omission of stop sounds
  - /tʃ/ may be substituted for /ʃ/ (e.g., *Chirley* for *Shirley*)
  - /d/ or /z/ may be substituted for /ð/, which does not exist in Spanish (e.g., *dis* for *this* or *zat* for *that*)
  - schwa may be inserted before word-initial consonant clusters (*eskate* for *skate* or *espend* for *spend*)
  - omission of many consonants at word-final positions
  - /r/ may be trapped (as in the English word *butter*) or trilled
  - word-initial /h/ may be silent (e.g., *old* for *hold* or *it* for *hit*)
  - /y/ may be substituted for /dʒ/, an absent sound in Spanish (e.g., *yulie* for *Julie*)
  - /s/ may be produced more frontally, giving the impression of a lisp

- In treating articulation and phonological disorders in other bilingual children (such as those whose primary language is one of many Asian languages):
  - use the general guidelines already specified for working with bilingual children
  - note that because of the diversity of Asian languages, a general description of phonological characteristics is neither practical nor meaningful
  - note that many descriptions in the literature under the heading of *Asian* children or speakers apply only to the Chinese, not to other Asian languages
  - note that Asian languages belong to different language families and hence are highly varied in their phonological and other characteristics

Kayser, H. (1995). *Bilingual speech-language pathology: An Hispanic focus*. San Diego: Singular Publishing Group.

Peña-Brooks, A., & Hegde, M. N. (2000). *Assessment and treatment of articulation and phonological disorders in children*. Austin, TX: Pro-Ed.

Roseberry-McKibbin, C. (1995). *Multicultural students with special needs*. Oceanside, CA: Academic Communication Associates.

Sound-Evoking Techniques for English Consonants.

Several procedures to evoke sounds during treatment are available; no systematic research has evaluated the relative effectiveness of these procedures; these techniques are based on clinical experience of many clinicians; therefore, use them with caution and modify or abandon procedures that do not produce results; generously reinforce any slight improvement in the client's target sound production or a movement in the right direction:

- Evocation of /p/, a bilabial, voiceless, stop-plosive:
  - model the sound production several times; draw attention to the lip closure, building up of air pressure in the mouth, and air explosion as the sound is produced

- with a piece of paper, show the plosive characteristic that can move the paper held in front of the mouth
- manually guide the two lips to the required articulatory posture; ask the child to forcefully expel the air from the mouth
- shape the /p/ from the explosive airstream
- Evocation of /b/, a bilabial, voiced stop-plosive:
  - use the same procedures as those described for /p/ except that, as the child forcefully releases the air, ask him or her to add voice or to turn on the voice box; let the child feel the vocal fold vibrations as you produce the sound; ask the child to produce those vibrations as the air is released from the mouth; shape the /b/ out of these manipulations
- Evocation of /t/, a lingua-alveolar, voiceless stop-plosive:
  - model the sound production several times, drawing attention to the placement of the tongue tip against the alveolar ridge; with the help of a moving feather, draw attention to the air that escapes through the mouth as the sound is produced
  - ask the child to place the tongue tip firmly against the alveolar ridge; if necessary, place a piece of food on the alveolar ridge with a Q-tip to teach the exact tongue tip placement; hold the breath briefly, lower the tip slightly, and release the air as the tongue tip is lowered
  - shape /t/ with such manipulations
- Evocation of /d/, a lingua-alveolar, voiced stop-plosive:
  - use the same procedures as those described for /t/; in addition, teach the child to add voicing by helping the child feel the vocal fold vibrations; ask the child to turn on the voice box
- Evocation of /k/, a lingua-velar, voiceless stop-plosive:
  - model the sound production several times, demonstrate the tongue tip placement behind the front teeth

and the raised back portion of the tongue that makes firm contact with the soft palate; build up air pressure in the mouth and suddenly lower the back of the mouth to release the air in a plosive manner

- shape the sound with this manipulation

- Evocation of /g/, a lingua-velar, voiced stop-plosive:
  - use the procedure as described for /k/ and ask the child to add voice or turn on the voice; let the child feel the vocal fold vibrations

- Evocation of /f/, a labiodental, voiceless fricative:
  - model the production of the sound several times; draw attention to the lower lip position under the front upper teeth; manually guide the lips and the teeth to the right placement
  - ask the child to blow air through the teeth and the lip when they are still in contact with each other; ask the child to turn off the voice box
  - use a feather or a piece of paper to demonstrate the air flow out of the mouth
  - shape the sound out of such manipulations

- Evocation of /v/, a labiodental, voiced fricative:
  - use the same procedure as described for /f/ and ask the child to add voice or turn on the voice box; let the child feel the vocal fold vibrations

- Evocation of /θ/, linguadental voiceless fricative:
  - model the sound production several times; draw attention to the slightly protruded tongue tip between the upper and lower front teeth and the air being blown over the tongue and through the constriction between the tongue tip and the teeth
  - instruct the child to position the tongue as demonstrated; if necessary, ask the child to stick the tongue out of the mouth, then draw it slowly in until it is correctly positioned; use manual guidance with a tongue depressor

- ask the child to blow the air over the tongue and through the constriction between the tongue tip and the teeth; shape the sound through these manipulations
- alternatively, shape the sound while the child produces /f/; ask the child to push the tongue tip forward to come in contact with the teeth as the /f/ is being produced
- alternatively, shape the sound while the child produces /s/; ask the child to move the tongue tip to position as the /s/ is being produced

- Evocation of /ð/, a lingua-dental voiced fricative:
  - use the same procedure as described for /θ/ and ask the child to add voice or turn on the voice box; let the child feel the vocal fold vibrations

- Evocation of /s/, a lingua-alveolar voiceless fricative:
  - model the sound production several times; draw attention to either the tongue-tip-up position or the tongue-tip-down position with which this sound can be produced
  - teach the child to place the tip of the tongue behind the upper teeth and groove the tongue-midline
  - teach the child to bring the upper and lower teeth together
  - teach the child to blow the air out along the groove of the tongue
  - alternatively, shape an /s/ out of /θ/ by asking the child to draw the tongue inward until the sound approximates the /s/

- Evocation of /z/, a lingua-alveolar voiced fricative:
  - use the procedures described for /s/ and ask the child to add voice by turning on the voice box; let the client feel the vocal fold vibrations
  - alternatively, shape /z/ out of /ð/ or from /θ/ to which the child adds voice

- Evocation of /ʃ/, lingua-palatal voiceless fricative:

- model the sound production several times; draw attention to the articulatory position
- shape /ʃ/ out of /s/; while the child is producing /s/, ask the child to pucker the lips and to move the tongue back until /ʃ/ results
- ask the child to produce "shh" (the "be quiet" sound) and shape /ʃ/ out of this production
- Evocation of /ʒ/, a lingua-palatal voiced fricative:
  - use the procedures described for /ʃ/ and ask the child to add voice or turn on the voice box
  - alternatively, shape /ʒ/ out of /z/
- Evocation of /tʃ/, alveo-palatal voiceless affricate:
  - model the sound production several times; draw attention to the articulatory positions
  - shape /tʃ/ out of an initial /t/ the child is asked to hold and then explode into an /ʃ/, which may result in /tʃ/
  - alternatively, have the child place the tip of the tongue right behind the front teeth; then ask the child to move the tip slightly back; ask the child to make the sneezing sound (*choo!*) while puckering the lips
  - alternatively, have the child say phrases in which the first word ends with /t/ and the second word begins with /ʃ/ (e.g., *that ship*); bring the production of the two sounds together to achieve /tʃ/
  - shape the sound with these manipulations
- Evocation of /dʒ/, alveo-palatal, voiced affricate:
  - use procedures described for /tʃ/ and ask the child to add voice or turn the voice box on
  - alternatively, have the child produce phrases in which the first word ends with /t/ and the second word starts with /j/ (e.g., *meet you* and *found you*); bring the /t/ and the /j/ sounds closer to achieve /dʒ/
- Evocation of /m/, a bilabial, voiced nasal:
  - model the sound production several times; draw attention to the articulatory positions; emphasize the nasal resonance; have the client feel the nasal vibrations

- instruct the child to hum continuously and, while doing this, open the mouth; this might result in *ma,* from which you can shape /m/
- alternatively, teach the child to breathe in deeply through the nose, close the mouth, and let the air come out of the nose while saying "Ah"; this might result in /m/
- shape /m/ out of these manipulations
- Evocation of /n/, a lingua-alveolar, voiced nasal:
  - model the sound production several times; draw attention to the articulatory positions; emphasize the nasal resonance; let the child feel the nasal vibrations
  - shape /n/ from /d/; teach the child to let the air out through the nose while producing /d/
  - alternatively, ask the child to breathe out through the nose with voice added while keeping the tongue tip positioned for /n/
  - shape /n/ with such manipulations
- Evocation of /ŋ/, a lingua-velar, voiced nasal:
  - model the sound production several times; draw attention to the articulatory positions; emphasize the nasal resonance; let the child feel the nasal vibrations
  - shape /ŋ/out of /g/ by teaching the child to produce /g/ while keeping the mouth closed to direct the air through the nose
  - alternatively, ask the child to produce a prolonged [i] and, while doing this, ask the child to raise the back of the tongue to make a firm contact with the roof of the mouth
  - shape /ŋ/ out of these manipulations
- Evocation of [j], a lingua-palatal voiced glide:
  - model the sound production several times; draw attention to the articulatory positions
  - shape [j] with a prolonged [i]; teach the client to prolong the [i] and quickly produce [u], resulting in [iju]; teach the client to shorten or unvoice the [i], resulting in [j]

- shape [j] with /ʒ/; ask the child to produce /ʒ/ in quick succession, resulting in [ʒ]
- shape [ʒ] with these manipulations
- Evocation of [w], a bilabial, voiced glide:
  - model the sound production several times; draw attention to the articulatory positions
  - shape [w] with [u]; ask the child to produce a prolonged [u] and then quickly add the schwa, resulting in [uwa]; teach the child to shorten the [u] or turn the voice off on it, resulting in [wa]
  - alternatively, teach the child to raise the back of the tongue without touching the roof of the mouth, round the lips and bring them closer, and breathe out with voicing
  - shape [w] with such manipulations
- Evocation of [r], an alveo-palatal voiced glide:
  - model the sound production several times; draw attention to the articulatory positions
  - ask the child to place the tongue tip slightly behind the upper front teeth; ask the child then to "curl the tongue backward" without making contact with the roof of the mouth; round the lips slightly, and breathe out with voice on; this should result in [r]
  - alternatively, shape [r] from [d]; from the [d] position, ask the child to lower the tongue tip; retract the tongue, round the lips slightly, and breathe out with voice on; this should result in [r]
  - alternatively, ask the child to growl like a tiger and shape [r] from that growl
  - shape [r] with such manipulations
- Evocation of [l], an alveolar voiced lateral:
  - model the sound production several times; draw attention to the articulatory positions
  - with a tongue depressor, lift the tip of the tongue and position it for [l]; ask the child to breathe out and turn on the voice, resulting in [l]

- alternatively, ask the child to produce a prolonged [a] and, while producing this, ask the child to raise the tongue tip to the alveolar ridge, resulting in [l]
- shape [l] by such manipulations

Treatment of Articulation and Phonological Disorders: Specific Techniques or Programs

Behavioral Approaches. Articulation treatment techniques based on the use of Behavioral Contingencies of stimulus-response-consequence in shaping or teaching sound production in words, sentences, and conversational speech; also may use a programmed learning approach; elements of behavioral approaches are found in almost all programs of articulation and phonological treatment, including those that that are not typically described as behavioral.

Programmed Conditioning for Articulation. A behavioral treatment method that uses behavioral principles and programmed learning concepts; developed by R. Baker and B. Ryan.

- Criterion of Performance: Ten correct responses in a row.

Establishment Phase: Training Sequence
Sound in Isolation
- Sound in isolation with Continuous Reinforcement (crf)

Nonsense Syllable Level
- Sound in initial position of nonsense syllables (crf)
- Sound in final position of nonsense syllables (crf)
- Sound in medial position of nonsense syllables (crf)

Word Level
- Sound in word-initial position (50% rf)
- Sound in word-final position (50% rf)
- Sound in word-medial position (50% rf)

Phrase Level
- Sound in word-initial position produced in two- or three-word phrases (50% rf)

- Sound in word-final position produced in two- or three-word phrases (50% rf)
- Sound in word-medial position produced in two- or three-word phrases (50% rf)

Sentence Level
- Sound in word-initial position produced in four- to six-word sentences (50% rf)
- Sound in word-final position produced in four- or six-word sentences (50% rf)
- Sound in word-medial position produced in four- to six-word sentences (50% rf)

Contextual Reading Level
(Go to the next level if the client is a nonreader)
- Sound in orally read sentences (crf)

Story Narration Level
- Sound in story retelling (after silently reading a story) (crf)

Picture Description Level
- Sound in sentences and phrases produced to describe a story (crf)

Conversational Speech Level
- Sound in conversational speech (crf)
- Sound in conversational speech (10% rf)

Administer the criterion test

Move to the Transfer Phase and begin training on new sounds

Transfer Phase: Training Sequence
Home Training
- Sound in words, repeats the words (crf)
- Sound in phrases, repeats the phrases (crf)
- Sound in sentences, repeats the sentences (crf)
- Sound in oral reading or picture description (crf)
- Sound in conversation (crf)

Clinician Training in Different Settings
- Conversation outside the clinic room door (crf)
- Conversation down the hall (crf)

- Conversation outside the clinic building or in another room (crf)
- Conversation in playground, cafeteria, or away from school or clinic (crf)
- Conversation outside classroom (crf)

Training in Classroom

- Conversation with clinician in classroom (crf)
- Conversation with clinician and teacher in classroom (crf)
- Conversation in small-group activity (crf)
- Conversation in large-group activity (crf)
- Speech or "show and tell" in front of the class (crf)

Administer the transfer criterion test

Maintenance Phase: Training Sequence

- Conversation during weekly meetings for the first 4 weeks (crf)
- Conversation during one monthly meeting (crf)
- Dismiss the client

Baker, R. D., & Ryan, B. P. (1971). *Programmed conditioning for articulation.* Monterey, CA: Monterey Learning Systems.

Peña-Brooks, A., & Hegde, M. N. (2000). *Assessment and treatment of articulation and phonological disorders in children.* Austin, TX: Pro-Ed.

Contrast Approach. A cognitive-linguistic approach to treatment of articulation disorders; often used in remediating phonological processes; uses contrasting pairs of words that contain **minimal** or **maximal** differences between the target sounds and those contrasted; the actual training of sounds may involve behavioral contingencies; researched by multiple investigators.

Minimal Pair Contrast Method. Uses word pairs that have minimal phonemic contrast (e.g., *b*at-*p*at).

- Analyze the client's misarticulations
- Write minimal contrast word pairs; for instance, to remediate deletion of final consonants, write such pairs as *boat-bow, bee-bead,* and *tee-teeth*; to remediate

fronting, write such pairs as *can-tan, key-tea,* and *gate-date.*
- Obtain pictures for words in selected pairs
- Begin treatment by modeling both the target and the contrast words; ask the child to imitate both
- Provide extensive trials on imitative production of the target and contrast words
- Ask the client to spontaneously name the picture pairs
- Ask the client to name the pictures and then sort them into separate piles
- Alternatively, ask the client to say the target word as you pick the correct picture (the client says *boat* and you pick up the picture of *boat*; if the client says *bow,* you pick-up the picture of *bow* and then correct the client)
- Ask the client to match two pictures by first picking a picture from several displayed and then selecting its minimal pair match

Maximal Pair Contrast Method. Uses word pairs that have multiple (maximal) phonemic contrasts or maximal opposition.
- Select word pairs that contrast maximally; for instance, select such word pairs as *chain-main; can-man; gear-fear* (the initial phoneme in the first word of each pair is the target of treatment; the initial phoneme in the second word in each pair is the phoneme with maximal opposition)
- Use the general procedure outlined for Minimal Pair Contrast Method

Cycles Approach. A phonological pattern approach designed to treat children with multiple misarticulations and highly unintelligible speech; approach consists of treatment cycles which vary between 5 weeks and 16 weeks; includes auditory stimulation and production practices; developed by B. Hodson and E. Paden.

- Assess the client's phonological performance with 50 spontaneous naming responses and continuous speech samples; may use Hodson's *Assessment of Phonological Processes—Revised*
- Arrange a hierarchy of stimulable phonological patterns that occur in at least 40% of the relevant contexts
- Treat the most stimulable pattern first, then the next most stimulable pattern, and so on
- Target only one phonological pattern in any single session
- Treat each phoneme within a target pattern for about 60 minutes per cycle (one 60-minute, two 30-minute, or three 20-minute sessions) before moving to other phonemes within the pattern or to other patterns
- Review the prior week's production practice word cards (*see below*); skip this step if introducing a new pattern for treatment
- Begin treatment with auditory bombardment:
  - ask the client to listen attentively for about 2 minutes as you produce 12 words with the target sound and sentences containing those words
  - slightly amplify your presentation with an auditory trainer
  - do not ask the client to produce the sounds
  - periodically contrast the correct and the incorrect production of the target sound
- Use five production-practice word cards: Ask the client to first say a target word and then draw, color, or paste the picture of the word on 5×8 index cards; write the word on the card
- Begin production practice:
  - ask the client to name about five target pictures (five words per sound)

- model the target word; use auditory, tactual, and visual cues
- engage the client in conversation
- use a game format
- Probe for stimulability of next session's target sounds
- Repeat the amplified auditory bombardment; present the same 12 words as before
- Ask the family members or teachers to read the same 12-word list to the client; ask the client to name the five picture cards used in production practice during the week
- Recycle a pattern that persists in conversational speech

Hodson, B., & Paden, E. (1983). *Targeting intelligible speech: A phonological approach to remediation.* San Diego: College-Hill Press.

Peña-Brooks, A., & Hegde, M. N. (2000). *Assessment and treatment of articulation and phonological disorders in children.* Austin, TX: Pro-Ed.

Distinctive Feature Approach. Articulation treatment approach based on a distinctive feature analysis; the goal is to establish missing <u>Distinctive Features</u> or feature contrasts by teaching relevant sounds; technically, not a treatment procedure; approach assumes that teaching a feature in the context of a few sounds will result in generalized production of other sounds with the same feature or features; more research is needed to fully support this assumption; approach is most useful with children who have multiple misarticulations that can be grouped on the basis of distinctive features, not useful for (a) treating distorted sounds as the analysis is not relevant to such errors; (b) treating a client with only a few errors that do not form patterns based on distinctive features; developed and researched by multiple investigators.

- Obtain an extended conversational speech sample

- Determine omitted and substituted sounds (phonemes in error)
- Score the distinctive features for all phonemes by assigning plus and minus values
- Select target features for treatment: select the features that are not produced at all (100% error rate) or those that have a high error rate
- Select the phonemes that represent those features for teaching
- Use the programmed approach of teaching the selected sounds at the level of isolated production and production of sounds in syllables, words, phrases, and sentences
- At all levels, except for the sentence level, model the correct production for the child to imitate
- Fade modeling when the client's imitative responses are consistent
- Probe untreated sounds that share the same features as the target sounds to see if generalized productions occur
- Select additional sounds for training when there is no generalized production
- Select new sounds that contain other target features for training when there is generalized production
- Shift treatment to conversational speech inside and outside the clinic and to speech produced in home, school, and other nonclinical settings
- Teach self-monitoring
- Teach family members to praise the client for correct productions

Costello, J. M., & Onstein, J. (1976). The modification of multiple articulation errors based on distinctive feature theory. *Journal of Speech and Hearing Disorders, 41,* 199–215.

McReynolds, L. V., & Bennet, S. (1972). Distinctive feature generalization in articulation training. *Journal of Speech and Hearing Disorders, 37,* 462–470.

Peña-Brooks, A., & Hegde, M. N. (2000). *Assessment and treatment of articulation and phonological disorders in children.* Austin, TX: Pro-Ed.

Multiple Phoneme Approach. A method of articulation remediation in which all errors are treated in all sessions; appropriate for children with six or more errors; based on behavioral principles; focuses on sound production in conversational speech; does not emphasize auditory discrimination training; consists of establishment, transfer, and maintenance phases; each phase has several steps; highly structured and carefully sequenced; developed and researched by R. McCabe and D. Bradley.

- Obtain conversational speech sample of about 150 words
- Mark each word that contains at least one error
- Calculate percentage of words spoken correctly (Whole Word Accuracy: WWA)
- Use WWA measure to supplement single-word articulation tests

Phase I, Step 1. Establishment. Goal: Production of consonants in response to a printed letter or phonetic symbol representing it.

- Show an upper- or lowercase letter and ask "Do you know what sound this letter makes?" (visual cue only)
  - Ask the client to produce the sound in isolation on five successive trials (record the correct responses)
  - If the client cannot do this, record the error and move to the next step
- Give verbal instructions along with auditory and tactile stimuli; use any other effective procedure (auditory, visual, and phonetic-placement); continue until four out of five attempts are correct; move to the next step

- Show the letter and model the sound for the child to imitate (auditory and visual stimuli only); seek five consecutively correct responses; then, move to the next step
- Present only the letter (visual stimulus only); ask the client to make the sound; seek five consecutively correct responses

(Skip *visual only step* for children under age 5)

- In the first session or two, include sounds produced correctly to give experience of success; omit these sounds in subsequent sessions
- Reinforce correct responses (verbal praise, tokens)

Phase I, Step 2. Holding Procedure. Designed to maintain the correct production of sounds produced in isolation when they are not yet advanced to syllable or word levels; other sounds are moved to these higher levels.

- Evoke one correct response by showing the letter once and asking the client to produce the sound (visual stimulus only)

Phase II. Transfer. Goal: Production of all target sounds in conversational speech; simultaneous training of five or more sounds; sounds may be at different levels.

Phase II, Step 1: Syllable. Used only when the client fails to produce the sound correctly in 6 out of 10 probe words (5 words with the sound in the initial position and 5 words with the sound in the final position)

- Provide one auditory-visual model or one visual-only stimulus
- Ask the client to produce the sound with a variety of vowels
- Ask the client to produce the sound in both initial and final positions

- Seek five productions for each stimulus presentation
- Use a criterion of 80% correct over two sessions or 90% correct in one session

Phase II, Step 2: Word. Goal: Accurate production of target sounds in 25 to 30 varied words to be later included in sentences (nouns, verbs, modifiers, and prepositions).

- Present printed words or picture stimuli
- Ask the client to produce the word
- Accept erred production of nontarget phonemes
- Move training to the sentence level when the sound in a given position (e.g., initial position) is produced with 80% accuracy over two sessions or 90% accuracy in one session
- Continue training at the word level when the sound in a given position (e.g., final position) does not meet the criterion
- Consider using another approach, such as the minimal contrast therapy or phonological process approach, to eliminate the final consonant deletion process

Phase II, Step 3: Phrase and Sentence. Goal: Correct production of all sounds in words; self-monitoring.

- Construct phrases and sentences (imperatives, declaratives, and interrogatives) with words already trained, adding new words as needed
- Present Rebuses, Blissymbolics, or pictures for nonreaders
- Model phrases and sentences
- Ask the client to imitate
- Note phonetic contexts in which errors occur; have the client practice the production in these contexts
- Have the client practice words in which sounds are produced incorrectly as well as those that precede or follow such words

- Vary stress, rhythm, timing, and accent patterns
- Seek 80% accuracy over two sessions or 90% accuracy in one session, calculating accuracy with target sounds only

Phase II. Step 4: Reading and Storytelling. Goal: Accurate production of target sounds in connected utterances containing four to six words.

- Select reading materials that are easy for the child
- For nonreaders, select comic books, picture books, and sequence cards
- Tell a story and ask the child to retell it
- Seek whole word accuracy and 80% correct production over two sessions or 90% in one session

Phase II. Step 5: Conversation. Goal: Accurate production of all sounds used in conversational speech.

- Begin to monitor conversational speech when even one or two sounds reach this level
- Encourage discussions, descriptions, comments, questions, state facts, identify cause-effect relations, talk about emotions and desires; do not just answer questions
- When multiple sounds need to be monitored, group sounds on the basis of manner or place of articulation; monitor sounds in one group for 3 to 5 minutes; then, monitor sounds in another group, and so on
- Count every spoken word as a response and calculate the whole word accuracy level
- Note the context in which certain sounds are misarticulated and use these contexts for additional practice
- Seek 80% correct production of all words over two sessions or 90% in one session for children 6 years and older; seek 69% criterion for younger children

Phase III: Maintenance. Goal: Maintenance of 90% whole word accuracy in conversational speech produced in various speaking situations without treatment or external monitoring.

- Have the client return to the clinic; assess and monitor sound productions
- Visit classrooms
- Maintain telephone contact with the client and the family
- Obtain reports from others
- Have others monitor accuracy in various speaking situations
- Monitor for 3 months

McCabe, R., & Bradley, D. (1975). Systematic multiple phonemic approach to articulation therapy. *Acta Symbolica, 6,* 1–18.

Peña-Brooks, A., & Hegde, M. N. (2000). *Assessment and treatment of articulation and phonological disorders in children.* Austin, TX: Pro-Ed.

Paired-Stimuli Approach. A method of articulation remediation that depends on identifying a Key Word in which a target sound appears only once in either initial or final position and is correctly produced 9 out of 10 times; uses key words to teach the production of sounds in other contexts; explicitly uses operant reinforcement contingencies; uses pictures to evoke the target words; highly structured and carefully sequenced; a single speech sound is the target at any one time; developed and researched by J. Irwin and A. Weston.

Word Level

Consult Weston and Irwin(1971/1975) for assigned key words, questions to be asked, and expected answers.

- Select the target phonemes for the client

- Find four key words; two containing the target sound in the initial position and two containing it in the final position
- When absent, create key words by teaching them
- Select at least 10 training words in which the target sound is misarticulated and the sound appears only once in the same position as in the key word
- Select pictures as stimuli to evoke the word productions
- Place the **first** key word (picture) with sound in the **initial position** in the center and arrange the 10 training words (pictures) around it
- Point to the key word (picture) and ask the client to, "Say this"
- Reinforce the likely correct production
- Ask the client to name one of the 10 target words
- Ask the child to name the key word again
- Ask the child to name another target word; alternate the key word and a training word in this manner
- Reinforce the client by giving a token for the correct production of the target sound in both the key and the training words; ignore misarticulations of other sounds
- Complete a *training string* by pairing each of the 10 target words with the key word
- Include three training strings in each session that lasts about 30 minutes
- Adhere to a training criterion of 8 correct out of 10 productions of the training words in two successive training strings without reinforcement
- Arrange the **second** key word with the same sound in the **final position** and pair it with 10 training words

- In the next stage of training, ask the child to say the **third** key word with the target sound in the **initial position** and a training word as a <u>Response Unit</u> with only a brief pause between the two (e.g., "said-salad"; *s* is the target; *said* is the key word and *salad* is the target word)
- Reinforce only if the sounds in both the words are correctly produced
- Adhere to a training criterion of 8 out of 10 correct *response units* over two successive training strings
- Ask the child to say the **fourth** key word with the target sound in the **final position** and a training word as a *response unit* with only a brief pause between the two
- Reinforce the correct productions in response units as before

Sentence Level

- Pair the **first** key word with its 10 training words; ask a question designed to evoke a response in the sentence form (e.g., "What do you see?" "I *see* a cat" with *see* as the key word for /s/).
- Reinforce with a token on a fixed ratio 3 (FR3) schedule of reinforcement
- Complete a training string of 10 questions
- Adhere to the training criterion of 8 out of 10 correct sentences over two training strings
- Alternately, ask two questions (e.g., "What do you see?" for key word *see* and "That's what?" for key word *that's*) as you present the **first** and the **second** key words and their 10 training words
- Reinforce with a token for three correct sentences (FR3)
- Adhere to the training criterion of 8 out of 10 correct sentences over two training strings

- Ask four questions (e.g., "What is this?" "What do you see?" "That's what?" and "What did you say that was?") as you present the first and the fourth key words and their 10 training words
- Adhere to the criterion of 8 out of 10 correct sentences over two successive training strings

Conversational Level
- Engage the child in conversation
- Stop the conversation (a) when the child correctly produces a target sound in four words or (b) when the child incorrectly produces a target sound in any word; model the correct production; ask the child to repeat it
- Reinforce the child verbally and by showing your scoring of correct responses
- Subsequently, require the correct production of a target sound in seven words; probe when the child can do this
- In subsequent stages, require the correct production of a target sound in 10 and 13 words: probe when the child can do this
- Give verbal praise and visual feedback of scoring only when all productions are correct
- For all probes, take a conversational speech sample; no feedback of any sort during probes
- Terminate training on a given sound when the child gives 15 consecutively correct productions of a target sound in conversation held on two successive treatment sessions separated by at least 1 day

Irwin, J. V., & Weston, A. J. (1971/1975). *Paired Stimuli Kit.* Milwaukee, WI: Fox Point.

Peña-Brooks, A., & Hegde, M. N. (2000). *Assessment and treatment of articulation and phonological disorders in children.* Austin, TX: Pro-Ed.

Weston, A. J., & Irwin, J. V. (1971). Use of paired stimuli in modification of articulation. *Perceptual Motor Skills, 32,* 947–957.

Phonological Knowledge Approach. An approach to treating phonological disorders in children; based on the assumption that children's knowledge of phonological rules of the adult system is reflected in their productions; the greater the consistency of correct productions in varied contexts, the higher the level of phonological knowledge and vice versa; treatment begins with sounds that reflect least knowledge and ends with those that reflect greater degrees of knowledge; proposed by M. Elbert and J. Gierut and researched by Gierut and associates.

- Obtain a representative, continuous, conversational speech sample
  - sample all sounds
  - sample sounds in all word positions
  - sample each sound in several different words
  - sample each word more than once
  - sample production of minimal pairs (cat/bat)
  - sample morphophonemic alterations (dog/doggie; run/running)
- Analyze the sample
  - create the child's phonetic inventory (all the sounds the child produces, correctly or incorrectly)
  - create the child's phonemic inventory (sounds the child uses contrastingly or those that signal meaning)
  - find out the distribution of sounds (distribution by word position and by morphemes)
  - create hierarchical arrangement of sound productions that reflect least knowledge (misarticulations in all word positions and in all morphemes) to most knowledge (no misarticulations)
- Treat the sounds that reflect the least knowledge first and move up through the hierarchy

- Use the Contrast Approach (described earlier in this section) in teaching sounds
  - use near-minimal pairs (words that differ by more than one sound) if necessary and initially
  - move from imitation to spontaneous productions
  - reinforce the child for correct productions
  - in spontaneous production training, ask the child to name and sort pictures into target and contrast piles (sorting)
  - present an array of pictures and ask the child to select a picture, name it, and find its minimal pair match (matching)
- Promote generalization and maintenance by varying the context of sound productions, selecting child-specific stimulus items, loosely structuring treatment in later stages, and so forth

Elbert, M., & Gierut, J. (1986). *Handbook of clinical phonology.* San Diego: College-Hill Press.

Phonological Process Approach. An approach to treating articulation disorders; technically, not a treatment procedure because it does not involve any unique treatment techniques; an approach to treatment based on the assumptions that multiple errors reflect the operation of certain phonological rules and that the problem is essentially phonemic, not phonetic; group errors based on Phonological Processes; targets the elimination of processes by teaching only a few individual phonemes within a process on the assumption that other, untreated phonemes within the same process will be produced without training—an assumption with mixed evidence; untrained phonemes may or may not be produced; uses several established methods of teaching sounds; researched by multiple investigators; includes multiple programs with varying degrees of empirical research, some with negligible controlled research base; the Cycles Approach and the

<u>Phonological Knowledge Approach</u> are examples of phonological process approaches to treatment.

- Obtain a conversational speech sample that reflects a variety of words and linguistic contexts in which all sounds are produced; may use one of the several available protocols of phonological analysis
- Identify the <u>Phonological Processes</u> that account for error patterns
- Select processes for elimination through teaching specific sounds or groups of sounds; for instance:
  - identify all phonemes that are misarticulated within a process (e.g., all final consonants a child omits—the final consonant deletion process)
  - teach only a few final consonants
  - use any effective procedure to teach the consonants
  - use the comprehensive treatment approach described at the beginning of this main entry with modeling, shaping, manual guidance (phonetic placement), positive reinforcement and corrective feedback
  - alternatively, use paired-stimuli approach, contrast approach, or any other technique supported by controlled evidence
  - teach sounds in syllables, words, phrases, and sentences
- When a few final consonant productions meet the training criterion, probe to see if other, *untreated sounds* within the pattern are produced correctly without training, based on generalization (e.g., other untreated final consonants that are omitted)
- If there is no generalized production of untreated phonemes, then treat them as well
- If untreated phonemes are produced on the basis of generalization, select another phonological process for elimination; teach selected phonemes within the process; administer probes

- Schedule maintenance activities as appropriate

Peña-Brooks, A., & Hegde, M. N. (2000). *Assessment and treatment of articulation and phonological disorders in children.* Austin, TX: Pro-Ed.

Sensory-Motor Approach. An articulation treatment approach based on the assumption that syllable is the basic unit of training; requires a context in which a misarticulated sound is correctly produced; focuses on increasing auditory, tactile, and proprioceptive awareness of motor patterns involved in speech sound production; does not include auditory discrimination training nor training at the sound level; developed and researched by E. McDonald.

- For each target sound, find a context in which the child produces it correctly
- If necessary, administer a deep test such as *McDonald's Deep Test of Articulation* to find a context in which an otherwise misarticulated sound is correctly produced (e.g., in the context of *watch-sun,* a child who generally misarticulates the /s/ may produce it correctly)

Practice With Sounds Produced Correctly

- Select a sound the child can produce **correctly** and combine it with vowels to create duplicated bisyllables (*kiki, koko, kaka, kuku,* etc.)
- Begin treatment by having the child imitate your production of the bisyllables; place equal stress on both the syllables
- Next, have the child imitate your production of bisyllables with primary stress on the first syllable
- Then, have the child imitate your production of bisyllables with primary stress on the second syllable
- Ask the child to describe the placement of the articulators and the direction of the articulatory movements

- Change the vowel and have the child imitate bi-syllables with the same consonant but different vowels (e.g., moving from *kiki* to *koko*); provide training such that a variety of articulatory movements are practiced for a given sound
- Give similar training with other consonants the child produces correctly
- Initiate training on trisyllables (e.g., *kukuku* or *lala-la*); follow the procedure used to train bisyllables

Training Correct Production of Misarticulated Sounds. Begin training on the typically misarticulated sound with a context in which it is correctly produced (e.g., /s/ is produced correctly in the context of *watch-sun,* a deep test item)

In successive stages, ask the child to say watch-sun:

- with slow motion
- with equal stress on both the syllables
- with primary stress on the first syllable
- with primary stress on the second syllable
- and prolong the /s/ until a signal is given to complete the word
- in sentences ("Watch, the sun will burn you.")
- in other and longer sentences and with different stress patterns
- use such a performance criterion as 20 consecutively correct productions to move from one level to the next

Next, vary the phonetic contexts (e.g., watch-sit, watch-saw)

- have the child practice correct production of the target sound in different phonetic contexts by varying the words in which the target sound appears)
- have the child practice correct production in the context of different first words (e.g., *teach-sand, reach-soon*)

- have the child practice the target sound in a totally different phonetic context (e.g., *mop-sun* or *book-sun*)
- implement generalization and maintenance activities

McDonald, E. T. (1964). *Articulation testing and treatment: A sensory motor approach.* Pittsburgh, PA: Stanwix House.

Peña-Brooks, A., & Hegde, M. N. (2000). *Assessment and treatment of articulation and phonological disorders in children.* Austin, TX: Pro-Ed.

Traditional Approach. An articulation treatment approach developed for the most part by Van Riper who included several techniques from various sources; sounds are trained in isolation, in syllables, in words, and in sentences; training includes four levels: (1) Perceptual Training or Ear Training; (2) Production Training: establishment; (3) production training: stabilizing the productions; and (4) production training: transferring the productions; used or researched by multiple investigators.

Perceptual Training (Ear Training)

- Demonstrate how the target sound is produced
- Ask the child to raise a hand when he or she hears the sound in isolation among sounds that are similar and among sounds that are dissimilar
- Ask the child to raise a hand when he or she hears the target sound in first words, then phrases, and finally in sentences
- Ask the child to identify the position of the sound in words (initial, medial, or final)
- Bombard the client with productions of the target sound
- Have the child judge your correct and incorrect productions of a target sound

Production Training

Sound Establishment

- Ask the child to imitate your correct productions of target sounds in isolation, in syllables, or in words
- Vary the phonetic contexts of such productions
- Use contexts in which the target sound is correctly produced
- Use such techniques as Phonetic Placement, Moto-Kinesthetic Method, and Shaping to teach the sound production

Stabilization

- Continue training the **sound in isolation** to encourage more consistent production
- Vary the number and intensity of productions
- Switch from one sound to the other
- Ask the child to respond to printed letters that represent the target sounds
- Have the child produce the sounds in nonsense syllables or clusters
- Begin training the sounds in **words** when the sounds are consistently produced correctly in nonsense syllables
- Move from simple to complex words; continue training until the sound productions are stabilized in a variety of words and in each word position (initial, medial, and final)
- Train at the **phrase** level if necessary
- Move to **sentences**; vary the sentence lengths; move from simpler and shorter to more complex and longer sentences and from those with single occurrence of the target sound to those with multiple occurrences
- Have the child produce sentences along with you in slow motion and at rapid rate

- Begin training at the **conversational level** when the child can fluently and easily produce the target sounds in sentences
- Structure the conversation initially to maximize opportunities for the production of target sounds
- Move to spontaneous conversational speech
- Have the child read to further stabilize sound productions

Transfer (Carry-over)

- Initiate carry-over activities when the child can produce the sounds correctly in unstructured conversational speech
- Give specific speech assignments for the child to complete at home
- Require reports from parents on assignments
- Teach self-monitoring
- Create varied speaking situations for the client to use the target sounds

Peña-Brooks, A., & Hegde, M. N. (2000). *Assessment and treatment of articulation and phonological disorders in children.* Austin, TX: Pro-Ed.

Van Riper, C. , & Emerick, L. (1984). *Speech correction: An introduction to speech pathology and audiology* (7th ed.). Englewood Cliffs, NJ: Prentice-Hall.

Artificial Larynx. Mechanical larynges used in the communicative rehabilitation of patients with laryngectomy; generates a mechanical sound that is articulated into speech with people whose larynges have been removed because of such life-threatening diseases as cancer; the same as Electronic Device for Alaryngeal Speech or Pneumatic Device for Alaryngeal Speech.

Aspiration. A condition in which food, fluid, and secretion penetrate below the true vocal folds; can cause asphyxiation and aspiration pneumonia; potential complications in patients with Dysphagia.

Aspiration Pneumonia

Aspiration Pneumonia. Lung infection due to aspiration; a complication often found in patients with Dysphagia.

Assessment. Procedures that include (a) description of a client's existing and nonexisting communicative behaviors, background variables, and associated factors to evaluate or diagnose a communicative problem; (b) clinical measurement of a person's communicative behaviors.

- Obtain case history
- Interview client, the caregivers, family members, and others concerned
- Conduct an orofacial examination
- Make client-specific judgments on use of standardized or nonstandardized measures
- Use measures appropriate to the client and his or her ethnic, cultural, and linguistic background
- Screen hearing
- Obtain a speech-language sample
- Analyze results
- Draw conclusions; make a diagnosis; recommend treatment; disseminate information to the client, the family, and the referring professional
- Consult books on assessment in speech-language pathology and *PGASLP*

Assimilation Processes. A group of Phonological Processes in which the productions of dissimilar phonemes sound more alike; in phonological treatment, the objective is to eliminate such processes; major assimilation processes include:

- *Alveolar assimilation:* substitution of an alveolar sound by a nonalveolar sound (e.g., substitution of /d/ for /p/)
- *Devoicing:* substitution of a voiceless final sound for a voiced (e.g., /k/ for /g/ in final positions)
- *Devoicing of final consonants:* substitution of a voiceless final consonant for a voiced (e.g., /t/ for /d/)
- *Labial assimilation:* substitution of a labial sound for a nonlabial (e.g., /b/ for /d/)

- *Nasal assimilation:* substitution of a nasal consonant for a nonnasal (e.g., /n/ for /d/)
- *Postvocalic voicing:* substitution of a voiceless sound for a voiced sound that follows a vowel (e.g., /t/ for /d/)
- *Prevocalic voicing:* substitution of a voiced sound for voiceless sound preceding a vowel (e.g., /b/ for /p/ in pre-vocalic positions)
- *Reduplication:* repetition of a syllable, resulting in substitution of one for another (e.g., *wawa* for *water*)
- *Velar assimilation:* substitution of a velar consonant for a nonvelar (e.g., /g/ for /d/)

Assimilative Nasality. Undesirable nasal resonance on vowels that are adjacent to nasal consonants.

Assistive Listening Devices. Devices other than the traditional hearing aids that help persons with hearing impairment in various communicative situations; used in situations in which the traditional hearing aids are less effective; most capable of transmitting speech signals directly from the mouth of the speaker to the ears of the listener; see also Aural Rehabilitation; include the following:

- **Frequency Modulated (FM) auditory trainers** that offer wireless connection between a speaker and a listener; consists of a transmitter with a microphone and a receiver with earphones; signal is transmitted to the receiver through radio frequency and is unaffected by noise in the room, a problem not solved by traditional hearing aids; may be used in group aural rehabilitation
- **Infrared listening systems** that include transmitters that send messages on pulses of light and receivers worn by individuals to receive and decode those messages; useful in large listening environments such as concert halls, theaters, houses of worship, and classrooms.
- **Signaling or alerting devices** (also known as environmental adaptations) that include mechanisms to amplify telephone ringing; flashing lights that alert a person with

hearing impairment to incoming phone calls, smoke or fire alarm, a baby's cry, ringing of a door bell, and so forth; vibratory mechanism that wakes up a person with hearing impairment from sleep

- **Television or radio amplifiers** that include a small amplifier, a microphone that is clipped to the television or radio, and ear phones the person needing extra amplification of signals wears; volume may be adjusted on the amplifier, thus allowing louder signals only for the person using the system

- **Text telephones (TTs)** and telecommunication devices for the deaf (TDDs) that allow two persons communicating over a phone to type their messages; allows display of typed messages on a small screen on the telephone; may be a part of a relay service that allows a hearing person without the special equipment to speak to a staff person who types in the message, which is transmitted to the TT used by the person with hearing impairment

Ataxia. A neurological disorder characterized by disturbed balance and movement due to injury to the cerebellum.

Ataxic Dysarthria. A type of motor speech disorder resulting from damage to the cerebellum. See Treatment of Dysarthria: Specific Types under Dysarthria.

Athetosis. A neurological disorder characterized by slow, writhing, worm-like movements due to injury to the extrapyramidal motor pathways.

Atrophy. Wasting away of tissues or organs.

Attention Disorders. Disorders that affect a person's reaction to stimuli in the environment; disorder that affects the duration of response to stimuli; attention is a prerequisite for all kinds of learning; disturbed attention makes learning difficult or impossible; compounds memory deficits; often found in persons with neurological disease or trauma;

attention is a treatment target for patients with aphasia, dementia, traumatic brain injury, mental retardation, autism, and similar disorders.

- Make a thorough assessment of attentional deficits; consult the cited sources and the *PGASLP*
- Integrate attentional training activities to other functional activities such as communication training
- Work directly on functional attentional tasks (e.g., paying attention to speech or instructions; to environmental cues; to treatment stimuli) instead of abstract and nonfunctional attentional tasks (e.g., showing a bunch of playing cards and asking the patient to indicate when a red card is shown; such mental exercises as counting backwards; listening to auditory clicks and signaling when there is a shift in the pattern of clicks)
- Consult with the family and health care staff in identifying attentional deficits of concern and functional treatment activities and goals
- Design a treatment program that is client-specific, functional, and helps pay attention to environmental events; as a speech-language pathologist, consider strategies to improve the patient's attention in all treatment tasks
- Work with the family and health care staff to ensure that they, too, use the same strategies as you do
- Select treatment stimuli that are relevant to the patient's interests and premorbid hobbies; prepare colorful and attention-getting stimuli for treatment
- Implement the treatment initially in a quiet, simple, clutter-free place with minimal stimuli; gradually broaden the treatment environment to include more natural settings in which you reinforce attentional behaviors
- Conduct treatment sessions sitting in front of the client; make sure there is enough lighting on your face and on the treatment stimuli and activities
- Give all treatment instructions in simple, brief, and direct language; repeat, if necessary; break down the instructions

to smaller steps; talk slowly; and make sure the patient understands your instructions by asking questions about them

- Draw the patient's attention before presenting all treatment stimuli by giving alerting signals and frequently using his or her name (e.g., "Watch for this now, Mr. Triumph"; "Here it comes, Mrs. Robinson"; "I am going to show you a picture now, Ms. Lopez"; "Mr. Rodriguez, look at me now"; "Mr. Woo, please pay close attention."); make sure the client has established eye contact with you or with the stimulus before you present the stimulus

- Verbally reinforce the client for maintaining eye contact, looking at the treatment stimuli, concentrating on treatment tasks, performing accurately on tasks on hand

- Give corrective feedback; stop the client as soon as you find his or her attention wandering; reinstruct, reorient, draw attention, and continue with treatment trials

- Experiment with the loudness of your voice; some clients may need a louder and more intoned voice; others may react better to soft voice and speech

- Limit choices offered in treatment tasks (e.g., put only a few stimulus item in front of a patient with brain injury)

- Use manual guidance in the case of severely impaired clients to orient their face toward the stimuli; use touch to draw attention; guide the patient's hand toward required manual tasks (e.g., pointing to a correct picture in a stimulus array)

- Give necessary intertribal interval time; do not rush stimulus presentations; but do not wait too long between stimulus presentations as this would give room for competing responses

- Judge the patient's physical endurance; hold brief sessions if the patient fatigues easily; take short breaks during treatment; hold sessions at times when the patient is well rested

- Shape attending behaviors; increase the duration of required attention gradually (e.g., initially set a realistic goal of attending to a task for only a few seconds and gradually increase the duration); reinforce for all on-task behaviors
- Teach the client to make appropriate requests that help him or her concentrate (e.g., requesting others to turn down the music, close a door or a window to reduce outside noise, speak louder or softer)
- Teach the client to organize his or her belongings into categories and keep them separately (e.g., writing and reading items in one place, such personal care items as toothbrush and razor in a different place)
- Use high probability behaviors to reinforce attending behaviors (e.g., good attending behavior in an earlier portion of treatment may mean that the patient can have a rest or watch TV)
- Teach the patient to assess and verify his or her work to promote self-correction (e.g., ask the client how she or he did in concentrating on a task on hand; give feedback; encourage realistic self-evaluations)
- Measure duration of attending behaviors and the frequency of inattentive behaviors to document changes and improvements; give this informational feedback to the patient (e.g., "Yesterday you could concentrate only for 2 minutes; today you concentrated for 3 minutes.")
- Teach the patient to cue himself or herself (e.g., by repeating instructions and reading a list of steps to be taken in completing a task before beginning the task)
- Teach family members to prompt and reinforce attending behaviors; to draw attention; to repeat instructions; and so forth

Lezak, M. D. (1995). *Neuropsychological assessment* (3rd ed.). New York: Oxford University Press.

Mateer, C. A., & Mapou, R. L. (1996). Understanding, evaluating, and mapping attention disorders following brain injury. *Journal of Head Trauma Rehabilitation, 11,* 1–16.

Meyer, M., Benton, A., & Diller, L. (Eds.). (1987). *Neuropsychological rehabilitation*. Edinburgh, Scotland: Churchill Livingstone.

Audience Generalization. Production of unreinforced responses in the presence of persons not involved in training; a strategy necessary in almost all cases to achieve generalized production of clinically established behaviors.

- Invite persons not involved in training to treatment sessions conducted in later stages of therapy
- Evoke behavior (e.g., fluency, correct production of speech sounds, naming, appropriate vocal qualities)
- Reinforce target behavior
- Have the visitor engage the client in conversational speech
- Have the visitor reinforce the target communication skills
- Take the client to nonclinical situations and evoke and reinforce target communication skills in the presence of other persons

Auditory Discrimination Training. Treatment designed to teach clients to distinguish between correct and incorrect articulation of speech produced by the clinician and other persons; used on the assumption that misarticulations are due to a failure to hear differences between different speech sounds and that auditory discrimination training is a precursor to speech sound production training; assumption questioned by some clinicians who cite experimental evidence showing that production training will induce discrimination as well; same as Perceptual Training, a part of several traditional articulation treatment programs; a clinically practical strategy is to train production first and then probe for discrimination and train discrimination only if sound discrimination problems persist and negatively affect communication; it is likely that in most cases, production training will be sufficient to generate auditory discrimination as well.

- Describe the target sound, how it is made, and how it sounds

- Produce words and phrases that contain the target sound as well as nontarget sounds
- Ask the client to respond in some way to the production of the target sound (by raising the right hand or by pointing to the drawing of a smiling face)
- Produce a word with the correct sound and a word with a sound the client substitutes for a correct sound (e.g., *radio* and *wadio*)
- Ask the client to respond to the correct production (/r/ in *radio*) in one manner (pointing to the drawing of a smiling face) and to the incorrect production (/w/ in *wadio*) in a different manner (pointing to the drawing of a frowning face)
- Produce many words and phrases that are loaded with the target sounds to provide intense auditory stimulation
- Move on to production training, as there is little or no evidence that auditory discrimination training will result in correct production of speech sounds

Augmentative and Alternative Communication. Augmentative communication includes methods of communication that enhance and expand extremely limited oral means of communication by nonvocal means; alternative communication includes methods that replace oral communication by teaching substitute modes of communication; augmentative alternative methods may be integrated in rehabilitation; some augmentative communication may involve speech generated mechanically; includes various means of communication, some of which are more technologically oriented than others; usually used for persons who have limited oral communication skills because of severe clinical conditions including aphasia, autism, cerebral palsy, and other neurological disorders, deafness, dementia, dysarthria, glossectomy, intubation, laryngectomy, mental retardation, tracheostomy, and traumatic head injury; for procedures, see Augmentative Communication, Gestural (Unaided); Augmentative Communication, Gestural-Assisted (Aided); Augmentative Communication, Neuro-Assisted (Aided).

Basic Principles of Selecting an Augmentative Communication Mode or System

- Assess the client's speech as well as nonspeech communication potential
- Consider the client's strengths and limitations
  - cognitive level
  - sensory disabilities
  - motor status
  - language comprehension
- Select a mode or system that gives the maximum advantage to the client
- Consider cost
- Consider the client's acceptance of the mode or system
- Consider the communicative demands the client faces
- Consider the amount of training required
- Consider how the client and the family will use the mode or system

Augmentative Communication, Aided. Methods of communication that enhance or expand (and rarely substitute) vocal communication by such external aids as an alphabet letter board or a computer.

Augmentative Communication, Gestural (Unaided). Methods of communication that use patterned muscle movements (gestures) to enhance oral communication but do not use instruments or external aids; gestures play a crucial role in conveying the speaker's message; appropriate for all persons with severely impaired oral, expressive communication.

- Teach gestures for *Yes* and *No* to all speakers with extremely limited expressive oral communication because of severely impaired motor performance but relatively intact receptive language
  - teach the client to gesture *Yes* or *No* in response to a series of common questions with a carrier phrase "Do you want _____?"
  - shape a clear gesture that all communication partners can understand

- model the gesture if necessary
- reinforce consistently discriminated responding (client always gives the gesture that is meant)
- consider the following gestures: head movements (side to side for *No* and up and down for *Yes*); eye movements (looking up for *Yes* and down for *No*; blinking once for *Yes* and twice for *No*; blinking the right eye for *Yes* and the left eye for *No*); hand movements (thumbs up for *Yes* and thumbs down for *No*;) feet movements (right foot movement for *Yes* and the left foot movement for *No*)

- Teach a pattern of eye-blinks that convey certain basic messages; for instance, beyond the *Yes* and *No* teach the client to:
  - blink three times to say *I am hungry*
  - blink four times to say *I am thirsty*
  - blink five times to say *I need to go to bathroom*
- Teach pointing to objects needed
  - teach finger pointing
  - teach pointing by directing gaze
- Teach the Left-Hand Manual Alphabet
  - consider teaching the left-hand manual alphabet for clients whose right hand is paralyzed
  - consider teaching the Manual Shorthand, which combines gestures with letters from the left-hand manual alphabet (*talking hand system*)
- Teach Pantomime
  - teach the client to use pantomime along with speech
  - teach initially a few mimed concepts that help communicative basic needs
  - expand the mimed repertoire as the client becomes more competent in its use
  - fade mimes if and when the client regains or improves oral speech
- Teach American Indian Hand Talk (AMER-IND)
  - teach first the signs that express mands (basic needs, requests)

- teach the one-hand version for those with one paralyzed hand
- teach signs that express concrete ideas first and those that express abstract ideas later
- Teach American Sign Language (ASL or AMESLAN)
  - select initially the signs that express Mands (basic needs, requests)
  - teach signs that express concrete ideas first and those that express abstract ideas later

Beukelman, D. R., & Mirenda, P. (1998). *Augmentative and alternative communication: Management of severe communication disorders in children and adults* (2nd ed.). Baltimore, MD: Paul H. Brookes.

Glennen, S. L., & DeCoste, D. (1997). *Handbook of augmentative and alternative communication.* San Diego: Singular Publishing Group.

Silverman, F. H. (1995). *Communication for the speechless* (3rd ed.). Boston: Allyn and Bacon.

Augmentative Communication, Gestural-Assisted (Aided).
Methods of communication in which gestures are used to (a) select or scan messages displayed on a non-mechanical device (e.g., a communication board) or (b) display messages on a mechanical device (e.g., a computer monitor); used with many persons with minimal expressive language; the initial use of gestural-assisted means may promote appropriate vocalization or word productions in many clients; the emergent vocal productions may be strengthened and expanded; includes a variety of nonmechanical and mechanical methods.

Use Pictures and Symbols to Teach Functional Communication
- Teach the client to communicate with photographs and drawings that may be displayed on a communication board
  - teach the client with limited cognitive functions to communicate basic needs with regular or miniaturized objects (e.g., the client points to a fork to indicate he or she wants to eat)

- teach the client to express a particular message through a picture (e.g., teach the client to point to or look at a picture of a person sleeping to communicate that he or she is tired or sleepy)
- teach the client to express bodily states (e.g., pain in a certain part) by pointing to or looking at specific body parts on a line drawing

- Teach the client to communicate with various symbols that may be displayed on a communication board; select among many symbol systems that are available on the market; for instance:
  - <u>Picsyms,</u> a set of graphic symbols that represent nouns, verbs, and prepositions
  - <u>Pic Symbols</u> (Pictogram Ideogram Communication), which are white drawings on a black background
  - <u>Sig Symbols</u> which are based on <u>American Sign Language (ASL);</u> use them especially in conjunction with ASL
  - <u>Blissymbolics</u> which are a set of semi-<u>iconic</u> and abstract symbols that can be taught to persons of any language; teach the client to combine symbols to form more complex messages
  - <u>Premack-type Symbols,</u> or the <u>Carrier Symbols</u> which are abstract plastic shapes; associate words and phrases with each shape; teach the client to arrange and rearrange the plastic shapes like printed words
  - traditional orthography (e.g., the English alphabet); teach the client to spell out the word (by pointing to or scanning) along with the alphabet, display digits 1 through 10 and a set of common phrases or sentences so that not every word has to be spelled out or scanned (<u>Scanning in Augmentative Communication</u>)
- Teach the client to communicate with <u>Rebuses</u>
  - use rebuses (pictures that represent objects or events along with words, grammatic morphemes, or both)

123

- teach the client to add grammatic morphemes to a picture or a word (e.g., adding s to the picture of a book to suggest *books*)
- combine rebuses to form more complex utterances

Use Nonelectronic Communication Boards to Teach Functional Communication

- Teach the client to communicate with messages on a nonelectronic communication board
  - design a board of paper, cardboard, fabric, wood, or cork; if practical, prepare a book of symbols and written messages; select a board that all conversational partners can see simultaneously; portable, if necessary; attractive to look at; big enough to contain critical elements of the system; not overwhelmingly big or complex
  - write symbols (alphabets, orthographic messages, pictures, various kinds of symbols) on separate cards that can be mounted on the board
  - teach the client who cannot point (because of extremely limited motoric performance) to scan the message: you offer selections and the client indicates *Yes* to the right selection (e.g., You point to the word "food," or a symbol for it, or a picture of a food item; the client indicates *Yes* or *No*)
  - teach the client to encode a message by pointing to a number printed on a separate, smaller, portable selection chart; have the messages on a larger communication board numbered: let the client point to a number on the selection chart; decode the number into the message on the board (e.g., if the client points to #5, it may mean "I am hungry" as per the communication board)
  - teach the client to directly select the message: teach the client to select the actual message on the board, instead of a number which stands for a message; teach clients to select by means of pointing and other

124

hand gestures, finger movements, eye gestures, gaze, headpointers, or headsticks.
- Teach the client to communicate by drawing symbols or pictures
  - teach the client to draw simple line drawings to communicate
  - let the client use paper, magic slate, or any other convenient surface
- Teach the client to communicate by writing (<u>Traditional Orthography</u>)
  - teach conventional writing to nonverbal children who can master it
  - teach them initially to write simple, functional messages
  - teach them to write more complex messages

Use Electronic Communication Systems to Teach Functional Communication

- Select an appropriate system for the client; consider the cost, ease of use, and efficiency of the system
- Select an appropriate and practical switching mechanism that the client can use with little effort and learn to generate signals for the electronic device (such as those that are specially constructed or a modified or regular microcomputer); consider push switches, push plates (plate-like structures that when touched will generate a signal), large and specially designed keyboards, joy sticks, squeeze bulbs, and several other available types of selection devices
- Select an appropriate display system to show messages when the client activates the switching mechanism; these may be computer screens, liquid-crystal displays (found on calculators), printed outputs (as with a computer printer), and many other kinds of special displays
- Select an appropriate control electronic unit (a dedicated augmentative communication unit or a computer)
- Teach the client to use the device; start with simpler messages; give plenty of practice in using the switching

mechanism; increase the complexity of messages in gradual steps; train the communicative partners in the environment

Beukelman, D. R., & Mirenda, P. (1998). *Augmentative and alternative communication: Management of severe communication disorders in children and adults* (2nd ed.). Baltimore, MD: Paul H. Brookes.

Silverman, F. H. (1995). *Communication for the speechless* (3rd ed.). Boston: Allyn and Bacon.

Augmentative Communication, High Technology.

Methods of communication that enhance or expand (and rarely substitute for) vocal communication by external means that use sophisticated electronic technology, including computers; generate speech or printed messages; usually software run; more versatile than low-technology augmentative communication.

Augmentative Communication, Low Technology.

Methods of communication that enhance or expand (and rarely substitute) vocal communication by external means that use no or limited electronic technology; there is no message storage, printed output, or speech output; a communication board with letters and words on it is an example.

Augmentative Communication, Neuro-Assisted (Aided).

Methods of communication that use such bioelectrical signals as muscle action potentials to activate and display messages on a computer monitor; technically, a variety of switching devices; used for persons who are so profoundly impaired motorically that they cannot use a manual switching device; the communicator needs to have electrodes attached to the skin surface to pick-up and transmit muscle action potential signals to the device; this technology is not well developed.

- Train the client to use muscle action potentials to generate signals to an electronic communication device

- teach the client to vary muscle action potentials through biofeedback training
- use a myoswitch that picks up muscle action potential from contracting muscles and transmits the impulse to an electronic device
- use any of the several electronic devices available that have been modified for this purpose

Beukelman, D. R., & Mirenda, P. (1992). *Augmentative and alternative communication: Management of severe communication disorders in children and adults.* Baltimore, MD: Paul H. Brookes.

Silverman, F. H. (1995). *Communication for the speechless* (3rd ed.). Boston: Allyn and Bacon.

Augmentative Communication, Unaided.   Methods of communication that enhance or expand (and rarely substitute for) vocal communication without external or mechanical aids; includes a more formal, systematic, intensive, or extensive use of gestures, signs, and facial expressions to supplement oral (speech) communication.

Aural Rehabilitation.   An educational and clinical program implemented, for the most part, by audiologists; includes the assessment of hearing impairment in adults and children; counseling; selection and fitting of hearing aids and auditory training; use of group amplification systems in educational and communication training sessions; often implemented by a team of specialists including audiologist, otologist, special education specialists, psychologists, and speech-language pathologists; for speech-language pathologists' treatment of communication disorders in persons with hearing problems, see Hearing Impairment; also see Hard of Hearing; and Hearing Loss; note that in an aural rehabilitation program, the following are an audiologist's responsibilities:

- Counseling clients with hearing impairment
  - giving information to persons with hearing impairment on available services

- helping clients make appropriate decisions regarding services
- educating them about different types of hearing aids and assistive listening devices
- answering questions the clients may have about their problems and needs
- educating them about available sources of financial help to meet the cost of hearing rehabilitation
- informing clients about the nature of services offered by other professionals and making referrals to appropriate selected professionals (e.g., otologists, speech-language pathologists, educators of the deaf)
- Counseling parents of children with hearing impairment
  - giving information on hearing impairment, its causes, and its effects on the child's communication, education, and eventual occupation
  - informing them about the various services needed and available to them and to their hearing impaired child
  - helping them with their search for private and public sources of financial help
  - helping the family develop an aural rehabilitation program for the child through such counseling
- Hearing evaluation
  - testing hearing and establishing thresholds
  - testing speech reception and discrimination skills
  - evaluating such complex functions as central auditory processing
  - making an accurate assessment of the type and degree of hearing loss, impairment, or disability it causes
- Hearing aid selection and fitting
  - trying different hearing aids on the patient to evaluate their suitability
  - selecting a hearing aid that is most suitable to the client's pattern of hearing loss
- Hearing aid orientation

- educating the client about the use of the selected hearing aid (e.g., wearing it, adjusting the volume)
- letting the client experience various amplified sounds so he or she can get used to it
- helping the client discriminate amplified sounds
- educating the client on taking care of the hearing aid (e.g., changing battery, keeping the ear mold clean)
- Working with other professionals on interdisciplinary teams
  - helping speech-language pathologists design and implement appropriate oral communication training programs and serving as a resource and consultant
  - helping educators of the deaf in designing and implementing appropriate educational goals and serving as a resource and consultant
  - working with otologists and helping make decisions about surgical or medical interventions
  - working with pediatricians, psychologists, and other professionals as found necessary in individual cases
- Prescription of <u>Assistive Listening Devices</u>
  - counseling clients about the availability of various assistive listening devices
  - helping the client select one or more device that best improves the client's communication in social situations
  - helping the client understand use and care of devices
- Follow-up and continued support
  - keeping in touch with the clients and their families
  - periodically evaluating the client's hearing status and communication needs
  - updating hearing aids or assistive listening devices
  - helping the client and the family meet the changing needs of aural rehabilitation

Autism.   A pervasive developmental disorder that in a majority of clients persists into adulthood; often associated with mental retardation; communication disorders are a significant characteristic; lack of interest in people and communication is a dominant characteristic; many of the treatment procedures for Language Disorders in Children are applicable, with the following special considerations:

Treatment of Autism: General Guidelines

- Note that behavioral methods of teaching appropriate behaviors, including communicative behaviors, have received extensive experimental support
- Note also that such popular procedures as sensory integration therapy, auditory integration training, and facilitated communication have not proved effective and should be avoided
- Integrate communication training with other skill training by working with behavior analysts, special educators, and other professionals
- Use a consistent set of goals that all members of an interdisciplinary team will support
- Let other professionals know the target skills you will be teaching and ask them to incorporate your goals into their treatment (e.g., if you are teaching a set of basic words, give the list to other professionals so that they can prompt and reinforce the production of those words)
- Seek information on what other professionals are doing and support their efforts by integrating their goals into your work (e.g., if the educator is teaching the child to answer questions appropriately, teach question comprehension and giving correct responses to questions in language therapy)
- Make language therapy relevant to the child's educational program; select language therapy goals in consultation with the regular and special education teachers
- Teach observable, measurable skills so the progress or lack of it can be evident
- Consider the three types of teaching, all known to be effective in teaching skills to autistic children: di-

rect teaching, activity-based teaching, and incidental teaching

- Use direct teaching to establish initial communication skills (e.g., words and phrases; grammatic morphemes; articulation of speech sounds); use the discrete trial methods in which target skills are taught with massed trials; use modeling, prompting, shaping, fading, and similar behavioral techniques; positively reinforce correct responses
- Use activity-based instruction to teach more advanced language skills or to have the child expand established language skills; in a play-oriented setup, teach advanced language skills as you engage the child in conversation (e.g., the production of plural or other grammatic morphemes in sentences)
- Use incidental teaching to promote even more naturalistic language production; reinforce a child's attempt to communicate in naturalistic contexts (e.g., when a child points to banana on top of the refrigerator, say the word *banana* several times and give it to the child); see Language Disorders in Children; Treatment of Language Disorders: Specific Techniques for details on incidental teaching
- Expect resistance, interfering behaviors, aggressive behaviors, self-stimulation, inattention, stereotypic behaviors—all interrupting and disrupting your planned communication treatment
- Keep the child motivated and on-task by structuring short sessions; positively reinforcing even small improvements in behaviors, keeping quiet, sitting even for as short a duration as 1 minute; allowing frequent breaks in which the child is free to play; demanding less and demanding what the child is capable of doing
- Increase gradually the task complexity, the demand level, and session durations; decrease gradually the

frequency and duration of breaks; begin to control what the child does during breaks
- Sit in front of the child, with the child's legs between yours; gradually, move the chairs closer to the table and begin working off the table top
- Select appropriate and strong reinforcers because motivating children with autism is extremely important; much of the success may depend on whether you have a functional reinforcer for the child; use tokens and have a variety of back-up reinforcers available; select activities the child chooses on his or her own; make access to those activities the back-up reinforcer for tokens

Teaching Language and Communication to Autistic Children
- Use objects, not pictures, as stimuli to promote generalized production of target skills in natural settings
- Teach in a variety of linguistic contexts (e.g., teach grammatic morphemes in several phrases and sentences with varied linguistic contexts)
- Teach in a variety of environments (e.g., extend treatment to home, school, and other settings)
- Reduce Echolalia (find out if echolalia is functional; some evidence suggests that teaching autistic children to make requests may reduce echolalia)
- Give direct, intensive training (repeat trials and provide frequent training; target useful skills and teach them directly)
- Reinforce any attempt at appropriate communication (e.g., words, phrases, gestures, functional echolalia); gradually shift the reinforcement contingency to more precise, socially appropriate, complex, verbal responses
- Reduce autistic leading (tendency to grasp an adult's hand and leading to a desired object) by teaching them to point to things desired

- Target eye contact during conversation and reinforce this systematically
- Reduce pronoun reversal by teaching the correct use of *I* and *you*; to teach the pronoun *I*, ask the child to perform an action such as clapping the hands; ask "What are you doing?," prompt the correct response "*I* am clapping," and fade the modeling; to teach the pronoun *you*, perform a similar action, and ask "What am I doing?," prompt the response "You are clapping," and then fade the modeling
- Teach turn taking by stopping interruptions and by teaching the child to pay attention to such verbal prompts as "It is my turn" and "It is your turn" (to talk)
- Teach topic maintenance by having the child talk about an event or a weekend activity and prompting the child to say "more" about the topic or requiring the child to say three or four new things about the topic and then extending the required number of new pieces of information
- Consider Augmentative and Alternative Communication (AAC) options if systematic language treatment efforts have failed
- Reduce undesirable behaviors by positively reinforcing alternative, incompatible, desirable behaviors that will replace the undesirable behaviors (e.g., teach the child to request help or nod his or her head to indicate *yes* instead of throwing a tantrum); see Differential Reinforcement to teach alternative behaviors that replace undesirable behaviors
- Pay special attention to generalization and maintenance strategies; extend treatment to home settings; train parents to prompt and reinforce desirable behaviors at home
- Teach nonverbal communication (e.g., American Sign Language) if necessary

- Work closely with other specialists and family members

Hegde, M. N. (1996). *A coursebook on language disorders in children.* San Diego: Singular Publishing Group.

Maurice, C. (Ed.). (1996). *Behavioral intervention for young children with autism: A manual for parents and professionals.* Austin, TX: Pro-Ed.

Automatic Reinforcers.   Sensory consequences of responses that reinforce those responses (e.g., the sensation a child with autism derives from banging his or her head).

Autosomal Dominant.   Any chromosome apart from the sex chromosome is autosomal; not sex-linked; dominant indicates that the defective gene dominates its normal partner in its phenotypic expression.

Aversive Stimuli.   Events that people work hard to avoid or move away from; reduction in aversive stimulation is the essence of negative reinforcement; a behavior that reduces negative experiences tends to increase in frequency; in treatment, positive reinforcement is preferable to negative reinforcement.

Avoidance.   A behavior that prevents the occurrence of an aversive event and hence is reinforced; negatively reinforced behavior; in treatment, target is to reduce avoidance if judged undesirable; a typical target in persons who stutter; typically, the client is made to face previously avoided situations with appropriate clinical support; for instance, in reducing avoidance of certain speaking situations by persons who stutter:

- Build a hierarchy of most to least frequently avoided speaking situations or tasks
- As the client becomes more fluent during treatment, introduce the client to least frequently avoided situations first and move up the hierarchy
- Offer training in situations the clients avoids; for instance:
  - take the client to a restaurant and have him or her order food (an avoided responses); monitor fluency and provide subtle reinforcement and corrective feedback

- have the client make phone calls as you monitor fluency (e.g., prompt the person to slow down)
- arrange group situations in which the client will speak or make brief presentations
- introduce strangers to the treatment setting and let the client practice fluency skills in front of them
- Generally, reinforce the client for facing previously avoided situations and tasks

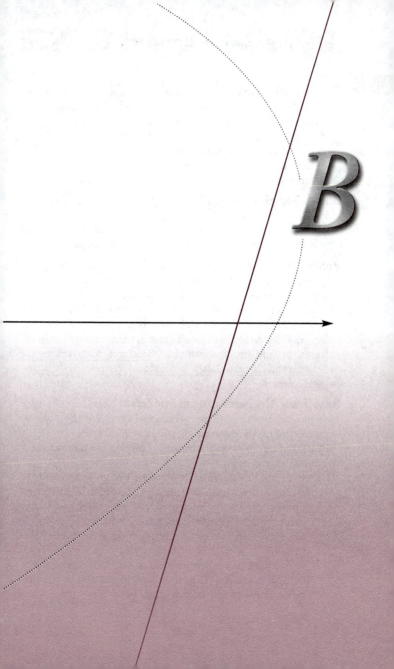

B

Backup Reinforcers.   Events, objects, and opportunities for selected behaviors that become available to clients who exchange their earned tokens in treatment sessions.
- Have a collection of backup reinforcers
- Give tokens to reinforce target responses
- Exchange tokens for selected events, objects, or opportunities for certain behaviors

Basal Ganglia.   Structures located deep within the brain and just above midbrain that are important for movement control; part of the extrapyramidal system; include the caudate nucleus, the putamen nucleus, and globus pallidus.

Baselines.   Recorded rates of responses in the absence of planned intervention; also known as the operant level of a response; reliability or stability of repeated measures is a required characteristic; help establish the clinician accountability; in treatment research, help rule out extraneous variables; a necessary measure before starting treatment in all cases; should be established in <u>Baselines, Conversational Speech</u> and <u>Discrete Trials, Evoked</u> and <u>Discrete Trials, Modeled</u> formats.

Baselines, Conversational Speech.   Measures of target behaviors produced in conversational speech in the absence of treatment; an important pretreatment measure.
- Record a conversational speech sample in as naturalistic a manner as possible
  - with children, have toys, pictures, books, and other materials to evoke speech; engage the child in conversational speech with the help of the materials; if necessary, focus on the target features to be measured (e.g., drawing the child's attention to actions you perform to evoke the *ing*)
  - with adults, conduct conversation on their favorite topics
  - in most cases, the client interview might also be used to measure the production of target behaviors

- measure the correct and incorrect productions of the target behaviors in the sample
- calculate the percent correct baseline response rate

Baseline, Discrete Trials.   Baselines of target behaviors established in discrete trials in which a client's multiple attempts to produce a target response are counted separately; trials are separated in time; should be established in both the evoked trials and modeled trials format.

- Select target behaviors (phoneme productions, grammatic morphemes, sentence structures, pragmatic skills, fluent productions, naming skills, etc.)
- Specify target behaviors in measurable terms; for instance
  - production of /s/ in word initial positions
  - production of present progressive *ing*
  - naming pictures
  - reduced rate of speech
  - elimination of hard glottal attacks
- Prepare stimulus items to evoke target responses; in the case of speech and language targets, prepare 20 stimulus items for each target response; for instance
  - twenty pictures that help evoke 20 words with /s/ in the initial position
  - twenty sentences with the present progressive feature in them (e.g., The boy is walk*ing*.)
- Prepare questions to be asked to evoke the response, and the exact way of modeling the response
- Prepare recording sheet
- Select type: Baseline Evoked Trials or Baseline Modeled Trials
- Analyze data to calculate percentage of correct responses (e.g., 50% correct production of the /s/ in word initial positions; 75% correct production of *ing* in sentences)
- Repeat measures; compare the discrete trial and conversational speech measures
- When measures are stable, begin treatment

B

Baseline Evoked Trials.   Discrete baseline trials that are temporally separated; each attempt to produce a target behavior is discretely measured; no modeling of the target response; no consequences for the correct or incorrect responses.

- Place stimulus item in front of client (e.g., a picture of a *ball*) or demonstrate an action (e.g., moving a toy car)
- Ask the relevant predetermined question (e.g., "What is this?" "What am I doing?" or "What is happening?")
- Wait a few seconds for the client to respond
- Record the client's response on the recording sheet
- Remove the stimulus item (move it toward you, away from the client)
- Wait 2–3 seconds to signify the end of a trial
- Begin the next trial with a different item

Baseline Modeled Trials.   A discrete baseline trial in which the clinician models the correct response for the client to imitate; no consequences for the correct or incorrect responses.

- Place a stimulus item in front of the client or demonstrate an action
- Ask the predetermined question (e.g., "What is this?") Immediately model the correct response (e.g., "Johnny, say *ball.*")
- Wait a few seconds for the client to respond
- Record the client's response on the recording sheet
- Remove the stimulus item (move it toward you, away from the client)
- Wait 2–3 seconds to signify the end of a trial
- Begin the next trial with a different stimulus item

Behavioral Contingency.   In behavioral analysis and treatment, a dependent relationship between Antecedents, responses, and Consequences; in behavioral treatment, clinician manages this contingency by:

- Providing antecedents (stimuli, modeling, instruction, demonstration, etc.)

- Requiring a specified response
- Providing immediate consequences in the form of positive reinforcers or corrective feedback

Behavioral Momentum. A behavioral treatment procedure in which the clinician rapidly and repeatedly evokes a high-probability response and then immediately commands a low-probability response; often used to reduce noncompliance; in increasing the frequency of a low-probability response:
- Find a response the client readily performs (e.g., hand clapping)
- Model and have the child imitate that high-probability response repeatedly and in rapid succession
- Immediately, ask the child to open his or her mouth (an example of a low-probability response)
- Reinforce the occurrence of the low-probability response

Biofeedback. A method used to reduce incorrect responses or shape and increase desirable responses in treatment; includes mechanical feedback given to the client on vocal pitch and intensity, respiration, galvanic skin response, and muscle action potential level.

Bite Block. A small block of acrylic or putty custom-made for a client who holds it between the lateral upper and lower teeth; observed to improve speech intelligibility in clients who have abnormal jaw movements; recommended for some clients with dysarthria.

Blissymbolics. A set of symbols used to communicate nonorally; meant to be an international language; more widely applied and researched than other symbol systems in teaching communication to severely handicapped clients; symbols may be combined to form complex expressions; developed by C. Bliss; see Augmentative Communication, Gestural-Assisted (Aided).

Bolus. A mass of chewed or otherwise prepared food moved as a unit in the act of swallowing.

B

Booster Treatment.   Treatment given any time after the client was dismissed from the original treatment; part of response maintenance strategy.
- Conduct periodic follow-ups
- If the follow-up measures show decline in response rate, give booster treatment
- Use the original or newer, more effective procedures

Botulinum Toxin Injection.   A medical treatment procedure for neurogenic or idiopathic adductor spasmodic dysphonia and adductor spasmodic dysphonia that does not respond to behavioral treatment; botulinum toxin is injected into the thyroarytenoid muscle unilaterally or bilaterally; effects last about 3 months.

Bradykinesia.   Slowness of movements; difficulty in stopping movement once initiated; freezing of movement.

Breathiness.   A voice quality that results when there is excessive air leakage during phonation because of inadequate approximation of the vocal folds; caused by various factors; treatment varies by cause.

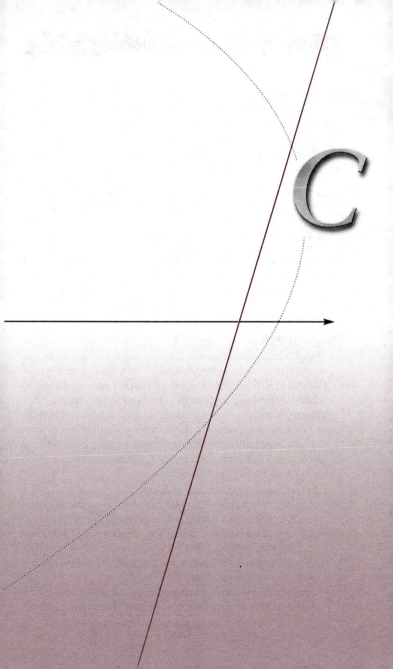

C

Carrier Symbols. A set of plastic symbols (adapted from the Premack symbols) used in teaching nonverbal communication; used as a part of the Non-SLIP (Non-Speech Language Initiation Program); once learned, the program helps initiate oral speech training; developed and researched by J. Carrier.

Carry-over. Generalized production of any behavior taught in a special setting in natural and untreated settings and in relation to novel stimuli; an important goal of clinical intervention; the same as Generalization.

Cathode-ray Display (CRT). A video display system used in many desktop computers; more easily read under varied lighting conditions than the Liquid Crystal Display; used in some devices of Augmentative and Alternative Communication (ACC).

Cerebral Palsy. A congenital, nonprogressive neurological disorder that affects motor control; caused by injury to the cerebral levels during the prenatal or perinatal period; symptoms tend to improve with growth; causes speech disorders, mostly dysarthria; symptoms related to speech include respiratory control problems, laryngeal dysfunction resulting in voice problems, possible velopharyngeal inadequacy, potential language disorders, and significant articulation problems (dysarthria); may involve cognitive functions; may be associated with feeding problems.

Classification of Cerebral Palsy

- *Ataxic Cerebral Palsy:* Ataxia, disturbed balance and movement, is the main characteristic; injury to the cerebellum.
- *Athetoid Cerebral Palsy:* Athetosis, characterized by slow, involuntary, writhing movements, is the distinguishing feature; injury to the extrapyramidal motor pathways, especially to the basal ganglia.
- *Spastic Cerebral Palsy:* Increased tone or rigidity of muscles is the distinguishing feature; the most common type; in-

jury to the pyramidal motor pathways and the higher cortical centers of motor control.

Treatment of Cerebral Palsy

General Principles

- Work closely with the team of specialists serving children with cerebral palsy
- Counsel parents about the effects of cerebral palsy on communication and their role in stimulating language at home
- Work closely with parents throughout the treatment duration
- Make a thorough assessment of communication problems and design treatment to suit the child's problems, needs, and strengths
- Consider educational demands made or to be made on the child in planning treatment; work closely with educators
- Borrow techniques from other communicative disorders in children (e.g., language disorders, articulation and phonological disorders, dysarthria, voice disorders) as cerebral palsy is not the name of a unique speech disorder; modify the standard techniques to suit the individual child and his or her specific symptom complex

Treatment Procedures

- Treatment of language disorders
  - train parents to stimulate language at home; see Parent Training and Language Stimulation by Parents
  - assess the child's language development periodically to determine the need for formal clinical treatment
  - implement formal language treatment if necessary
  - use the treatment procedures described under Language Disorders in Children and modify the procedures to suit the individual child with cerebral palsy
- Treatment of voice disorders
  - diagnose the specific voice disorder; when appropriate, use one or more treatment techniques described

C

under Voice Disorders techniques with suitable modifications; be aware that voice disorders may be due to respiratory problems associated with cerebral palsy
- treat associated respiratory problems; prescribe exercises to improve breath support for speech; use techniques described under Dysarthria, Treatment
- treat velopharyngeal incompetence only if there is enough tissue mass, and behavioral training thus is likely to be effective; see Treatment of Voice Disorders and Treatment of Disorders of Resonance
  - Treatment of articulation and phonological disorders
    - assess the child's specific sound errors and error patterns
    - assess the compensatory articulatory postures the child uses
    - modify or eliminate inappropriate and ineffective compensatory postures
    - teach the specific phonemes or classes of phonemes based on distinctive features or phonological patterns
    - use the treatment techniques described under Articulation and Phonological Disorders with appropriate modifications

Chaining. A behavioral technique of linking elements of a complex skill; similar to shaping; useful in teaching a variety of nonverbal and verbal skills, although most frequently employed in teaching self-help skills; includes forward chaining and backward chaining.
- Initially, make a task analysis and identify the steps involved in achieving a complex task (e.g., in teaching a child to tie his or her shoe lace, identify such different individual tasks as: 1. inserting the foot in to a shoe, 2. pulling the lace ends together, 3. making a bow, and 4. making the final knot)
- Use backward chaining to teach the skills in the reverse order and then practice the skill in an integrated manner:

C

- prompt and manually guide the child through skill 3; stop direct assistance and prompt the child to take the final step of making a knot (skill 4)
- starting all over, prompt and manually guide the child through skill 2; prompt the child to perform skill 3, making a bow out of the two lace ends
- starting over, prompt and manually guide the child to perform skill 1; stop and prompt the child to perform skill 2
- starting over, prompt the child to perform all four skills, ending in a knotted shoe lace
- Use forward chaining to teach skills in their sequence of first skill component to the last skill and practice the total skills in an integrated manner
  - use essentially the same procedure as in backward chaining except begin with skill 1 and move through the sequence

Changing Criterion, Research Design.   A single-subject research design to evaluate treatment effects; effectiveness of a treatment is demonstrated by effecting changes in target behaviors that approximate a changing criterion of performance; in successive stages of treatment, the behavior is held to a lower or higher criterion.

Changing Criterion, Treatment Procedure.   A method of shaping desirable behaviors by using performance criteria that change every time the client meets a certain criterion; the criterion may change in either direction (lower or higher) depending on the target behavior; in reducing the speech rate of clients with certain communicative disorders, the criteria are progressively lower; in shaping longer utterances, the criteria are progressively higher.

Chant-Talk.   A voice therapy technique characterized by speech that resembles chanting; consists of soft glottal attacks; raised pitch, prolonged syllables, even stress, and smooth

C

blending of words; considered appropriate for hyperfunctional voice problems; helps reduce excessive muscular effort and tension associated with voice production; for procedures, see Specific Normal Voice Facilitating Techniques under Voice Disorders.

Chewing Method. A voice therapy technique used to reduce vocal hyperfunction; helps reduce excessive tension and muscular effort associated with voice production; for procedures, see Specific Normal Voice Facilitating Techniques under Voice Disorders.

Child-Centered Approach. A child language intervention approach that assigns a more active role to the child; play-oriented and indirect treatment method; clinician takes the child's lead in targeting language structures for intervention; see Language Disorders in Children; Treatment of Language Disorders: Specific Techniques or Programs.

Childhood Aphasia (Congenital Aphasia). A controversial and somewhat dated term used to describe certain children's language disorders that could not be explained on the basis of other known variables including neurological problems, hearing impairment, mental retardation, environmental deficit, and so forth; a diagnosis made on negative evidence; questioned or rejected by many clinicians.

Choreiform Movements. Jerky, irregular, involuntary, and rapid movements; caused by damage to the caudate and the putamen; major symptom of Huntington's Disease.

Circumlocutions. Talking around a theme or failing to use specific terms.

Cleft. An opening in a structure that is normally closed.

Cleft Lip. Opening in the upper lip; may be on one (unilateral) or both (bilateral) sides of the lip; due to failure in embryonic growth processes.

Cleft Palate. Opening in the palate, the structure that separates the oral and nasal cavities; varies in extent and severity and may extend from the upper lip to the soft palate; due to failures in embryonic growth processes.

Surgical Management of the Clefts

- *Lip Surgery.* Surgical methods to close unilateral or bilateral clefts; usually done when the baby is about 3 months old or weighs about 10 pounds.

- *Palatal Surgery.* Surgical procedures performed to close the cleft or clefts of the palate; done when the baby is between 9 and 24 months, many between 9 and 12 months; the earlier the closure of the cleft, the better the speech development.

- *V-Y Retroposition.* A surgical method to repair the cleft of the palate; also known as Veau-Wardill-Kilner procedure; clefts are closed by raising from the bone single-based flaps of palatal mucoperiosteum on either side of the cleft and closing the cleft with the flaps as they are pushed back to lengthen the palate; improves chances of better speech production.

- *von Langenbeck Method.* A surgical method to repair the cleft of the palate by raising two bipedicled (attached on both ends) flaps of mucoperiosteum, bringing them together, and attaching them; leaves denuded bone on either side; does not lengthen the palate.

- *Delayed Hard Palate Closure.* A surgical sequence to close the cleft in which the soft palatal cleft is closed first and the hard palatal cleft is closed later.

- *Primary Surgery for the Clefts.* The initial surgery in which the clefts are closed.

- *Pharyngeal Flap.* A secondary palatal surgical procedure designed to improve the velopharyngeal functioning for speech; a muscular flap is cut from the posterior pharyngeal wall, raised, and attached to the velum; the flap is open on either side to allow for nasal breathing, nasal drainage,

C

and production of nasal speech sounds; helps close the velopharyngeal port and thus reduce hypernasality.

- *Pharyngoplasty.* A surgical procedure designed to improve velopharyngeal incompetence; such substances as Teflon, silicone, dacron wool/silicone gel bag, and cartilage may be implanted or injected into the posterior pharyngeal wall to make it bulge and thus help close the velopharyngeal port.
- *Secondary Surgeries for Clefts.* Surgical procedures done after the primary surgery to improve functioning and appearance.

Bzoch, K. R. (1997). *Communication disorders related to cleft lip and palate* (4th ed.). Austin, TX: Pro-Ed.

McWilliams, B. J., Morris, H. L., & Shelton, R. L. (1990). *Cleft palate speech* (2nd ed.). Philadelphia: B. C. Decker.

Peterson-Falzone, S. J., Hardin-Jones, M. A., & Kernell, M. P. (Eds.). (2001). *Cleft palate speech.* St. Louis, MO: Mosby.

Shprintzen, R. J., & Bardach, J. (1995). *Cleft palate speech management.* St. Louis, MO: Mosby.

Cleft Lip and Palate: Treatment for Articulation and Phonological Disorders
General Principles

- A thorough assessment of articulation skills and velopharyngeal function is necessary before starting treatment
- Treatment is effective if the child has at least a marginal velopharyngeal competence
- Children with significant velopharyngeal incompetence need surgery, prosthetic assistance, or both
- Treatment should be offered as early as possible
- Treatment should emphasize production and not auditory discrimination
- Trial therapy may be needed to determine prognosis
- Behavioral principles and procedures are effective in teaching correct articulation
- Phonological approach may be appropriate in certain children with repaired cleft

Cleft Palate: Articulation Disorders

- Many techniques used to treat Articulation and Phonological Disorders in children without clefts are appropriate in teaching sound production to children with repaired clefts

Treatment Procedures: Articulation and Phonological Disorders

Use the procedures of treating Articulation and Phonological Disorders; consider the following suggestions, some of which are unique to children with repaired clefts.

- Educate parents about the speech mechanism
- Withhold reinforcement for undesirable compensatory behaviors, the need for which has been eliminated by medical treatment
- Teach the more visible sounds before the less visible except for the linguadentals
- Teach stops and fricatives before other class of sounds
- Avoid or postpone training on /k/ and /g/ if the velopharyngeal functioning is inadequate
- Teach fricatives, affricates, or both if they are stimulable or after stops are mastered
- Teach linguapalatal sounds, lingua-alveolars, and linguadentals in that order
- Progress from syllables to words, phrases, and sentences
- Give auditory and visual cues; model frequently
- Provide systematic practice and reinforce correct productions
- Introduce compensatory articulatory positioning where appropriate
- Teach the client to direct the breath stream orally; let the child feel the airstream on hand or see the movement of a piece of tissue
- Teach the child to avoid posterior articulatory placements

C

- Teach the child to articulate with less effort and facial grimacing
- Give tactile cues and instruction to improve tongue positioning
- Work on generalization and maintenance; train parents to reinforce correct articulation at home

Bzoch, K. R. (1997). *Communication disorders related to cleft lip and palate* (4th ed.). Austin, TX: Pro-Ed.

McWilliams, B. J., Morris, H. L., & Shelton, R. L. (1990). *Cleft palate speech* (2nd ed.). Philadelphia: B. C. Decker.

Peterson-Falzone, S. J., Hardin-Jones, M. A., & Kernell, M. P. (Eds.). (2001). *Cleft palate speech*. St. Louis, MO: Mosby.

Shprintzen, R. J., & Bardach, J. (1995). *Cleft palate speech management*. St. Louis, MO: Mosby.

Cleft Lip and Palate: Treatment of Language Disorders

General Principles

- Language stimulation by parents may be all that is needed in some cases
- Formal language treatment may be necessary in some cases
- Need to work with the parents from early infancy to establish a long-term rapport
- Counseling parents about language development is essential
- The basic language treatment procedures are not much different from those used with Language Disorders in Children without clefts

Treatment Procedures: Language Disorders

Use the procedures of treating Language Disorders in Children without clefts; consider the following suggestions, some of which are unique to children with clefts.

- Teach patients to stimulate language at home
- Ask parents to encourage free verbal expression in their child

C

- Ask parents to integrate stimulation for articulation and language
- Integrate information about all aspects of rehabilitation in your discussion with the parents
- Ask parents to socially reinforce the child's spontaneous verbal productions
- Teach parents to reduce negative feedback, and make more positive statements about the child's communicative attempts
- Meet with parents regularly to review progress and modify their home language stimulation program
- Periodically assess the child's language skills
- Start formal language treatment when one of the periodic assessments warrant it
- Consider the imminent educational demands and plan language intervention to help meet them

Cleft Lip and Palate: Treatment of Phonatory Disorders

General Principles

- Phonatory problems may be due to compensatory behaviors or may be independent of velopharyngeal insufficiency
- Use techniques described under Voice Disorders if the problems are independent of velopharyngeal insufficiency (and due to vocal abuse)
- Consider phonatory treatment as diagnostic; discontinue if there is no improvement in phonatory problems or other speech symptoms worsen
- Do not try to eliminate nasal escape and hypernasality
- Do not offer phonatory treatment for children with a clear diagnosis of velopharyngeal incompetence
- Follow treated children because some improve, some deteriorate, and some stay the same

Treatment Procedures for Hyperfunctional Voice

- Describe how voice is produced to the child and the parents

- Reduce <u>Vocally Abusive Behaviors</u> in the child and in other members of the family
- Counsel the family about good vocal behaviors (e.g., talking less in noisy environments, practicing soft speech, good conversational turn taking, clapping instead of shouting or yelling)
- Use auditory discrimination training by helping the child to discriminate his or her voice from that of other children without vocal nodules or other vocal pathology
- Use such biofeedback instruments as the Visi-Pitch in training
- Train healthy voice production by teaching the child to
  - reduce vocal loudness
  - eliminate hard glottal attacks
  - initiate words that start with vowels
  - use easy, gentle onset of phonation
  - self-monitor voice

McWilliams, B. J., Morris, H. L., & Shelton, R. L. (1990). *Cleft palate speech* (2nd. ed.). Philadelphia: B. C. Decker.

Cleft Lip and Palate: Treatment for Resonance Disorders

General Principles

- Do not treat <u>Hypernasality</u> if it is a result of velopharyngeal incompetence
- Treat hypernasality only if the child is capable of achieving velopharyngeal closure
- See if surgery reduces or eliminates hypernasality; improvement may continue for up to a year following surgery

Treatment Procedures: Resonance Disorders

- Use techniques described under <u>Voice Disorders</u> to reduce hypernasality including increased loudness, discrimination training to distinguish oral and nasal resonance, lowered pitch, encouraging increased oral opening
- Use respiratory training to improve loudness
- Attempt articulation with the nares occluded

- Decrease intra-oral breath pressure on stop consonants and fricatives, while simultaneously using loose articulatory contacts
- Use such biofeedback instruments as Tonar II to reduce hypernasality
- Use the whistle-blowing technique of R. J. Shprintzen and his associates to promote velopharyngeal closure during speech
  - teach whistling and blowing at the same time
  - reinforce when nasal airflow is absent
  - continue until there is no nasal escape during whistling or blowing
  - eliminate whistling or blowing, and introduce phonation
  - continue until no nasal escape is evident
  - introduce vowels /i/ or /u/ while blowing or whistling
  - continue until there is no longer nasal escape
  - eliminate blowing or whistling, and produce only the vowels
  - form monosyllables by using non-nasal consonants with vowels
  - move to words, sentences, and conversations
  - teach self-monitoring skills

Boone, D. R., & McFarlane, S. C. (1988). *The voice and voice therapy* (4th ed). Englewood Cliffs, NJ: Prentice-Hall.

McWilliams, B. J., Morris, H. L., & Shelton, R. L. (1990). *Cleft palate speech* (2nd. ed.). Philadelphia: B. C. Decker.

Peterson-Falzone, S. J., Hardin-Jones, M. A., & Kernell, M. P. (Eds.). (2001). *Cleft palate speech*. St. Louis, MO: Mosby.

Wilson, D. K. (1972). *Voice problems in children.* Baltimore, MD: Williams & Wilkins.

Client-Specific Strategy. A method of selecting target behaviors that are relevant, useful, and functional for the individual client.

- Observe the client's environment for clues to functional targets

- Study the educational, occupational, and social demands made on the client
- Select targets that are useful and relevant to the particular client
- Select targets that will immediately enhance the client's communication in natural settings
- Select targets that have potential for generalized productions
- Select targets that serve as building blocks for more complex communicative behaviors

Closed-Head Injury. The same as <u>Nonpenetrating Head Injury;</u> injury to the brain when the meninges are intact although the skull may or may not be fractured.

Cloze Procedure. Modeling parts of an utterance and pausing for the child to produce words and phrases to complete the utterance; the same as <u>Partial Modeling</u> and <u>Completion.</u>
- Model only the initial portion of a target response (e.g., say "The boy is . . ." and wait for the response)
- Let the child complete the partial model (e.g., the child says "walking")
- Reinforce the child's response

Cluttering. A speech-language disorder characterized by rapid speech rate, irregular speech rate, or both; a fluency disorder related to, but different from, stuttering; may co-exist with stuttering; also defined as a fluency disorder with rapid rate, indistinct articulation, and impaired language formulation possibly suggesting poor organization of thought with reduced or absent awareness or concern about the problems; certain elements of treatment are common to stuttering and cluttering.
- Make a thorough assessment of the overall symptoms; determine the extent of fluency, articulation, and language problems; consult the cited sources and *PGASLP*
- Teach a slower rate of speech

Cluttering

- Teach syllable prolongation
- Use <u>Metronome-Paced Speech</u> or <u>Delayed Auditory Feedback</u> (both described under <u>Stuttering; Treatment of Stuttering: Specific Techniques or Programs</u>) if necessary to slow the rate and induce prolongation
- Use <u>Shadowing</u> (described under <u>Stuttering; Treatment of Stuttering: Specific Techniques or Programs</u>)
- Teach slow and distinct articulation
- Teach pausing between clauses and sentences
- Ask the client to increase the rate beyond baseline and then slow down to encourage discrimination
- Correct any phoneme-specific misarticulations through methods of treating <u>Articulation and Phonological Disorders</u>
- Teach the client to produce syllables with deliberate stress, especially the final and unstressed syllables of words
- Tape-record the client's cluttered speech and play it back to increase awareness
- Give prompt, contingent feedback on cluttered speech to increase awareness
- Heighten clutterers' awareness of their listeners' difficulty in understanding them; sensitize the clients to the listeners' facial expressions and gestures that signal difficulty in understanding
- Treat word finding difficulties by having the client name rapidly and learn words in semantically varied categories
- Teach conversational turn taking, organized expressions, and coherent talking
- Teach <u>Self-Control (Self-Monitoring) Skills</u>
- Implement a maintenance program
- Follow up and give booster treatment

Myers, F. L., & St. Louis, K. O. (1992). *Cluttering: A clinical perspective*. Kibworth, England: Far Communications.

Rate Reduction in Treating Cluttering

A speech rate slower than the normal or below a client-specific baserate; a typical target to improve speech intelligibility and to reduce dysfluencies of persons who clutter; may use <u>Delayed Auditory Feedback (DAF)</u> to induce rate reduction.

- Establish a baserate of speech rate measured either in syllables or words per minute
- Instruct the client in rate reduction and describe its desirable effects
- Reassure the client that a more acceptable rate is the final target of treatment
- Model a slow rate of speech for the client
- Model pausing at appropriate junctures
- Experiment with slower rates and increased frequency or duration of pauses that result in reduced or eliminated dysfluencies and improved intelligibility
- Model the effective rate selected for the client
- Ask the client to imitate the reduced rate
- Use delayed auditory feedback if instructions and modeling are not effective
- Start with words and phrases and move on to controlled and spontaneous sentences
- Add other targets (distinct articulation, increased stress, prolonged vowels)
- Fade excessively slow rate while maintaining distinct articulation and decreased dysfluencies
- Teach self-monitoring skills
- Follow up and arrange for booster treatment

Collaborative Model.   A service delivery model used in public schools; the speech-language pathologist works with the classroom teacher in identifying clinical activities that promote academic learning in a child with communication disorders; the clinician works in the classroom along with the teacher.

Collagen Injection.   A medical treatment procedure for clients with paralyzed vocal folds; injected into the middle third of the fold, collagen increases the bulk and the chances of adduction.

Communication.   Exchange of information through various verbal or nonverbal actions; more or less organized; target of treatment in clients with communicative disorders; its various forms include:

- Aided communication: Communication achieved through the assistance of such external devices as paper and pencil, communication boards, and computers.
- Alternative communication: Communication achieved by nonoral means; all modes others than the verbal.
- Augmentative communication: Oral or verbal communication that is in some way limited but enhanced or expanded by aided or unaided alternative communication means including speech synthesizers, communication boards, and paper and pencil.
- Manual communication: Communication achieved by signs, gestures, and symbols and without oral speech.
- Nonverbal communication: Communication achieved without oral speech; may be in the form of signs, gestures, facial expressions, and symbols.
- Simultaneous communication: Communication achieved through multiple means including oral speech, signs, symbols, and gestures.
- Total communication: Communication achieved through the simultaneous use of verbal expressions as well as a sign language (e.g., American Sign Language).
- Unaided communication: Communication achieved without the help of external means; normal oral communication that is accompanied by typical gestures and expressions.
- Verbal communication: Communication achieved through spoken words and language; may be accompanied by culturally appropriate normal gestures and facial expression

Communication Boards.   An augmentative/alternative communication system; boards on which letters, words, phrases, sentences, symbols, or pictures are pasted for the

C

client to point to, touch, or select in any manner possible to communicate.

Compensatory Strategies. Means of achieving communication in unusual or atypical means; achieving communication in spite of organic, intellectual, or other kinds of deficiency that may be expected to affect communication; in articulation, methods of producing speech sounds in atypical means because of neuroanatomic deficiencies; in adult communication rehabilitation (such as in patients with dementia), communication through strategies that help adapt to deficiencies.

Completion. The same as Cloze Procedure and Partial Modeling.

Concurrent Stimulus-Response Generalization. Production of new and unreinforced responses in relation to new stimuli; the most complex form of generalized production.

Conditioned Generalized Reinforcers. Tokens, money, and other reinforcers that are effective in a wide range of conditions; Secondary Reinforcers that have a generalized effect; use them to:
- Promote generalized productions of target behaviors
- Enhance the effectiveness of the reinforces used in treatment

Conditioned Reinforcers. Events that reinforce behaviors because of past learning experiences (e.g., verbal praise or tokens); the same as Secondary Reinforcers; see Unconditioned Reinforcers.

Conditioned Response. A learned response reliably elicited or evoked by a conditioned stimulus; in clinical terms, a target response elicited or evoked and then reinforced; see Unconditioned Response.

Conditioned Stimulus. A stimulus that elicits or evokes a response only because of a learning history; stimuli clinicians use in treatment sessions; see Unconditioned Stimulus.

Conditioning and Learning. A behavioral method of selecting and strengthening behaviors in individuals; technique of teaching new behaviors; changing the probability of existing behaviors by arranging different consequences for behaviors:

- *Avoidance conditioning:* Learning or teaching behaviors that help avoid aversive conditions, stimuli, and persons; once learned, hard to extinguish; often found in persons who stutter; modifying such avoidance behaviors as not talking on the phone is a treatment target.
- *Classical conditioning:* Also known as Pavlovian conditioning, classical conditioning involves systematic pairing of two stimuli—one, an unconditioned stimulus(UCS) and the other a conditioned stimulus (CS) so that the CS begins to elicit the response typically given to the UCS.
- *Operant conditioning:* Creating, shaping, selecting, strengthening, or weakening behaviors of an individual by arranging different consequences for those behaviors; the most researched and effective techniques known to teach new skills, including communicative skills.

Conductive Hearing Loss. Inefficient conductance of sound to the middle or inner ear due to the abnormalities of the external auditory canal, the ear drum, or the ossicular chain of the middle ear.

Conduction Aphasia. A type of fluent aphasia characterized by markedly impaired repetition skills; caused by lesions in the supramarginal gyrus, the superior temporal lobe, and regions between Broca's and Wernicke's areas. See Aphasia.

Confrontation Naming. Naming a stimulus when asked to do so; a correct response to such questions as "What is this?"; typically impaired in patients with aphasia and hence a treatment target for clients with Aphasia.

Congenital Disorder.　Any clinical condition a person is born with; a condition noticed at the time of or soon after birth; may or may not be inherited.

Congenital Aphasia.　Aphasia noticed early in childhood; a disorder that affects the acquisition of language as against aphasia in adults that disrupts acquired language. The same as Childhood Aphasia.

Congenital Palatopharyngeal Incompetence.　An inadequate velopharyngeal mechanism that cannot close the velopharyngeal port for the production of nonnasal speech sounds; not due to clefts; the person is presumably born with a deficient velopharyngeal mechanism; hard palate may be too short or the nasopharynx may be too deep; speech is hypernasal; depending on the degree of incompetence, resonance (voice) therapy may be ineffective without surgical or prosthetic help.

Consequences.　Events that follow a response and thus increase or decrease the future probability of those responses; in treatment, clinician's differential response to client's correct, incorrect, and no response; technically known as reinforcers (both positive and negative) that typically increase behaviors and punishers (corrective feedback) that decrease them.

Constituent Definitions.　Dictionary definitions of terms with no reference to how what is defined is measured (e.g., *The goal of treatment is to reduce stuttering.*) contrasted with Operational Definitions (e.g., *The goal of treatment is to reduce specified dysfluencies to below 3% of the words spoken.*).

Consultant Model.　A service delivery model; the speech-language pathologist selects the training targets and procedures; trains teachers, parents, siblings, aides, and others who actually provide the service; the clinician evaluates the results and modifies the procedures.

Contact Ulcers (Contact Granuloma). Benign lesions on the posterior third of the glottal margin; possibly due to trauma, reflux, or vocally abusive behaviors; voice symptoms include low pitch, effortful phonation, and vocal fatigue.

* Do not recommend complete vocal rest or surgical treatment
* Do not recommend forced whispering
* Ask the patient to talk less
* Reduce <u>Vocally Abusive Behaviors</u>
* Teach the client to speak with less effort and force
* Teach relaxed phonation and speaking
* Teach the client to speak more softly
* Eliminate glottal attacks

Contingency. An interdependent relation between events or factors; in behavioral analysis and treatment, a dependent relation between antecedents, responses, and the clinician's feedback to the client; the most important element in behavioral treatment; includes <u>Environmental Contingency</u> and <u>Genetic/Neurophysiological Contingency.</u>

Contingent Consequences. Consequences that closely follow behaviors and thus change their frequency; in treatment, the feedback clinicians give their clients immediately after the clients produce correct or incorrect responses; consequences that depend on the nature of responses (correct or incorrect); reinforcers and punishers that depend on the responses.

Contingent Queries. Questions the clinician asks immediately following an unclear statement from the client in language therapy; lead to more specific or elaborate responses from the client.

* Ask a question immediately following an unclear response from the child (e.g., the child says "kick ball"; you ask,

"Who is kicking the ball?"); such contingent queries may lead to a more clear and perhaps elaborate response from the child.

Continuous Airflow.   A stuttering treatment target; maintaining uninterrupted airflow throughout an utterance; for procedures see Stuttering, Treatment; Treatment of Stuttering: Specific Techniques or Programs.

Continuous Reinforcement.   A schedule in which every occurrence of a response is reinforced; effective in establishing new skills; inefficient in maintaining already established skills; therefore:
- Use this schedule only in initial stage of treatment
- Gradually shift from continuous to Intermittent Reinforcement

Contrast Effect.   Increase in the frequency of an undesirable response that has been kept under check by an aversive stimulus when the aversive stimulus is absent.

Contrastive Stress Drills.   A treatment method used to promote both articulatory proficiency and natural prosody, especially the stress and rhythm aspects of spoken language; used in treating Apraxia of Speech (AOS) in Adults; different phrases and sentences are used to teach placing stress on different words; stressed words or terms may be used to promote articulatory proficiency or simply to vary prosodic features of speech.

In Teaching Articulatory Proficiency
- Construct phrases and sentences preferably with a single target sound in them (e.g., "My name is *Peter*" for /p/; "*S*am did it" for /s/)
- Ask a series of questions such that the client will respond with the target phrase placing extra stress on the target word (e.g., "Is your name Tom?"; client will respond "No, my name is *Peter*"; the client is likely to stress the word

Peter, especially the initial sound, and thus improve the articulatory precision of /p/; similarly, ask "Tom did it?"; the client will respond "*Sam* did it.")

- Reinforce the client for articulatory proficiency

In Teaching Prosodic Features

- Create a series of phrases and sentences (e.g., "Tom does not read mystery novels.")
- Ask questions that will force stress on different words in target phrases and sentences (e.g., "Does Tom read *romance* novels?" may evoke "No, Tom reads *mystery* novels." "Does Tom *never* read mystery novels?" may evoke "Tom *reads* them all the time.")
- Reinforce the client for varying stress on different words

Control Group.   The group that does not receive treatment and hence shows no change in the target disorder or disease; part of the Group Design Strategy that helps evaluate treatment effects and efficacy.

- Select subjects randomly (Random Selection)
- Assign subjects into control and experimental groups randomly
- Alternatively, match subjects in the experimental and control groups (see Matching)
- Assess the control group
- Withhold treatment to the control group while the experimental group receives treatment.
- Demonstrate that the control group did not change (improve) while the experimental group did

Controlled Evidence.   Data that show that a particular treatment, not some other factor, was responsible for the positive changes in a client's behavior; evidence gathered through controlled experimentation with either group or single-subject design strategy; data that show that treatment is significantly better than no treatment; evidence that supports the use of a treatment technique; one of several Treatment Selection Criteria.

C

Controlled Sentences. Specific sentences that contain target language features the clinician asks the child or an adult to produce; may be modeled; use of pictures and other clinical stimuli may be used to evoke them; less spontaneous.

Conversational Probes. Methods to assess generalized production of clinically established behaviors in conversational speech and language.
* Take a naturalistic conversational speech sample
* Direct it minimally to adequately sample the production of speech or language behaviors under probe
* Count the number of opportunities for producing the skill under probe
* Calculate the percent correct production of probed behaviors
* Give additional training at the conversational level if the adopted probe criterion is not met (e.g., 90% accuracy)
* Dismiss the client only after the criterion is met

Conversational Turn Taking. A pragmatic language skill and treatment target; often deficient in a client with language disorders; involves appropriate exchange of speaker and listener roles during conversation; for procedures, see Language Disorders in Children; Treatment of Language Disorders: Specific Techniques or Programs.

Corrective Feedback. Response-contingent feedback from the clinician that reduces the frequency of undesirable responses of clients; frequently used in treatment.
* Give corrective feedback as soon as you detect an incorrect response
* Give Verbal Corrective Feedback ("No." or "That is not correct.") for all incorrect responses
* Give Nonverbal Corrective Feedback when appropriate (gestures that show disapproval of a response)
* Give Mechanical Corrective Feedback or Biofeedback whenever possible

- Measure the frequency of incorrect responses to see if the feedback is effective
- Replace ineffective forms of corrective feedback with other, potentially more effective forms
- Minimize the use of corrective feedback by giving more positive feedback for correct responses and by Shaping complex skills

Craniocerebral Trauma. The same as Traumatic Brain Injury.

Criteria for Making Clinical Decisions. Rules to make various clinical judgments; includes such treatment-related rules as when to model, when to stop modeling, and when a behavior is considered trained.

- Model most target behaviors for most clients, especially in the initial stages
- Discontinue modeling when the client gives five consecutively correct, imitated responses
- Reinstate modeling if errors persist
- Consider an exemplar of a target behavior trained when the client gives 10 consecutively correct responses
- Consider a behavior tentatively trained when the client gives 90% correct responses on untrained exemplars on an intermixed probe
- Consider a behavior trained when the client gives 90% or better correct responses in conversational speech produced in extraclinical situations

Cued Speech. A system of nonverbal communication that is used as a supplement to speech reading; consists of eight hand shapes that represent categories of consonants and four positions about the face that represent categories of vowels; these hand shapes and positions suggest speech sounds in running speech; known to promote better reading skills in children who are deaf.

Cultural Diversity and Treatment Procedures. Factors related to ethnic background, culture, and linguistic

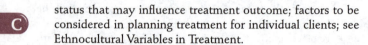

C

status that may influence treatment outcome; factors to be considered in planning treatment for individual clients; see <u>Ethnocultural Variables in Treatment.</u>

Cysts.   Acquired or congenital, fluid-filled lesions of the larynx caused by trauma; can occur contralaterally to a unilateral <u>Vocal Nodule;</u> usually unilateral; treatment is surgery.

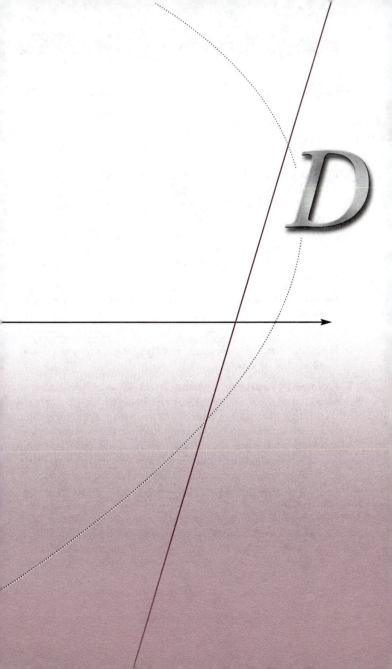

D

Deaf. A person whose hearing impairment is severe enough to prevent normal oral language acquisition, production, and comprehension with the help of audition; profound hearing loss that exceeds 90 dB HL; see Hearing Impairment for rehabilitation.

Deblocking. A technique used in treating clients with aphasia; uses an intact response to one kind of stimulus to deblock a deficient or absent response to another kind of stimulus (e.g., visual stimuli to which the client responds appropriately may be used in promoting a deficient or non-existent response to auditory stimuli; for the procedure, see Aphasia, Treatment; Treatment of Naming: Targets and Techniques.

Dedicated Systems of Augmentative Communication. Computers designed and built exclusively for augmentative communication; see Augmentative Communication.

Deglutition. Swallowing; see Dysphagia for normal and abnormal swallow.

Delayed Auditory Feedback (DAF). A procedure in which a speaker's speech is fed back to his or her ears through headphones after a delay; most speakers slow their speech down under DAF; technique is used in reducing the speech rate in persons who stutter or clutter and those who have dysarthria; see Cluttering; Dysarthria; Stuttering; Treatment of Stuttering: Specific Techniques or Programs.
- Select one of the several DAF machines available on the market
- Experiment with different durations of delay that induce speech that is free from stuttering or cluttering or speech rate that improves intelligibility in dysarthric speakers
- Train and stabilize the target speech skills with the selected delay
- Fade DAF and shape the normal rate and prosody

Deletion Processes.   A group of phonological processes in which one or more consonants or a syllable in a word is deleted or omitted; in phonological treatment, the target is to eliminate such processes; major deletion processes include:

- *Cluster reduction:* one or more consonants are deleted in a cluster of consonants (e.g., bu for *blue*)
- *Initial consonant deletion:* omission of an initial consonant of a syllable (e.g., ink for *sink*)
- *Final consonant deletion:* omission of a final consonant (e.g., goo for *good*)
- *Unstressed syllable deletion:* omission of a syllable (e.g., medo for *tomato,* nana for *banana*)

Demands and Capacities Model (DCM).   A theory of stuttering which states that when the environmental demands made on a child to produce and sustain fluency exceeds the child's capacity to do so, stuttering results; treatment involves reducing the demands and gradually increasing the child's fluency skills; for procedures see Stuttering, Treatment; Treatment of Stuttering: Specific Techniques or Programs; Stuttering Prevention: A Clinical Method.

Dementia.   An acquired neurological Syndrome associated in most cases with persistent or progressive deterioration in intellectual and communicative functions and general behavior; sustained over a period of months or years; examples include dementia due to Alzheimer's Disease, Huntington's Disease, Parkinson's Disease, or vascular disease; dementia is static in a few cases and reversible in 10 to 20% of the cases; in most cases, treatment is concerned with behavioral and clinical management because the disease is progressive and the effects irreversible; both the client and his or her family need treatment.

Counsel and Educate the Family Members
Dementia affects family as much as it affects the persons who have it; therefore, counseling the family and finding

them emotional, financial, and professional support are important.

- Educate the family members about:
  - the causes, symptoms, and course of dementia
  - the specific type of dementia and its neurological basis
  - general medical and behavioral management procedures
- Give family members a realistic picture of what is ahead; discuss with them the need to cope with a difficult, prolonged, and expensive problem, the nature or even existence of which may not be understood by the patient himself or herself, especially in later stages
- Tell them that that as time passes, they are most likely to be concerned with and troubled by the patient's:
  - physical violence
  - memory deficits
  - catastrophic reactions
  - incontinence
  - delusions and hallucinations
  - making accusations and suspiciousness
  - uncooperative at bathing and at mealtime
  - communication problems
  - demanding, critical behaviors
  - unsafe driving, cooking
  - hiding things
  - daytime wandering and night walking
- Let them understand that patients with dementia, especially in the beginning states, are frustrated, worried, anxious, and angry
- Let them understand that in due course, the patient is likely to be depressed and may withdraw from the family
- Prepare the family members for:
  - potential emotional outbursts and angry exchanges over trivial matters

- abusive, aggressive, and violent behaviors in later stages
- constant supervision or institutionalization of the patient in the later stages of dementia
- the eventual need to feed, clothe, and take care of the person in all respects, including oral hygiene
- the eventual incontinence that will increase the burden of care tremendously
- extended period of home care (1 to 2 years to 10 to 15 years)
- needing emotional, social, financial, and psychological help for themselves, not just the patient

- Impress upon the family members that rehabilitative efforts are still very important to slow down the process of deterioration in the physical, social, and intellectual status of the person with dementia
- Help the family members cope financially with the long-term care of the patient with dementia:
  - let them appreciate the long-term cost and efforts involved in managing a person with dementia
  - discuss the family's available resources to care for and pay for the services
  - help them find and contact local, state, and federal agencies along with private sources that offer financial support to families who have a patient with dementia
- Offer them help in finding appropriate nursing home placement when the time comes
- Give them consumer-oriented printed information on dementia and its management
- Give them names and addresses of local professional and social associations and organizations concerned with aging and dementia
- Introduce them to local support groups
- Give them information on any accessible specialty clinics, research centers, and universities where unique programs are being evaluated

D

- Give them information on websites that offer suggestions, newsletters, and information on new developments in medically or behaviorally managing persons with dementia
- If not already served by a team of specialists, including those who can counsel the family members (e.g., psychiatrists, psychologists, and social workers), make referrals
- Arrange for the team to help the family members make rational and acceptable decisions about making or not making heroic efforts to sustain life in the terminal stage of dementia
- Arrange for continued counseling after the demise of the patient to help the family members regain their energies, rebuild deteriorated relationships among surviving members, deal with grief and loss, and manage financial burden of extended care

Clinical Management of Patients With Dementia. Design a program to help the person with dementia sustain skills and behaviors to the extent possible; cope with progressive deterioration in skills and behaviors; teach compensatory strategies.

- Establish a simple routine for the patient and the family
- Manage the patient's memory problems; design such stimulus control procedures as reminders, prompters, pictures, lists, and other devices to manage the memory problems; but include systematic training to use them; note that differential reinforcement is important to make stimulus manipulations work for the patients; see also Memory Impairments:
  - note that external cues are more effective than internal cues (self-monitored) in improving memory skills, although teaching self-monitoring skills is recommended
  - note that any kind of prompt that reminds the patient of an activity or encourages a patient to do something is better than no prompts

- give verbal prompts that remind patients of scheduled activities (e.g., a social gathering, a game, a party), which may be more effective than other kinds of reminders (e.g., a bright poster printed in large letters)
- note that just making materials and opportunities for activities may not be sufficient to prompt actions and activities; patients need verbal prompts and reinforcement for following through
- reinforce institutionalized patients for paying attention to reminders, signs, posters, announcements, and scheduled activities as these may not be effective without such reinforcement
- train patients by reinforcing them to use, and prompt them to consult, a diary that they keep about appointments and schedules of events because it is not sufficient to have them simply write them down on a piece of paper
- have caregivers in an institution wear name tags printed in larger letters, train the caregivers to draw attention to their name tags, and have patients read them or caregivers read them aloud; train the caregivers to reinforce the patients for saying the name or reading it aloud
- have patients keep a list of activities that are more immediate (i.e., *today's* activities as against this *month's* activity), and train caregivers to prompt the patient to consult the list at appropriate times
- teach the client to use portable alarms that remind him or her of appointments and scheduled activities; monitor the use of the devices and reinforce the patient for maintaining this skill
- give written instructions on daily living chores (closing the windows, locking the doors, turning the stove off); teach the client to follow the instructions and reinforce him or her for doing so

D

- train staff members in health care facilities to give frequent and systematic reminders to the clients and to reinforce the client in appropriate ways for exhibiting the required skills or following directions
- teach the client to rehearse information (e.g., just before leaving, rehearsing the names of people to be encountered in a party or class reunion; visualizing the faces of people to be encountered)
- teach the client to self-monitor; reinforce the client for doing this and evaluate its maintenance
- create a naming wallet containing pictures of family members, their names, and sentences and phrases about them, and train the patient to carry it and use it
- Teach clients to make a written list of *what to do* every day; train the client to use the list by frequent prompts and positive reinforcements
- Teach the client to keep personal belongings (keys, clothing items, eye glasses, pens) in a specific, invariable place; frequently monitor and reinforce this skill
- Teach the client to keep related objects together (e.g., paper and pencil; socks and shoes; coffee and sugar); frequently monitor and reinforce this skill
- Train the client to carry a card that contains the name, address, telephone number of a family member and a health care professional; frequently check the client to see if this is maintained
- Teach the client to wear a bracelet that contains personal identification; check its continued use
- Instruct the client to exploit his or her strengths to compensate for weaknesses (e.g., writing down everything when memory tends to fail)
- Teach clients to ignore relatively minor problems (e.g., word-finding difficulties)
- Teach the client to take enough rest so fatigue will not further complicate the condition
- Control disorientation and confusion

D

- place a large calendar in the patient's bedroom and cross off the current date every night; draw the patient's attention to this activity and tell the patient what you are doing (remember, that you are not doing it for your benefit)
- make the patient wear a digital calendar watch with large display of AM and PM, date and day; frequently draw attention to it; have the client use it in realistic situations (e.g., instructing the patient to look at the watch and saying that it is now 12 noon and time to have lunch)
- provide maps of frequently visited places (e.g., homes of relatives or friends, doctor's office, shops, favorite restaurants); before visiting the places, prompt the patient to consult the maps
- In treating communication disorders in early stages of dementia, provide cues to evoke words and then teach self-cueing techniques; see Aphasia for details and additional examples:
  - give phonemic cues for words (e.g., the clinician says "The word starts with an s" to evoke *spoon*)
  - give such semantic cues as a generic class (e.g., the clinician says "woman" to evoke the word "wife"); a synonym (e.g., the clinician says "dwelling" to evoke "house"); an antonym (e.g., the clinician says "good" to evoke "bad"); a category name (e.g., the clinician says "it is a fruit" to evoke "apple"); or an associated word (e.g., the clinician says "cup" to evoke "plate")
  - train the patient to use description as cues in which he or she describes an object before naming it
  - teach self-cueing by having the client produce the successful cues to generate the intended word
  - note that contingent consequences (positive reinforcement and corrective feedback) are known to be effective in modifying communicative behaviors in patients with dementia

D

- ask orientation questions (questions about time and place), model the correct responses, and verbally reinforce the patient for imitating the correct responses; gradually fade the modeling and have the patient respond to questions
- train the patients to initiate conversation and reinforce them for doing so
- ignore inappropriate, irrelevant, vulgar, delusional, and any other type of unacceptable or bizarre verbal behaviors and reinforce any appropriate verbal responses (differential reinforcement)
- reinforce the patients continuously (reinforcement for all desirable responses); if needed, reinforce the patients with tangible reinforcers
- To sustain social and communicative skills as long as possible, arrange group therapy sessions involving family members or other patients with similar problems; direct the sessions and manage the behavioral contingencies to promote the selected goals of the group session; provide refreshments during these sessions, as some data suggest their potentially positive effects on interaction; arrange the sessions to have the patients:
  - tell stories in group sessions
  - maintain topics of conversation
  - take appropriate turns in conversation
  - express their own feelings and thoughts about their disease
  - arrange for generous verbal reinforcers for all targeted expressions and any other appropriate expressions
  - ignore and teach the group members to ignore inappropriate responses
- Sustain skills as long as possible, even if they have to be progressively simplified:
  - encourage the patient to continue to cook but with support
  - arrange for cooking simpler foods

Dementia: Caregiver Strategies

- sustain reading skills with routine materials (e.g., TV listings, newspapers, labels on packaged foods, restaurant menus)
- get the patient involved in social activities and family group activities as long as possible
- provide plenty of verbal reinforcement for the patient's effort to sustain skills and social behaviors

Management Strategies for Patient's Caregivers, Including Family Members. Family members and other caregivers need help in managing persons with dementia; ask all those who care for and regularly interact with the client to:

- Be observant about changes in the patient's behavior that might signal a significant change in health status
- Take steps to sustain the patient's physical health by making sure that the patient:
  - regularly takes the prescribed medications
  - eats properly
  - exercises regularly
- Be consistent
- Reduce distractions
- Design and maintain a consistent routine for the patient
- Reassign household chores the patient cannot perform anymore, but do not expropriate the patient's responsibilities too soon
- Design and maintain a constant and simplified environment
- Make environmental modifications that support communication and help prevent social isolation and more rapid deterioration in behavior, including communication:
  - create and maintain communication opportunities for the patient
  - incorporate as much relevant speech as possible with daily routines
  - do not restrict expression and communication with the fear that the patient may be irrelevant

179

D

- remove unduly restrictive rules against talking and social interactions in institutional settings
- find regular conversational partners for the patient at home and in institutional settings; recruit friends, grandchildren, family members who do not see the client regularly, neighbors, former colleagues, and volunteers (especially in an institution)
- help the patient maintain contact with grandchildren and other younger acquaintances; work with both the younger persons and the patient to foster this relationship
- encourage patients to observe social activities even if they do not participate in them
- encourage patients in the early stage of dementia to offer help in some designated activities to their spouses and other family members at home or other patients in institutions (e.g., helping spouses in cooking, cleaning, or shopping; helping new patients with routines in an institution)
- arrange regular small group activities at home; facilitate and reinforce the patient's participation
- let the patient have a say in arranging or rearranging his or her personal space (room design, color, furniture, decorations)
- encourage the patient to be responsible for maintaining his or her personal space for as long as possible
- allow the patient some privacy (do not relentlessly supervise when it is unnecessary)
- use contrasting colors to enhance orientation to hand rails, hallways, communication boards, table settings, and room decorations; note that just these measures may not promote appropriate behaviors; train the patient to make use of them
- pay attention to the patient's ethnocultural background in arranging his or her environment

- pay attention to the patient's ethnocultural background in arranging conversational partners and topics
- pay attention to a bilingual patient's primary language or the dominant language in arranging communication opportunities and topics; find interpreters or similarly bilingual conversational partners
- have family members regularly visit the institutionalized patient
- have family members participate in social events at the institution
- have family members take part in social activities arranged at the institution
- Attend to the sensory needs of the patient, especially in the early and middle stages of dementia:
  - have the client's vision checked and provide new glasses if need
  - provide magnifying glasses and printed material with larger print to sustain reading skills
  - place all visual information at the patient's eye level
  - keep the patient's living environment visually attractive
  - have the client examined by an otologist and take necessary steps to maintain the patient's otological health
  - have the client's hearing checked by an audiologist and provide hearing aids as recommended
  - monitor the use of hearing aids on a daily basis, as assistance may be needed in inserting and removing the hearing aids and in volume adjustments
  - discuss with an audiologist the need for Assistive Listening Devices described under Aural Rehabilitation and follow the recommendations
  - reduce or eliminate noise in situations where communication takes place (e.g., turn off the TV or radio while talking to the client; monitor such mechanical noises as those of air conditioners and fans)

D

- evaluate whether the patient whose visual and auditory acuity is diminished reacts better to improved tactile and olfactory cues
- Approach the client slowly, with calm and inviting expressions, and within his or her visual field (do not surprise the patient)
- Establish eye contact before speaking
- Let the patient see your face clearly while talking (stoop down if the patient is in a wheelchair)
- Supplement speech with gestures, smiles, and posture
- Speak clearly and directly
- Speak in simple terms
- Use requests instead of commands (e.g., "Should we do this together?" or "Would you give me a hand and help?")
- Specify referents for speech (e.g., "We need to go to the dining hall" instead of "We need to go over there."); use proper names (e.g., your wife Jane, physical therapist Tom) instead of pronouns (e.g., *he, she, they*)
- Have only one or two people engage the client in conversation at any one time
- Do not argue with the patient; instead rearrange the environment (e.g., do not try to convince a suspicious person with arguments that no one has taken his or her possessions; instead, make sure that the possessions are always kept in one predictable, easily accessible place)
- Record problems that occur with a view to find patterns in them; design strategies to control them (e.g., an episode of aggressive behavior may have been triggered by physical pain that may need medical attention)
- Ask yes/no questions
- Ask either/or questions
- Ask short questions
- Ask simple questions

Dementia: Caregiver Strategies

- Be specific in your communication with the patient
- Avoid vague references, sarcasm, indefinite referents, proverbs and such other abstract statements, and humor
- Say only a little at a time and make sure the patient understands before saying more
- Repeat questions if necessary
- Avoid asking open-ended questions
- Be redundant, repeat, and restate
- Talk about familiar and concrete topics and directly observable objects
- Use photographs and drawings to improve understanding
- Avoid the use of analogies
- Restate and paraphrase when the client has not comprehended
- Use touch
- Praise the patient frequently for appropriate behaviors
- Say good-bye or other departing signals
- Always use the same phrase to suggest daily routines (e.g., "Let's eat" or "Let's go to bed now.")
- Observe what conditions aggravate the client's behavioral problems and try to avoid or reduce those conditions
- Look for physical reasons for emotional outbursts (e.g., pain, side effects of medication)
- Look for early warning signs of emotional or aggressive outbursts (e.g., body rigidity, a certain look, crying)
- Eliminate stimuli and situations that trigger emotional and aggressive responses; engage the client in a distracting activity
- Reduce difficult demands; do not insist on remembering useless facts
- Limit choices about food and clothing so that the client has fewer choices to make and reduced chances to get confused

- Control feeding problems some patients exhibit by:
  - feeding all meals in a constant place with no distractions
  - placing food in clear view of the patient
  - placing the eating utensils in the patient's hand
  - getting the patient's attention and modeling eating
  - manually guiding the act of eating (use touch and hand guidance)
  - teaching the client to pace eating (same time between bites)
  - routinely providing the patient's preferred beverage
  - offering finger foods as often as practical and nutritionally appropriate
  - offering plenty of social reinforcers for eating behaviors
- Install sensors under the rug in the house to monitor patient roaming at inappropriate times
- Install complicated locks on doors to prevent the patient from leaving the house and getting lost
- Control the patient's hostility and emotional outbursts by:
  - taking note of conditions under which the patient exhibits such reactions (e.g., the patient becomes angry when the spouse takes over bill payment, financial management, grocery shopping, business activities)
  - modify those conditions to the extent possible (e.g., ask the spouse to pay the bills when the patient is not in sight or take the patient to the store even if only the spouse manages shopping)
- Control the patient's sleep disturbances by:
  - controlling the frequency and duration of daytime naps
  - putting the patient to bed at the same hour every night
  - requiring and encouraging the patient to exercise every day for about 30 minutes

Demonstration

- feeding the patient a light snack an hour before the regular bedtime
- having the patient wear sleep wear that does not disturb the sleep by twisting or binding around the body
- keeping the bedroom quiet by closing the widows and doors
- maintaining a night light to avoid confusion or anxiety in the night when the patient wakes up

- Sustain themselves (especially family members) by:
  - joining support groups for families who have patients with dementia
  - taking breaks from caregiving to renew themselves
  - maintaining certain hobbies and recreational activities
  - recognizing their own need for professional counseling
  - seeking financial support to meet the cost of caring for the individual at home and to be able to take a break from their demanding caregiver duties

Bayles, K. A., & Kaszniak, A. W. (1987). *Communication and cognition in normal aging and dementia.* Austin, TX: Pro-Ed.

Bourgeois, M. S. (1991). Communication treatment for adults with dementia. *Journal of Speech and Hearing Research, 34,* 831–844.

Brookshire, R. H. (1997). *An introduction to neurogenic communication disorders* (5th ed.). St. Louis, MO: Mosby Year Book.

Halpern, H. (2000). *Language and motor disorders in adults* (2nd ed.). Austin, TX: Pro-Ed.

Lubinski, R. (1995). *Dementia and communication.* San Diego: Singular Publishing Group.

Shekim, L. O. (1997). Dementia. In L. L. LaPointe (Ed.), *Aphasia and related neurogenic language disorders* (2nd ed., pp. 238–249). New York: Thieme.

Demonstration. A stimulus procedure used in treatment; usually preceded by instructions on how to produce a target response.

- Describe the target behavior the client is expected to produce

D

- Model the response for the client
- Show how the response is produced (e.g., how /k/ is produced)
- Give maximum feedback (use a mirror if necessary)
- Reinforce the correct response or an approximation of it

Denasality (Hyponasality). Lack of nasal resonance on nasal sounds; a disorder of resonance associated with various voice disorders and cleft palate; see treatment procedures under Voice Disorders and Cleft Palate.

Dependent Variables. Effects of causes studied by scientists; target behaviors taught to clients and pupils; contrasted with Independent Variables.

Deteriorating Baselines. Baselines of a progressively worsening problem; desirable behaviors (e.g., fluency) that are lower each time they are measured; require immediate treatment; an exception to the rule that in a treatment evaluation study, intervention should be started only after baselines are stable.

- Measure baselines repeatedly
- If the desirable behavior shows a consistent worsening (or the undesirable behavior shows a consistent increase) across baseline sessions, initiate treatment immediately

Determinism. A philosophical position that nothing happens without a cause; basis of modern science, whose goal is to explain events by finding their causes.

Developmental Apraxia of Speech (DAS). A speech disorder in children that shares some common characteristics with Apraxia of Speech (AOS) in Adults, but without documented neuropathology; primarily an articulatory (phonologic) disorder characterized by sensorimotor problems in positioning and sequentially moving muscles for the volitional production of speech; associated with prosodic problems; not caused by muscle weakness or neuromuscular slowness; presumed to be a disorder of motor programming for speech; controversial because of the absence of neuro-pathology; little or no controlled treatment efficacy data; most treatment programs are only suggestive.

Motor-Programming Approaches

* Plan on providing intensive treatment to children with DAS
* Use multiple repetitions of speech movements
* Use extensive drill; stress sequence of movements in-volved in speech production
* Determine the need for auditory discrimination training
* Progress hierarchically from easy to difficult tasks
  * determine at what level the child will respond (pho-nemes, syllables, words)
  * concentrate on vowels and consonants that children produce early
  * teach consonants that are visible
  * teach phonemes that occur often
  * teach voiceless consonants before voiced consonants
* Provide multimodality input on sound productions (visual, auditory, kinesthetic, tactile)
* Teach <u>Self-Control (Self-Monitoring) Skills</u>
* Reduce the speech rate if necessary
* Manipulate prosodic features within the treatment pro-gram; use such programs as <u>Contrastive Stress Drills</u>; if necessary increase pause durations between words
* Use techniques of treating <u>Articulation and Phonological Disorders</u>

Hall, P. K., Jordan, L. S., & Robin, D. A. (1993). *Developmental apraxia of speech: Theory and clinical practice.* Austin, TX: Pro-Ed.

Diagnosis.   A clinical activity designed to find causes of dis-eases or disorders, especially in medicine; in communicative disorders, diagnosis often is aimed at describing and assessing the degree of severity of disorders; requires precise and reli-able measurement of communicative behaviors; often means the same as <u>Assessment</u>; see the cited sources and *PGASLP* for details on assessing various disorders of communication.

- Take a case history
- Interview the client
- Screen hearing
- Conduct an orofacial examination
- Administer standardized tests that are culturally and linguistically appropriate for the client
- Design and use client-specific procedures
- Take a comprehensive speech-language sample
- Analyze the results and make a clinical judgment
- Write a diagnostic report that includes recommendations

Shipley, K. G., & McAfee, J. G. (1998). *Assessment in speech-language pathology: A resource manual* (2nd ed.). San Diego: Singular Publishing Group.

Tomblin, J. B., Morris, H. L., & Spriestersbach, D. C. (2000). *Diagnosis in speech-language pathology* (2nd ed.). San Diego: Singular Publishing Group.

Dialect. A spoken form of a language with its own phonologic, semantic, grammatic, and pragmatic properties and rules; any variation of a language; a variation may be considered standard although all variations are acceptable forms of communication; in a bilingual speaker, may be influenced by the primary language; not a basis to diagnose a disorder; see Ethnocultural Variables in Treatment.

Differential Reinforcement. (a) The method of establishing discriminated responding by reinforcing a response in the presence of one stimulus and not reinforcing the same response in the presence of another stimulus; (b) an indirect method of response reduction by increasing another, desirable behavior; specific techniques include Differential Reinforcement of Alternative Behaviors (DRA), Differential Reinforcement of Incompatible Behaviors (DRI), Differential Reinforcement of Low Rates of Behaviors (DRL), and Differential Reinforcement of Other Behaviors (DRO).

Differential Reinforcement of Alternative Behaviors (DRA). One of the Indirect Methods of Response

Reduction in which an undesirable behavior is reduced by reinforcing a specified desirable behavior that serves the same function as the one to be reduced; also known as Functional Equivalence Training.

- Find out what function (purpose) the undesirable behavior to be reduced seems to serve (e.g., fussing in treatment sessions may mean that the child finds the task too difficult and cannot request help)
- Select a behavior that is a desirable alternative to the behavior to be reduced (e.g., the response "help me," if the child could make it, may serve the same function as fussing)
- Reinforce the production of the alternative, desirable response (e.g., teach the child to say "help me" instead of fussing)

Differential Reinforcement of Incompatible Behaviors (DRI).

One of the Indirect Methods of Response Reduction in which an undesirable behavior is reduced by reinforcing a behavior that is incompatible with the behavior targeted for reduction.

- Specify the behavior to be reduced (e.g., leaving the chair and walking in the therapy room)
- Specify a behavior that is incompatible (e.g., sitting quietly and looking at the stimulus items presented)
- Systematically reinforce the child (for sitting quietly and looking at the stimulus items)
- Suspend training on the target communicative skill for a while if necessary and until the sitting behavior is stabilized

Differential Reinforcement of Low Rates of Responding (DRL).

One of the Indirect Methods of Response Reduction in which an undesirable behavior is reduced by reinforcing its progressively lower frequency of occurrence; the method shapes down an undesirable behavior.

- Specify the undesirable behavior to be reduced (e.g., interrupting treatment by irrelevant questions)
- Specify an acceptable level of the undesirable behavior (e.g., two questions in a 10-minute period)
- Reinforce the client for not exceeding the set level ("Good! You asked only two questions during the last 10 minutes!")
- Specify a new, more stringent criterion in successive stages until the behavior is eliminated or kept to a minimum

Differential Reinforcement of Other Behaviors (DRO). One of the Indirect Methods of Response Reduction in which an undesirable behavior is reduced by reinforcing any one of many unspecified behaviors; the behavior that will not receive reinforcement is clearly stated.

- Specify the undesirable behavior to be reduced (e.g., leaving the chair and walking around)
- Tell the client that he or she will not receive reinforcers for that behavior; also say that he or she will receive a reinforcer as long as the undesirable behavior is not exhibited
- Periodically reinforce the child for not exhibiting the undesirable behavior (perhaps for sitting quietly, reading, coloring, working on other assignments, but none specified as the response to be reinforced)

Digital Manipulation. Physical manipulation of the larynx during voice therapy; for the procedure, see Voice Disorders: Specific Normal Voice Facilitating Techniques.

Diplophonia. Double voice resulting from differential vibration of the two vocal folds or vibration of both the true and false vocal folds.

Direct Language Treatment Approaches. Clinician-planned and implemented language treatment with specified target behaviors; structured treatment sessions; requirement that the child first imitate and then spontaneously produce the selected target behaviors; described under Language Disorders in Children; Treatment of Language Disorders: Specific Techniques or Programs.

Direct Methods of Response Reduction.   Procedures to reduce undesirable behaviors by directly placing a contingency on them; contrasted with Indirect Methods of Response Reduction.

- Specify the undesirable behavior to be reduced
- Place one of the following contingencies on it:
  - Corrective Feedback (e.g., say "No")
  - Time-Out (say "Stop," turn your face away for 5 seconds and then reestablish eye contact and resume conversation)
  - Response-Cost (take back a token contingent on every incorrect response)
  - Extinction (ignore the response)
  - Imposition of Work (ask a child who disrupts your stimulus materials to organize them for you)

Direct Stuttering Reduction Strategies.   Treatment techniques that reduce stuttering by placing behavioral contingencies directly on stuttering itself; includes time-out (pause-and-talk) and response cost; see Stuttering.

Direct Treatment for Swallowing Disorders.   Treatment of swallowing disorders by feeding the patient small amounts of food or liquid; see Indirect Treatment for Swallowing Disorders.

Disability.   A person's inability to perform an action that is normally expected of that person; a term so defined in the World Health Organization's International Classification of Impairments, Disabilities, and Handicaps.

Discrete Trials.   Structured treatment or probe trials that are temporally separated providing discretely measured opportunities for producing responses; useful in establishing target skills but not efficient in promoting generalized and maintained production; include Baseline Evoked Trials, Baseline Modeled Trials, Treatment Evoked Trials, and Treatment Modeled Trials; the general structure of a discrete trial includes the following steps:

Discrimination

- Present a physical stimulus to evoke a response (e.g., a picture, an object)
- Ask a question that evokes a response (e.g., "What is this?")
- Model the correct response initially; fade the modeling gradually (e.g., "Johnny, say I see a *rabbit*" on the initial trials and just the question on later trials)
- Reinforce the correct response and give corrective feedback for incorrect responses
- Move the stimulus away from the client
- Record the response as correct, incorrect, absent, and so forth
- Wait for a few seconds to mark the end of a trial
- Represent the stimulus and start a new trial
- Adapt this basic structure to suit the different target behaviors that are taught with discrete trials

Discrimination. A behavioral process of establishing different responses to different stimuli; opposite of generalization; needed to teach such discriminated responding as plural words to plural stimuli and singular words to singular stimuli.

Distinctive Features. Unique characteristics of phonemes that distinguish one phoneme from the other; the system is binary in that a feature is scored as 1 if it is a characteristic of a phoneme and as 0 if it is not; may be used in economically describing errors of articulation and their changes in treatment (see treatment of Articulation and Phonological Disorders: Treatment of Articulation and Phonological Disorders: Specific Techniques or Programs); Chomsky-Halle's major distinctive features include the following:

- **Vocalic:** Sounds produced without a marked constriction of the vocal tract; all vowels and the consonants /l/ and /r/
- **Consonantal:** Sounds produced by vocal tract constriction; all consonants except for /h/, /w/, and /j/
- **High:** Sounds produced with elevated tongue position; include /ʃ/, /ʒ/, /tʃ/, /dʒ/, /k/, /g/, and /ŋ/

- **Back:** Sounds produced with tongue retracted; include /k/, /g/, and /ŋ/
- **Low:** Sounds produced with lowered tongue position; only /h/ in English
- **Anterior:** Sounds produced with point of constriction being relatively anterior; include /w/, /f/, /v/, /θ/, /ð/, /t/, /d/, /s/, /z/, /n/, /l/, /p/, /b/, and /m/
- **Coronal:** Sounds produced with raised tongue blade; include /θ/, /ð/, /t/, /d/, /s/, /z/, /n/, /l/, /r/, /ʃ/, /ʒ/, /tʃ/, and /dʒ/
- **Rounded:** Sounds produced with lips rounded; include only /r/ and /w/
- **Tensed:** Sounds produced with relatively greater muscle tension; include /p/, /t/, /k/, /tʃ/, /dʒ/, /f/, /θ/, /ʃ/, and /l/
- **Voiced:** Sounds produced with vocal fold vibration; all voiced sounds
- **Continuant:** Sounds that can be produced in a continuous manner; include /w/, /f/, /v/, /θ/, /ð/, /s/, /z/, /l/, /ʃ/, /ʒ/, /j/, /r/, and /h/
- **Nasal:** Sounds produced with nasal resonance; include /m/, /n/, and /ŋ/
- **Sonorant:** Sounds produced with unimpeded airstream passing through the oral or nasal cavity; include /w/, /j/, /l/, /r/, /m/,/n/, and /ŋ/
- **Interrupted:** Sounds produced with a complete blockage of the airstream at the point of constriction; include /t/, /d/, /k/, /g/, p/, /b/, /tʃ/, and /dʒ/
- **Strident:** Sounds produced by forcing airstream through a small opening; include /f/, /v/, /s/, /z/, /ʃ/, /ʒ/, /tʃ/, and /dʒ/
- **Lateral:** Sounds produced with the front of the tongue against the alveolar ridge with lateral opening; includes only the /l/

Dysarthria. A group of motor speech disorders resulting from disturbed muscular control of the speech mechanism due to damage of the peripheral or central nervous system;

D

oral communication problems due to weakness, incoordination, or paralysis of speech musculature; classified into types including Ataxic Dysarthria, Flaccid Dysarthria, Hyperkinetic Dysarthria, Hypokinetic Dysarthria, Mixed Dysarthria, Spastic Dysarthria, and Unilateral Upper Motor Neuron Dysarthria; treatment of specific type of dysarthria follows the general guidelines, goals, and procedures.

Treatment of Dysarthria: General Guidelines

- Conduct a thorough assessment of dysarthria and its type; consult the cited sources and *PGASLP.*
- Set the treatment goal as increased efficiency, effectiveness, and naturalness of communication; select goals that are appropriate for the client
- Be fully knowledgeable about medical, surgical, pharmacological, and prosthetic management, their limitations, and how they affect communication training
- Consider the complicating medical condition, associated conditions, and their prognosis in planning treatment
- Finalize the treatment plan only after a thorough discussion with family members
- Consider the client's environment and typical communication partners in planning treatment goals and procedures
- Exploit the client's strengths (e.g., residual physiological support)
- Start management early
- Provide treatment frequently
- Organize sessions to move from easy to difficult tasks
- End sessions with success
- Spend time on activities that focus on improvement of communication
- Increase physiologic support for speech initially
- Use intensive, systematic, and extensive drill
- Use modeling (followed by imitation), shaping, prompting, fading, differential reinforcement, and other proven behavioral management procedures
- Use phonetic placement and its variations

Dysarthria: Treatment Goals

- Provide instruction and demonstration
- Teach self correction, self-evaluation, and self-monitoring skills
- Provide immediate, specific, and social and natural feedback
- Use instrumental feedback or biofeedback when necessary
- Use consistent and variable practice
- Emphasize accuracy initially
- As accuracy is achieved, emphasize rate increase
- Restore lost function to the extent possible
- Teach compensatory behaviors for lost or reduced functions
- Reduce dependence on lost or reduced function
- Increase muscle strength
- Consider not recommending treatment if the motor speech disorder creates no disability or handicap
- Implement alternative or augmentative communication systems, if necessary

  Provide Counseling and Support
  - Teach client to inform the listener at the outset of an interaction how to effectively communicate with him or her (e.g., demonstrating use of an Alphabet Board)
  - Train client to set the context and topic before beginning a conversation
  - Train client to modify content and length of utterances
  - Teach client to monitor listener comprehension
  - Teach significant others to modify physical environment, be active listeners, and maximize their own hearing and visual acuity
  - Teach client and significant others to maintain eye contact, establish effective communication strategies, and determine methods of feedback

General Treatment Goals for Clients With Dysarthria
  - Modification of respiration
  - Modification of phonation
  - Modification of resonance

195

Dysarthria: General Treatment

- Modification of articulation
- Modification of prosody

General Treatment Procedures. Because of the variability of dysarthria, its subclassifications, and varied neuropathology, select a particular treatment target and strategy only when a careful assessment of the client's clinical problems justifies it; some techniques produce temporary effects; others are contraindicated for certain clients; many are suggested based on clinical experience and lack controlled experimental evidence to support their routine use; continue to use a technique only when it produces a clear and positive effect on the client's behavior; abandon ineffective procedures and modify those that seem to hold promise.

Modification of Respiration

- Train consistent production of subglottal air pressure; use manometer or air pressure transducer
- Train maximum vowel prolongation
- Shape production of longer phrases and sentences
- Teach controlled exhalation
- Teach sustained exhalation throughout utterances
- Teach pausing and breathing at appropriate junctures in speech
- Teach client to push, pull, or bear down during speech or nonspeech tasks
- Use manual push on abdomen
- Find a normal or an unusual posture that promotes respiratory support and teach it (e.g., some clients' speech improves in supine position)
- Let the client use neck and trunk braces if helpful
- Use adjustable beds and wheelchairs to make postural adjustments
- Use girdles and wraps around the abdominal area to increase muscle strength for respiration
- Use an Expiratory Board to stabilize the abdominal muscles for respiration

Dysarthria: General Treatment

- Teach the client to inhale more deeply and exhale slowly and with greater force during speech
- Train the client to terminate speech earlier during exhalation

Modification of Phonation

- Discuss with medical staff the need, effects, and effectiveness of medical treatments including Laryngoplasty, Teflon or Collagen Injection, Recurrent Laryngeal Nerve Resection, Botulinum Toxin Injection, and pharmacological measures; consider them in the total management of the client and in treating communication disorders
- Use biofeedback devices to give the client immediate feedback on vocal intensity to effect changes in excessive or too little loudness
- Train the client with a too soft voice in using a portable amplification system
- Train aphonic clients in the use of Artificial Larynx
- Ask clients with aberrant neck movements or neck muscle weakness to wear Neck Braces
- Teach Effortful Closure Techniques for clients with vocal fold paralysis (e.g., pulling or pushing while phonating)
- Teach the client to initiate phonation at beginning of exhalation
- Teach the client to turn head toward weak side during speech; try digital manipulation of the thyroid cartilage to increase loudness; be aware of temporary effects of these
- Try relaxation exercises and laryngeal massage to increase loudness
- Teach the client to tilt head back, initiate speech after a deep inhalation, and increase pitch to reduce strained voice quality
- Teach the client with vocal fold hyperadduction to initiate phonation with breathy onset or a sigh

Dysarthria: General Treatment

Modification of Resonance

- Discuss with medical staff the need, effects, and effectiveness of medical treatments including pharyngeal flap surgery, Teflon injection into the posterior pharyngeal wall, and palatal lift prosthesis to treat velopharyngeal incompetence
- Provide feedback on nasal airflow and hypernasality by using a mirror, nasal flow transducer, or a Nasendoscope
- Train the client to open the mouth wider to increase oral resonance and vocal intensity
- Use nasal obturator or nose clip; have the client speak in the supine position; be aware of temporary improvement.

Modification of Articulation

- Discuss with medical staff the need, effects, and effectiveness of medical treatments including Neural Anastomosis, botulinum toxin (Botox) injection to orofacial or mandibular muscles to decrease abnormal movements, and pharmacological treatment in relation to communication training.
- Analyze the error patterns and their potential reasons before developing a treatment program
- Encourage the client to assume the best posture for good articulation
- Use bite block to improve jaw control and strength
- Use behavioral methods to treat articulation disorders with clients for whom articulatory modification is a main target
  - provide instructions and demonstrations
  - simplify the task, use shaping
  - model frequently
  - use phonetic placement techniques
  - reduce speech rate to improve intelligibility
  - ask the client to exaggerate the production of medial and final consonants
  - give immediate feedback

- use minimal contrast pairs (e.g., *peet-beet; stop-top*)
- teach self-monitoring skills
- modify techniques in light of data
- move from simpler level of training to more complex levels

- Experiment with such stretching exercises as sustained jaw opening and maximum tongue protrusion to see if they help improve articulation
- Use electromyographic biofeedback to reduce hypertonicity and spasm of speech muscles
- Teach compensatory articulatory movements (e.g., use of tongue blade to make sounds normally made with tongue tip)
- Use of meaningful stimuli when possible
- Use intelligibility drills
  - ask the client to read texts or describe pictures you are not familiar with
  - retell what you hear
  - let the client work on improving his or her articulation to promote better understanding on your part

To Improve Speech Rate

- Use such prosthetic devices as <u>Delayed Auditory Feedback (DAF),</u> a <u>Pacing Board,</u> an <u>Alphabet Board,</u> or a metronome
- Use hand or finger tapping
- Provide visual feedback from computer or storage oscilloscope
- Use rhythmic or metered cueing; clinician points to words in a passage in rhythmic or metered fashion
- Modify pauses in speech

Modification of Prosody

- Reduce the speech rate
  - use <u>Delayed Auditory Feedback</u>
  - use computer programs that generate cursor movements to pace the rate of speech

D

- experiment with hand or finger tapping; be aware that some clients accelerate their tapping and the speech rate
  - use a Pacing Board to reduce the rate
  - use Alphabet Board Supplementation (ask the client to point to the first letter of each word to be spoken on an alphabet board)
  - use instructions, modeling, shaping, and differential reinforcement to slow the rate
- Modify pitch with the help of instruction, modeling, differential feedback, or with the help of such instruments as VisiPitch; be aware that direct work on pitch modification may not be needed in many cases because of successful modification of rate, intonation, and stress
- Shape louder speech through behavioral methods of modeling, shaping, and differential reinforcement of greater inhalation, increased laryngeal adduction, and wider mouth opening
- Teach the client to chunk utterances into natural syntactic units to promote more natural sounding speech
- Increase breath control to extend breath groups
- Use Contrastive Stress Tasks (sentences with the same words that change meaning when different words are stressed)
- Teach the client to signal stress by using other means (e.g., prolongation of syllables or pausing before a stressed word)
- Teach the client to vary the number of words per breath group
- Begin treatment with structured tasks and make transition to conversational speech
- Teach the client to self-monitor

Duffy, J. R. (1995). *Motor speech disorders.* St. Louis, MO: C. V. Mosby.

Freed, D. (2000). *Motor speech disorders: Diagnosis and treatment.* San Diego: Singular Publishing Group.

Dysarthria: Ataxic

Halpern, H. (2000). *Language and motor speech disorders in adults.* Austin, TX: Pro-Ed.

Johns, D. F. (Ed.). (1985). *Clinical management of neurogenic communicative disorders.* Boston: Little, Brown.

Yorkston, K. M., Beukelman, D. R., Strand, E. A., & Bell, K. R. (1999). *Management of motor speech disorders in children and adults.* Austin, TX: Pro-Ed.

D

Treatment of Dysarthria: Specific Types.   In planning treatment for a client with dysarthria, consider first the general guidelines and procedures described in the previous section along with those that follow for specific types. If a definitive diagnosis of a particular type is not made, carefully evaluate the communicative deficits and design a treatment program to remediate or modify targeted deficits.

Ataxic Dysarthria.   A type of motor speech disorder; its neuropathology is damage to the cerebellar system; characterized by slow, inaccurate movement and <u>Hypotonia;</u> all aspects of speech may be involved, but articulatory and prosodic problems dominate; specific symptoms include imprecise consonants, excess and equal linguistic stress, and irregular articulatory breakdowns; select appropriate treatment targets and procedures described under <u>Dysarthria;</u> in addition, consider the following that apply especially to ataxic dysarthria:

- Use behavioral methods of <u>Shaping</u> and <u>Differential Reinforcement</u> to improve control and coordination
- Do not concentrate on increasing muscle strength or reducing muscle tone
- Do not recommend prosthetic or surgical methods to improve phonation or resonance
- Modify respiratory problems associated with speech production:
  - teach the client to inhale more deeply and exhale in a slow and controlled manner to sustain speech

- measure the duration of exhalation and reinforce progressively longer (more controlled) exhalation
- teach the client to begin speaking soon after the start of exhalation to avoid wasting airflow; reinforce prompt phonation upon initiation of exhalation
- teach the client to end an utterance well before running out of air; stop the client when signs of airflow dissipation are evident, and ask the client to breathe in again
- teach the client to stop and inhale at natural junctures in a sentences (e.g., at the beginning of a grammatical clause)

- Modify prosodic problems that result mostly from irregular, slow, or even rapid rate of speech:
  - slow the rate of speech with the help of metronome beats
  - use finger or hand tapping to generate an even and appropriate rate of speech
  - provide such cues as pointing to a printed word to generate an appropriate and even oral reading rate
  - teach appropriate stress on words in sentences; use contrastive stress exercises
  - teach variations in pitch by using both printed sentences and conversational speech
  - control excess loudness variation by reinforcing normal variations

- Modify articulation problems that may persist even at slower rate of speech:
  - ask the client to produce words on a list while you judge their intelligibility while not looking at the list or the client's face
  - give corrective feedback to encourage appropriate production of sounds in words you do not understand

- teach correct production of sounds by using the Phonetic Placement Method
- reinforce overarticulation or exaggerated articulation of medial and final consonants
- use the Minimal Contrast Method, to improve intelligibility of words that differ by only one phoneme
- Reinforce more natural sounding conversational speech
- Implement a Maintenance Strategy to train family members and other caregivers who will help sustain treatment gains

Duffy, J. R. (1995). *Motor speech disorders.* St. Louis, MO: C. V. Mosby.

Freed, D. (2000). *Motor speech disorders: Diagnosis and treatment.* San Diego: Singular Publishing Group.

Halpern, H. (2000). *Language and motor speech disorders in adults.* Austin, TX: Pro-Ed.

Johns, D. F. (Ed.). (1985). *Clinical management of neurogenic communicative disorders.* Boston: Little, Brown.

Yorkston, K. M., Beukelman, D. R., Strand, E. A., & Bell, K. R. (1999). *Management of motor speech disorders dysarthric speakers.* Austin, TX: Pro-Ed.

Flaccid Dysarthria. A type of motor speech disorder; its neuropathology is damage to the motor units of cranial or spinal nerves that supply speech muscles (lower motor neuron involvement); flaccidity (hypotonia) and weak muscle contractions are dominant neurological symptoms; speech problems caused mostly by muscle weakness and Hypotonia; constellation of speech disorders dependent on the specific nerve or nerves that are affected, but include breathy and harsh voice quality, hypernasality, nasal emission, imprecise production of consonants, audible inspiration, monopitch and loudness, and short phrases; select appropriate treatment targets and procedures described under

<u>Dysarthria;</u> in addition, consider the following that apply especially to flaccid dysarthria:

- Make a thorough assessment of dysarthria and the associated neurological and physical conditions the client presents; consult the sources cited and the *PGASLP*
- Improve muscle strength and range of motion. Note that exercises to strengthen speech-related muscles are controversial; some recommend it whereas others consider it a waste of time because speech requires only a small amount of muscular force; may be recommended for clients with severe dysarthria; exercises that involve muscle movement (*isotonic* exercise) may be more beneficial than those that ask the client to exert force against stationary resistance (*isometric* exercise). Also, muscle strengthening work that involves speech production may be more effective than those that do not involve speech production. Nonetheless, various suggestions to strengthen muscles and their range of motion include the following:
  - try to increase muscle strength by asking the client to increase effort while speaking; may be sufficient in some cases
  - strengthen the jaw muscles by asking the client to several times open and close the jaw as fully as possible; manually push the jaw upward while the client tries to open it or hold the chin down while the client tries to close the jaw; these may be beneficial in the case of flaccid dysarthria caused by damage to trigeminal cranial nerve V
  - strengthen lip muscles by asking the client to resist as you pull a string attached to a button placed behind the client's closed lips and against the central incisors; ask the client to pucker the lips firmly and hold it for several seconds; ask the client to smile widely and hold it for several seconds; these

may be beneficial in the case of flaccid dysarthria caused by damage to facial cranial nerve VII

- increase overall muscle tone by asking the client to push down on the arms of a chair
- increase tongue strength (perhaps the most controversial of all muscle strengthening exercises) by having the client (a) push the tongue out; (b) push the tongue to one or the other side; (c) lift the tongue tip; and (d) lift the back of the tongue as you apply resistance with a tongue blade to oppose the client's effort in each case; may be beneficial in case of flaccid dysarthria caused by damage to hypoglossal cranial nerve XII

- Modify respiratory behaviors
  - use pushing/pulling exercises to increase respiratory support
  - make postural adjustments by asking the client to sit straight in the chair to increase breath support for speech
  - place a padded lap tray on the wheelchair, positioned next to the abdomen and ask the client to lean against it to increase breath support
  - teach the client to phonate at the beginning of exhalation to conserve air supply for speech
  - teach the client to inhale deeply and exhale in a controlled manner
  - increase breath group durations
  - increase the number of words per breath group
- Modify phonatory problems
  - increase loudness by modeling louder speech and reinforcing increase in client's vocal loudness; use computer programs to give feedback on loudness
  - consider Teflon/collagen injections to improve vocal fold adduction
  - teach pushing and pulling while speaking to promote better approximation of vocal folds

D

- ask the client to inhale deeply and hold the breath to promote firmer approximation of folds
- ask the client with a unilateral vocal fold weakness or paralysis to turn head toward the *affected* side or manually push the larynx toward the *unaffected* side to help achieve better closure

- Modify resonance problems
  - note that hypernasality is the main resonance problem caused by damage to the pharyngeal branch of the vagus nerve; the soft palate may be weak or paralyzed
  - discuss the suitability of the <u>Pharyngeal Flap Operation</u> with a surgeon to improve velopharyngeal closure; note that the results have been inconsistent
  - discuss the suitability of <u>Pharyngoplasty</u> with a surgeon to improve velopharyngeal closure; note that the results have been inconsistent
  - recommend <u>Palatal Lift Prosthesis,</u> as this has been more effective in reducing hypernasality than pharyngeal flap or pharyngoplasty; note that this device is most effective with clients who (a) are severely hypernasal and have not improved with behavioral treatment; (b) do not have spastic velopharyngeal mechanism which may dislodge the device; (c) have teeth for anchoring the device; (d) have good articulation and phonation without which the device will not improve speech intelligibility; (e) do not have hyperactive gag reflex or swallowing problems; and (f) are motivated to wear it and care for it
  - use behavioral methods if hypernasality is mild; shape progressively less hypernasal voice by modeling and positive reinforcement and corrective feedback

Dysarthria: Flaccid

- Modify articulatory problems
  - reduce the rate of speech to improve speech intelligibility (and to some extent, hypernasality); use finger tapping to cue a slower rate by having the client produce a syllable or a word per a tap; give frequent instructions to slow down and reinforce the desired rate
  - teach better articulatory skills by reinforcing improved articulation of speech sounds; use a systematic approach of modeling and reinforcing correct articulation in words, phrases, sentences, and conversational speech
  - if preferred, use the Intelligibility Drills in which the client reads aloud a list of words when the clinician has turned his or her back; when the clinician does not understand a word , he or she will turn around to face the client, analyze the errors, give suggestions on correct productions, and reinforce correct productions
  - use Phonetic Placement Method to teach correct placement of articulators in producing target sounds
  - teach exaggerated production of consonants to improve speech intelligibility; ask the client to fully articulate consonants, especially in medial and final positions of words
  - use the Minimal Contrast Method to further improve articulation
- Modify prosodic problems
  - note that pitch, stress, and rhythm deviations contribute to an abnormal prosody in clients with flaccid dysarthria
  - ask the client to discriminate pitch changes as you model different levels of pitch
  - ask the client to prolong an /a/ with lower and higher pitch

D

- have the client read printed sentences that indicate higher and lower pitch (arrows above and below words)
- model different and appropriate pitch levels in phrases and sentences and have the client imitate them
- monitor pitch in conversational speech and reinforce or give corrective feedback
- use Contrastive Stress Drills
- teach the client to chunk utterances into syntactic units; reinforce pauses (and inhale if necessary) at appropriate junctures in sentences

Duffy, J. R. (1995). *Motor speech disorders.* St. Louis, MO: C. V. Mosby.

Freed, D. (2000). *Motor speech disorders: Diagnosis and treatment.* San Diego: Singular Publishing Group.

Halpern, H. (2000). *Language and motor speech disorders in adults.* Austin, TX: Pro-Ed.

Johns, D. F. (Ed.). (1985). *Clinical management of neurogenic communicative disorders.* Boston: Little, Brown.

Yorkston, K. M., Beukelman, D. R., Strand, E. A., & Bell, K. R. (1999). *Management of motor speech disorders in children and adults.* Austin, TX: Pro-Ed.

Hyperkinetic Dysarthria. A type of motor speech disorder; its neuropathology is damage to basal ganglia (extrapyramidal system), resulting in rapid involuntary movements and variable muscle tone; may affect all aspects of speech, but a dominant symptom is prosodic disturbances; specific problems include prolonged intervals, variable rate, monopitch, loudness variations, inappropriate silences, imprecise consonants, and distorted vowels; most effective treatment is medical; various medications help control involuntary movements; for communication treatment, select appropriate treatment targets and procedures described under Dysarthria; in addition, consider the following that apply especially to hyperkinetic dysarthria:

- Make a thorough assessment of dysarthria and its specific symptoms that justify the diagnosis of the hyperkinetic variety; consult the cited sources and the *PGASLP*
- Be aware of the medications that control involuntary movements
  - haloperidol controls chorea and tics
  - clonazepam and valproic acid control myoclonic jerks
  - Botox injections control dystonia (more effective than other drugs listed in treating clients with hyperkinetic dysarthria)
  - note that medical treatment does not always eliminate the need for behavioral management of dysarthria
- Use a Bite Block (a small plastic cube the client bites down on) to inhibit or reduce interfering jaw movements during speech in clients with mandibular Dystonia
- Teach onset of speech, as this can help reduce involuntary movements that disrupt laryngeal movements especially in clients with mild hyperkinetic dysarthria
- Teach slower rate and increased vocal pitch when appropriate
- Try relaxation therapy to control involuntary movements
- Try habit reversal in which the client is taught competing voluntary behaviors to control involuntary behaviors (e.g., asking the client to blink slowly before the tics occur)

Duffy, J. R. (1995). *Motor speech disorders*. St. Louis, MO: C. V. Mosby.

Freed, D. (2000). *Motor speech disorders: Diagnosis and treatment*. San Diego: Singular Publishing Group.

Halpern, H. (2000). *Language and motor speech disorders in adults*. Austin, TX: Pro-Ed.

Johns, D. F. (Ed.). (1985). *Clinical management of neurogenic communicative disorders*. Boston: Little, Brown.

Yorkston, K. M., Beukelman, D. R., Strand, E. A., & Bell, K. R. (1999). *Management of motor speech disorders in children and adults*. Austin, TX: Pro-Ed.

Hypokinetic Dysarthria. A type of motor speech disorder; its neuropathology is damage to basal ganglia (extrapyramidal system) resulting in slow movement, limited range of movement, and rigidity; parkinsonism is the most frequent cause of this type of dysarthria; may affect all aspects of speech, but especially voice, articulation, and prosody; specific problems include monopitch, monoloudness, reduced stress, imprecise consonants, variable rate of speech, increased speech rate in some cases and a slower rate in a few, short rushes of speech, inappropriate silences, and harsh and breathy voice. Select appropriate treatment targets and procedures described under <u>Treatment of Dysarthria;</u> in addition, consider the following that apply especially to hypokinetic dysarthria:

- Make a thorough assessment of dysarthria and the symptom complex that justifies the diagnosis of hypokinetic dysarthria; consult the cited sources and *PGASLP*
- Modify respiratory behaviors by teaching the client to:
  - inhale deeply before speaking
  - start speaking when inhalation begins
  - exhale slowly and in a controlled manner
  - stop talking well before exhausting the air supply
  - gradually increase the number of words spoken per breath
- Modify phonatory problems
  - use voice therapy techniques to increase vocal loudness and to decrease breathiness; use various biofeedback instruments (e.g., the <u>VisiPitch</u>)

- use pushing and pulling techniques to increase the movement range of laryngeal muscles (e.g., having the client push down on the arm of the chair while phonating)
- use portable voice amplifiers to increase loudness
- Modify articulatory problems
  - use rate-control for clients who speak rapidly; use hand or finger tapping to cue-in production of syllables or words; use delayed auditory feedback to slow down the rate; use a metronome to have the client pace syllable or word productions; use a Pacing Board or an Alphabet Board if necessary
  - use Intelligibility Drills in which the client reads aloud printed words; judge the accuracy solely on the basis of phonatory cues and give corrective feedback or positive reinforcement
  - teach correct articulation by Phonetic Placement Method which shows correct placement of articulators for producing target sounds
  - improve speech intelligibility by asking the client to produce word-medial and final consonants with a certain degree of exaggeration
  - use the Minimal Contrast Method in which the client is taught to produce clearly pairs of words that differ by only one phoneme (e.g., *pat-bat*)
- Modify prosodic problems
  - note that a slower rate can improve the client's prosody
  - teach proper intonation through printed sentences that show rising and falling pitch by arrows
  - use Contrastive Stress Drills
  - teach appropriate chunking of words according to syntactic units (e.g., pausing at the end of a grammatic clause and a sentence)

Duffy, J. R. (1995). *Motor speech disorders.* St. Louis, MO: C. V. Mosby.

Freed, D. (2000). *Motor speech disorders: Diagnosis and treatment.* San Diego: Singular Publishing Group.

Halpern, H. (2000). *Language and motor speech disorders in adults.* Austin, TX: Pro-Ed.

Johns, D. F. (Ed.). (1985). *Clinical management of neurogenic communicative disorders.* Boston: Little, Brown.

Yorkston, K. M., Beukelman, D. R., Strand, E. A., & Bell, K. R. (1999). *Management of motor speech disorders in children and adults.* Austin, TX: Pro-Ed.

Mixed Dysarthria. A type of motor speech disorder that is a combination of two or more pure dysarthrias; the neuropathology is varied depending on the types of dysarthrias that are mixed; frequent causes include multiple strokes or multiple neurological diseases; speech disorders are varied and dependent on the types of pure dysarthrias that are mixed; select appropriate treatment targets and procedures described under Treatment of Dysarthria; in addition, consider the following that apply especially to mixed dysarthrias:

- Make a thorough assessment of the client's symptom complex of mixed dysarthria; consult the cited sources and the *PGASLP*
- Identify the dominant type, if any, and describe the major speech problems
- Select speech targets that when treated will immediately improve communication
- Treat those targets like you would in the case of pure dysarthrias
- Note that some clinicians recommend that problems of respiration, resonation, phonation, articulation, and prosody, if all present, be treated in that order
- Treat the most severe problem first if multiple problems exist in a single category (e.g., prosody); find out the client's preference to determine which problems should be addressed first in treatment
- Recommend Augmentative Communication devices for clients who need them; note that clients whose

mixed dysarthria is due to Amyotrophic Lateral Sclerosis (ASL) are likely candidates for augmentative communication.

Duffy, J. R. (1995). *Motor speech disorders.* St. Louis, MO: C. V. Mosby.

Freed, D. (2000). *Motor speech disorders: Diagnosis and treatment.* San Diego: Singular Publishing Group.

Halpern, H. (2000). *Language and motor speech disorders in adults.* Austin, TX: Pro-Ed.

Johns, D. F. (Ed.). (1985). *Clinical management of neurogenic communicative disorders.* Boston: Little, Brown.

Yorkston, K. M., Beukelman, D. R., Strand, E. A., & Bell, K. R. (1999). *Management of motor speech disorders in children and adults.* Austin, TX: Pro-Ed.

Spastic Dysarthria. A type of motor speech disorder caused by bilateral damage to the upper motor neuron (direct and indirect motor pathways) resulting in weakness, spastic paralysis, limited range of movement, and slowness of movement; may affect all aspects of speech; major speech problems include imprecisely produced consonants, monopitch, monoloudness, reduced stress, hypernasality, slow rate, strained-strangled-harsh voice, pitch breaks, and breathy voice; select appropriate treatment targets and procedures described under Treatment of Dysarthria; in addition, consider the following that apply especially to spastic dysarthria:

- Make a thorough assessment of dysarthria and the total symptom complex; make a differential diagnosis of spastic dysarthria; consult the cited sources and *PGASLP*

- Consult with the client's physician about medically controlling pathological crying, which might interfere with treatment

- Consider behaviorally modifying crying in treatment sessions by reinforcing noncrying (alternative) behaviors

D

- Do not teach pushing or pulling exercises that only aggravate hyperadduction
- Use relaxation and stretching exercises with caution because their effects on speech have not been documented
- Note that modification of respiratory behaviors is typically not a major concern in clients with spastic dysarthria; any apparent respiratory problems may be due largely to such phonatory problems as hyperadduction of vocal folds
- Modify phonatory problems
  - note that efforts to reduce hyperadduction of vocal folds have not been especially successful; nonetheless, these efforts may be made with caution
  - teach the client head and neck relaxation by instruction, modeling, and manual guidance; stand behind the client, take the client's head between the two hands, and gently tilt it back, move it forward, and to the sides; ask the client to move the head in the same manner without manual guidance
  - teach easy onset of phonation to a client who has learned to relax the neck and head muscles; model soft glottal closure and ask the client to imitate it; begin with an exhaled sigh and add a prolonged /a/; shape this relaxed production of /a/ into words, phrases, sentences, and spontaneous speech
  - teach the yawn-sigh motion before starting a gentle phonation; ask the client to inhale through open mouth, exhale, and begin phonation; shape the phonated speech into words, phrases, sentences, and spontaneous speech
- Modify resonance problems
  - increase vocal loudness to control the extent of hypernasality, as louder speech tends to be perceived less nasal

- discuss the usefulness of <u>Pharyngeal Flap Operation</u> with the client's physician or a <u>Palatal Lift Prosthesis</u> with a prosthodontist

D

- Modify articulatory problems
  - note that the effects of tongue and lip stretching exercises that some clinicians recommend have not been documented in controlled studies
  - use discretion in using such stretching exercises as gently pulling a client's lip or tongue out by holding it with a gauze pad; if used, carefully document the effects of such procedures and abandon them if data are negative
  - note that traditional articulation treatment may be more effective than stretching exercises; use <u>Intelligibility Drills</u> in which the client reads a list of words and the clinician judges the accuracy of production solely on the basis of phonetic cues and gives appropriate feedback on correct and incorrect productions
  - use <u>Phonetic Placement Method</u> to teach correct placement of articulators; show articulatory placements in a mirror if necessary; model and reinforce imitated and eventually evoked productions of target words, phrases, and sentences
  - teach the client to produce the medial and final consonants in words in an exaggerated manner
  - use <u>Minimal Contrast Drills</u> in which pairs of words that differ by only one phoneme are used to teach correct productions of target sounds
- Modify prosodic problems
  - ask the client to vary pitch on a prolonged vowel production (e.g., /a/); if necessary, model pitch variations as you prolong the target vowel; reinforce correct imitations; fade modeling and ask the client to vary his or her pitch

D

- teach the client to vary intonation in sentences; use printed sentences that indicate rising or falling intonation by arrows; model if necessary and fade modeling as the client becomes more successful in imitating suggested patterns of intonation; move on to conversational speech in which varied intonation is reinforced
- use Contrastive Stress Drills to place stress on different words in questions and answers; model stress on specific words in questions and sentences and ask the client to imitate; fade modeling; teach appropriate stress patterns in conversational speech
- teach the client to chunk utterances into syntactic units by modeling and reinforcing pauses at appropriate junctures in speech (e.g., at the end of grammatic clauses and sentences); ask the client to inhale at such junctures

Duffy, J. R. (1995). *Motor speech disorders.* St. Louis, MO: C. V. Mosby.

Freed, D. (2000). *Motor speech disorders: Diagnosis and treatment.* San Diego: Singular Publishing Group.

Halpern, H. (2000). *Language and motor speech disorders in adults.* Austin, TX: Pro-Ed.

Johns, D. F. (Ed.). (1985). *Clinical management of neurogenic communicative disorders.* Boston: Little, Brown.

Yorkston, K. M., Beukelman, D. R., Strand, E. A., & Bell, K. R. (1999). *Management of motor speech disorders in children and adults.* Austin, TX: Pro-Ed.

Unilateral Upper Motor Neuron Dysarthria. A type of motor speech disorder caused by damage to the upper motor neurons that supply cranial and spinal nerves involved in speech production; primarily a disorder of articulation in which the dominant speech problem is imprecise production of consonants; less significant speech symptoms include harsh voice quality, slow, imprecise, or irregular Alternating Motion Rates; generally slow rate of speech with increased rate in segments; mild hypernasality; excess and equal stress; select appropriate treatment targets and procedures described under Treatment of Dysarthria; in addition, consider the following that apply especially to unilateral upper motor neuron dysarthria:

- Make a thorough assessment of dysarthria and the specific symptom complex that justifies a differential diagnosis of unilateral upper motor neuron dysarthria; consult the cited sources and *PGASLP*
- Note that, in some cases, associated language deficits (aphasia) and apraxia may take treatment priority; dysarthria may or may not be treated, although it is recommended that it be treated
- Modify articulatory problems
  - use traditional methods to treat articulation disorders
  - use Intelligibility Drills in which the client reads a list of words and the clinician judges the accuracy of production solely on the basis of phonetic cues and gives appropriate feedback on correct and incorrect productions
  - use Phonetic Placement Method to teach correct placement of articulators; show articulatory placements in a mirror if necessary; model and reinforce imitated and eventually evoked productions of target words, phrases, and sentences
  - teach the client to produce the medial and final consonants in words in an exaggerated manner
  - use Minimal Contrast Drills in which pairs of words that differ by only one phoneme are used to teach correct productions of target sounds

Duffy, J. R. (1995). *Motor speech disorders.* St. Louis, MO: C. V. Mosby.

Freed, D. (2000). *Motor speech disorders: Diagnosis and treatment.* San Diego: Singular Publishing Group.

Halpern, H. (2000). *Language and motor speech disorders in adults.* Austin, TX: Pro-Ed.

Johns, D. F. (Ed.). (1985). *Clinical management of neurogenic communicative disorders.* Boston: Little, Brown.

Yorkston, K. M., Beukelman, D. R., Strand, E. A., & Bell, K. R. (1999). *Management of motor speech disorders in children and adults.* Austin, TX: Pro-Ed.

Dysfluencies.   Behaviors that interrupt fluency; measured in diagnosing Stuttering; specific forms include repetitions of sounds, syllables, words, and phrases; prolongations of sounds and articulatory postures; inter- and intralexical pauses; interjections of syllables, words, and phrases; revisions; and incomplete phrases; see *PGASLP* for examples and assessment procedures.

Dysphagia.   Disorders of swallowing, also known as disorders of deglutition; associated with many medical conditions including neuromuscular disorders and cancer of the larynx and the surgical removal of structures involved in swallowing; may occur at any age although more common in the elderly.

Disorders of Mastication.   Problems in chewing food; may be due to reduced range of movement by the tongue and the mandible, reduced buccal tension, and poor alignment of mandible and maxilla.

Disorders of the Preparatory Phase of the Swallow.   Problems in collecting the masticated food to form a bolus as a preparation for swallow; may be due to problems in labial closure, tongue movement and coordination, appropriate holding of the bolus in the mouth (e.g., holding it in the front of the mouth), and reduced oral sensitivity.

Disorders of the Oral Phase of the Swallow.   Problems in the tongue movement to initiate the voluntary aspect of the swallow and in passing the food over the base of the tongue; by the end of the phase, the bolus will have reached the faucial arch area; problems due to tongue thrust, reduced tongue tension and movement, and reduced buccal tension.

Disorders of the Pharyngeal Stage of the Swallow. Problems in propelling the bolus through the pharynx and into the P-E segment; may be due to delayed or absent swallowing reflex, inadequate velopharyngeal closure, reduced pharyngeal Peristalsis, pharyngeal paralysis, laryngeal movement disorders, and so forth.

Disorders of the Esophageal Phase of the Swallow. Problems in passing the bolus through the cricopharyngeus muscle and past the 7th cervical vertebra; due to many muscular and other problems including weak cricopharyngeus, esophageal Peristalsis, and esophageal obstruction (e.g., by a tumor).

Treatment of Dysphagia. Management of swallowing problems by a variety of medical and nonmedical procedures; speech-language pathologists may implement most of the nonmedical procedures.

General Guidelines

- Make a thorough assessment and diagnosis of the swallowing disorders of the client; consult the cited sources and the *PGASLP*
- Consider the following factors in deciding whether to treat and with what procedures:
  - diagnosis of the swallowing disorder and related medical condition of the client; if the disorder is likely to be cleared within a week or two, do not initiate an exercise program; teach a few compensatory strategies; if the patient has significant motor neuron disease, do not initiate range-of-motion exercises that may only tire the client; if the patient cannot follow directions because of dementia, do not select procedures that require the client to comprehend instructions

- prognosis for swallowing therapy is good for patients who have had strokes, traumatic brain injury, gun shot wounds, radiation therapy for neck and head cancer; hence, swallowing therapy is recommended; prognosis is not favorable for patients whose degenerative neurological disease has advanced to a stage where therapy is ineffective
- success in food intake with compensatory strategies suggests that an exercise program may not be needed
- very severe dysphagia exhibited during assessment suggests that the patient needs indirect therapy; exercises to increase muscle movements and their range in the absence of food in the mouth may be necessary
- poor respiratory function indicates a need to postpone certain therapy procedures until this function is improved
- caregiver support to help complete prescribed exercises at home; caregivers should be available and willing to remind the client to perform the exercises and supervise them when necessary
- patient's motivation and interest, without which no treatment program will work

- Discuss with the client and the family the swallowing process and the treatment procedure to be implemented
- Give written instructions to the patient and describe the steps to be followed
- Ask the patient to first practice swallow (without solid or liquid food)
- Note that patients are likely to reject or eat only a small amount of a variety of food if its bolus takes more than 10 seconds for pharyngeal and oral transit; such patients need to use at least a supplemental nonoral feeding program to sustain themselves

- Note that patients who aspirate 10% of each bolus and are aware of it will reject food that causes it
- Introduce only a small amount of food during direct treatment
- Show the client the amount of be swallowed
- Instruct the patient to cough to clear the airway and reinforce the client's coughs
- Initiate indirect treatment if the patient aspirates 10% of each bolus and the direct methods do not progressively reduce aspirations (intake of food into lungs); be aware that only radiographic data show aspiration
- Concentrate on increasing muscle control during indirect treatment
- Reduce distraction during treatment

Compensatory Treatment. Procedures that promote swallowing without modifying the physiological status of the patient; mostly clinician- or caregiver-managed; requires little or no patient effort and thus does not tire the patient; includes a variety of procedures.

- *Modification of patient's posture:* Use postural modification until swallowing improves or direct treatment may be initiated; instruct the patient to assume a posture that promotes better swallow and reduces or eliminates aspiration
  - the *chin-down posture* that widens the vallecullae; teach the client to tuck the chin to the chest during swallow while maintaining a straight cervical spine; recommended for patients with delayed triggering of the pharyngeal swallow; may be effective with patients who have reduced posterior motion of the tongue base; patients with inadequate laryngeal elevation, poor vocal fold closure, and absent cough reflex may not benefit from chin tuck
  - the *chin-up posture* that helps drain food from the oral cavity because of gravity; teach the patient to

D

tilt the head back by extending the neck by leaning the head back; most effective with patients in whom the oral transit of the bolus to the pharynx is difficult; not recommended for patients with neurogenic dysphagia

- *head rotation toward the weaker side* that helps direct food to a more efficient side of the pharynx; teach the patient to rotate the head during swallow toward the damaged, weaker, or hemiparetic side of the pharynx, which then gets narrowed; recommended for patients with unilateral laryngeal dysfunction resulting in aspiration

- *combined chin-down and head rotation* may reduce aspiration in some patients with inadequate laryngeal closure; teach this if a trial application supports this combination

- *head tilt to the stronger side,* which directs food to that side; teach this strategy to patients with unilateral oral and pharyngeal weakness; the patient may need consistent cues to do this

- *lying down on one side,* which helps control diffuse residue in the pharynx; teach this to patients in whom pharyngeal wall constrictions are bilaterally reduced, causing aspiration after the swallow; after eating lying down and before sitting up, teach the client to cough to clear the traces of food in the pharynx

- *Increased oral sensory awareness:* Procedures that enhance oral sensory awareness prior to swallow may be beneficial and include a variety of procedures; recommended for patients with swallow apraxia, delayed onset of the oral swallow, reduced oral sensation, delayed triggering of the pharyngeal swallow, and tactile agnosia for food; in all the techniques, a sensory stimulus is applied before an attempted swallow; presumably, the stimulus alerts the swallowing centers of the brain; use one or more of the following sensory enhancement techniques

- apply a downward pressure on the tongue while presenting food with a spoon
- present a sour bolus (50% lemon juice, 50% barium) before presenting the bolus
- present a cold bolus
- present a bolus that the patient needs to chew
- present a bolus of larger volume
- present a thermal-tactile stimulation before presenting a bolus; using a size 00 laryngeal mirror that has been dipped in crushed ice for several seconds, firmly rub the anterior faucial arch four or five times before presenting a bolus; this is expected to sensitize the system so that initiation of oral swallow will trigger pharyngeal swallow; note, however, there is controversy about its effectiveness

- *Modification of volume and speed of food presentation:* Procedures that change the amount of food presented and the rate of presentation that facilitate swallowing; use the following techniques
  - Try a larger bolus to trigger pharyngeal swallow in patients
  - Try a smaller bolus to trigger swallowing in some patients
  - Present smaller boluses at a slower rate to trigger swallowing in some patients
- *Modification of food consistency:* Procedures in which the food consistency or viscosity is changed to promote better swallow; try the following modifications
  - use thin liquids with patients who have oral tongue dysfunction, reduced tongue base retraction, reduced pharyngeal wall contraction, reduced laryngeal elevation, and reduced cricopharyngeal opening

D

- use thickened liquids with patients who have oral tongue dysfunction and delayed pharyngeal swallow
- use purees and thick foods (including thickened liquids) with patients who have delayed pharyngeal swallow, reduced laryngeal closure at the entrance, and reduced laryngeal closure throughout
- eliminate a certain food consistency only as a last resort
- *Use of intraoral prostheses:* Artificially fashioned devices that help compensate physiologic deficiencies; have them constructed with the help of a maxillofacial prosthodontist
  - use a palatal lift prosthesis, which helps lift a paralyzed soft palate to close the velopharyngeal port
  - use a palatal obturator, which closes a surgically resected soft palate in patients who have had oral cancer
  - use a palatal augmentation or reshaping prosthesis, which gives a new and more normal shape to the hard palate in patients who have had oral surgery

Swallow Maneuvers. Techniques designed to help patients gain voluntary control over certain involuntary aspects of swallow; to be effective, the patient should follow the directions and exert some muscular force, which may be impractical in some cases; use one of the four most commonly used maneuvers.

- the *supraglottic swallow,* which helps close the airway at the level of vocal folds before and during the swallow; it involves holding the breath during swallow to close the vocal folds: to implement this maneuver, place a bolus in the mouth of the patient and ask the patient to:
  - hold the food in the mouth
  - take a deep breath and hold the breath

- swallow while holding the breath
- cough soon after the swallow

Note that some patients may hold the breath by not closing the vocal folds, but by stopping the chest wall movement. Ask these patients to inhale deeply, exhale slightly, and then hold the breath and swallow while holding the breath; holding the breath on exhalation closes the folds more readily.

- the *super-supraglottic swallow,* which helps close the airway entrance before and during the swallow; it helps close the false vocal folds by tilting the arytenoid cartilage anteriorly to the base of the epiglottis before and during the swallow; arytenoids are tilted when the breath is held and the patient bears down; to implement this maneuver, ask the patient to:
  - inhale and hold the breath tightly by bearing down
  - swallow while holding the breath and bearing down
- the *effortful swallow,* which helps increase the posterior motion of the tongue base during the pharyngeal swallow; to implement this maneuver ask the patient to:
  - squeeze as hard as possible while swallowing
- the *Mendelsohn maneuver,* which helps elevate the larynx more and for longer duration, resulting in an increased width and duration of the cricopharyngeal opening; in implementing this maneuver:
  - educate the patient about the elevation of the larynx (tell them about the Adam's apple or voice box going up)
  - have the patient palpate the elevation of the larynx when he or she swallows saliva several times
  - instruct the patient to hold the larynx up for a longer duration (several seconds) as he or she swallows; give such instructions as "swallow long and strong" or "stretch out the swallow"

D

Direct Treatment of Dysphagia. Treating swallowing disorders by placing food or liquid in the patient's mouth and then shaping and reinforcing swallowing behaviors.

Disorders of Mastication

- Instruct the patient with limited lateral tongue movement to mash food by pressing the tongue against the hard palate or by keeping the food on the more mobile side of the tongue
- Teach the patient with reduced buccal tension to:
  - apply a gentle pressure with one hand on the damaged cheek to increase cheek tension
  - put food on the normal or stronger side
  - keep the head tilted to the stronger side to maintain food on that side
- Teach the patient with limited lateral movement of the mandible to mash food by pressing the tongue against the palate
- Design a Palate Reshaping Prosthesis for the patient with limited vertical tongue movement when indirect treatment (exercises) fail
- Gradually reshape the prosthesis by reducing its size as the patient's vertical tongue movements improve

Disorders of the Preparatory Phase of the Swallow

- Teach the patient with problems in forming and holding the bolus due to reduced tongue movement and coordination to
  - tilt the head forward to keep the food in front of the mouth until ready to swallow
  - tilt the head back to promote the swallow
  - consciously hold the bolus in the anterior or middle portion of the mouth
- Teach the patient with reduced oral sensitivity to
  - place food on the side of the oral cavity with better sensitivity

• better appreciate the placement of food by placing cold or spicy food in the mouth

Disorders of the Oral Phase of the Swallow

• Teach the patient who has developed a tongue thrust to:
  • place the tongue on the alveolar ridge and initiate a swallow with an upward and backward motion
  • compensate by placing food at the back of the tongue and then to initiate a swallow
• Teach the patient with reduced tongue elevation to:
  • compensate by placing food posteriorly in the oral cavity
  • place the straw almost at the level of the faucial arches to help swallow liquid
  • tilt the head back and let gravity push the food from the oral cavity into the pharynx
  • use the Supraglottic Swallow Maneuver to voluntarily protect the airway, if aspiration is a concern
• Teach the patient with disorganized anterior to posterior tongue movement to
  • hold the Bolus against the palate with the tongue
  • begin the swallow with a strong, single posterior motion of the tongue
• Teach the patient with a scarred tongue to:
  • place food behind the scarring
  • tilt the head posteriorly to allow gravity to help with oral transit

Disorders of the Pharyngeal Stage of the Swallow

• Teach the patient with delayed or absent swallowing reflex to compensate by:
  • tilting the head forward while swallowing
  • limiting the amount of Bolus that does not overflow into the open airway
  • counsel the family about the delay in initiating the swallow reflex; ask them to allow that much extra time for each swallow

Dysphagia: Direct Treatment

D

- Teach the patient with reduced peristalsis such compensatory behaviors as:
  - switching between liquid and semisolid swallows so that the liquid swallows help clear the pharynx
  - taking only liquids or semisolids
  - initiating dry swallows after each swallow of food to clear the pharynx
  - the Supraglottic Swallow Maneuver
- Teach the patient with unilateral pharyngeal paralysis such compensatory behaviors as:
  - turning the head toward the affected side to close the pyriform sinus on the affected side and to direct the food down the normal side
  - tilting the head toward the stronger side if the patient has a unilateral paralysis in lingual function and the pharynx
  - the Supraglottic Swallow Maneuver
  - washing away residual thicker food with liquid swallows
- Ask patients with cervical osteophyte to limit their diet to semisolid or liquid food until surgery corrects the problem and the patient recovers
- Teach the patient with a scarred pharyngeal wall the same compensatory behaviors used for the patient with unilateral pharyngeal paralysis
- Teach the patient with reduced laryngeal elevation to clear the throat after each swallow
- Use the Supraglottic Swallow Maneuver if residual material needs to be removed from the pharynx
- Teach the patient with reduced laryngeal closure to:
  - use the Supraglottic Swallow Maneuver
  - tilt the head forward while swallowing
  - turn the head to the side that is not functioning properly
  - place pressure on the thyroid cartilage on the damaged side to improve closure

Dysphagia: Indirect Treatment

Disorders of the Esophageal Phase of the Swallow
- Do not attempt to treat, as these are handled medically

Indirect Treatment for Dysphagia. Treatment of swallowing problems using exercises designed to improve the muscle functioning; does not involve food.

Oral-Motor Control Exercises
- Treat the patient with reduced range of tongue movements with such exercises as the following; ask the patient to:
  - open the mouth as wide as possible and raise the tongue in front as high as possible; hold the tongue for 1 second, and then lower it
  - raise the posterior part of the tongue as far as possible; hold it for 1 second, and then lower it
  - continue with the stretching exercises for 5–10 times in a session, for 3–4 minutes
  - repeat the set of exercises 5–10 times per day
- Increase the patient's buccal tension by asking the patient to:
  - stretch the lips as tightly as possible and say "e"
  - round the lips tightly and say "o"
  - rapidly alternate between "e" and "o"
- Instruct the patient with limited lateral movement of the mandible to:
  - keep the jaw open as widely as possible and hold this position for about 1 second
  - open and move the jaw sideways and hold the extended position for 1 second
  - make circular jaw movements
  - provide Manual Guidance to move the jaw in the desired directions
  - stop the task if any pain is experienced
- Treat the patient with limited tongue resistance by asking the patient to:
  - push the tongue against a tongue depressor and hold the pressure for 1 second

D

- push the tongue against the tongue blade, in an upward, forward, and sideways direction; hold the pressure for 1 second
- Shape more firm lip closure by asking the patient with problems in lip closure to:
  - stretch the lips for 1 second to stimulate the production /i/; increase the duration gradually
  - pucker the lips tightly for 1 second initially; increase duration gradually
  - close the lips tightly for 1 second; increase the duration gradually; provide Manual Guidance if necessary
  - close the lips around a spoon or an object; reduce the size of the object as the patient's lip closure improves
  - to hold the lips together for 1 minute once a lip seal is achieved; increase the duration gradually
  - repeat the exercises 10 times per day
  - ask the patient to close the lips around a tongue depressor
  - maintain lip closure when you or the patient tries to open them
- Treat the patient with bolus control problems by asking the person to grossly manipulate materials by:
  - holding a flexible licorice whip in the mouth, with one end on the patient's tongue and the other end in the clinician's hand
  - keeping the licorice stick between the palate and the tongue
  - moving the licorice stick from side to side with the tongue
  - moving the licorice stick forward and backward with the tongue, and then report where the licorice stick is
  - reporting when gross movement of the licorice stick is achieved

- moving the licorice stick in a circular motion starting from the center of the mouth
- chewing a piece of gum as manipulation capabilities improve

- Treat the patient with bolus control problems who has learned to grossly manipulate materials by:
  - placing a small bolus of paste consistency on the tongue
  - asking the patient to move the bolus around in the mouth
  - telling the patient not to spread the bolus around in the mouth
  - asking the patient not to lose the bolus
  - instructing the patient to cup the tongue around the bolus
  - expectorating the bolus once the task is complete (inspect the mouth for residue)
  - varying the consistency of the bolus, once success is achieved
  - introducing one-third of a teaspoon of liquid to the patient's mouth once success is achieved with the paste
- Treat the patient with bolus propulsion problems through posterior bolus propulsion exercises
  - place a long wad of gauze that is dipped in fruit juice in the patient's mouth
  - hold one end of the gauze
  - ask the patient to use the tongue to push the gauze up and back

Stimulating the Swallow Reflex
- Hold a small, long-handled laryngeal mirror in ice water for about 10 seconds
- Place the laryngeal mirror at the base of the anterior faucial arch
- Repeat this light contact 5–10 times

Dysphagia: Indirect Treatment

- Observe the likely rise of the thyroid cartilage, the twitching of the soft palate, and a slight movement of the faucial arches
- Ask the patient to swallow after the stimulation without food
- After repeating light contact stimulation some 5–10 times, release a small amount of liquid into the patient's mouth with a pipette and ask the patient to swallow by saying "Now"
- Repeat stimulation exercises four to five times daily for 3 weeks to a month in the case of patients with severely impaired swallow reflex
- Shape swallowing once the reflex begins to trigger by progressively larger amounts of food and food with greater consistency

Improving Adduction of Tissues at the Top of the Airway

- Teach lifting and pushing exercises to improve laryngeal adduction to protect the airway during swallowing; ask the patient to:
  - sit on a chair and hold his or her breath as tightly as possible
  - use both hands and push down, or pull up on the chair, while holding the breath for 5 seconds
  - use only one hand while pushing down or pulling up on the chair and to try and produce clear voice with each trial; repeat this exercise five times
  - use Hard Glottal Attack and repeat "ah" five times
  - repeat the exercises three times in succession, 5–10 times a day for 1 week
  - lift or push with simultaneous voicing; use both hands, pull on a chair, and use prolonged phonation
  - use Hard Glottal Attack, commence phonation on "ah," and sustain phonation with smooth voice quality for 5–10 seconds

- practice a <u>Pseudo Supraglottic Swallow</u>; instruct the patient to inhale, hold the breath, and use a strong cough

D

Medical Treatment of Dysphagia. Use of medical, mostly surgical, procedures to treat dysphagia; these procedures are designed to (a) improve a specific anatomic or physiologic deficiency related to swallow, (b) eliminate or reduce aspiration, and (c) provide food and liquid nonorally; medications are limited to treating esophageal swallowing disorders, not for improving oral or pharyngeal swallowing problems.

Botulinum Toxin Injection. A surgical procedure of injecting botulinum, a toxic substance, into cricopharyngeal muscle to improve swallowing; technically difficult because of the position of the target muscle (hidden behind the cricoid cartilage); misplaced botulinum can paralyze other muscles resulting in more serious dysphagia.

Cricopharyngeal Myotomy. A surgical procedure of splitting the cricopharyngeal muscle from top to bottom to keep a permanently open sphincter for swallowing; fibers of the inferior constrictor above and the esophageal musculature below also may be slit; eating may be resumed within about a week; recommended for patients with Parkinson's disease, amyotrophic lateral sclerosis, and oculopharyngeal dystrophy whose main problem is cricopharyngeal dysfunction; not to be performed in early phases of recovery from stroke, head injury, or spinal cord injury as these patients are likely to recover normal or near normal swallow.

Epiglottic Pull-Down. A surgical procedure designed to control unremitting aspiration; the epiglottis is sutured to the arytenoids by making incisions around the epiglottis, aryepiglottic folds, arytenoids,

D

and interarytenoid area; the procedure may fail in some cases, as the epiglottis tends to pull away from this attachment.

Esophagostomy. A nonoral, surgical feeding method for dysphagic patients who cannot tolerate oral feeding; insertion of a feeding tube into the esophagus and stomach through a hole (stoma) surgically created through cervical esophagus.

Gastrostomy (G-Tube). A nonoral, surgical feeding method for dysphagic patients who cannot tolerate oral feeding; insertion of a feeding tube into the stomach through an opening in the abdomen; may be inserted under general anesthetic (called operative gastrostomy) or precutaneously with local anesthetic with the help of an endoscope (called precutaneous endoscopic gastrostomy); blended table food is directly transported to the stomach; recommended when long-term (more than 30 days) nonoral feeding is required; may be more or less permanent; can be removed when no longer needed.

Jejunostomy. A nonoral, surgical feeding method for dysphagic patients who cannot tolerate oral feeding; insertion of a feeding tube into the jejunum through the abdominal wall; *jejunum* is that portion of the small intestine that extends from duodenum to the ileum; often recommended to reduce reflux; the food needs to be prepared because it enters the body below the stomach.

Laryngeal Bypass or Tracheoesophageal Diversion. A surgical procedure designed to separate the air and food passages to prevent or reduce aspiration; recommended for severely neurologically involved patients with life-threatening aspiration; the trachea is cut at the third or fourth tracheal ring; the proximal end is sutured into the cervical esophagus, and the distal end is bent forward to bring it up to the skin where an opening is made and sutured to it; prevents phonation; a tracheoesophageal stunt voice prosthesis will help develop esophageal speech.

Laryngeal Closures. A surgical procedure to minimize or eliminate unremitting aspiration; in one procedure, the vocal folds are sutured together to prevent aspiration; in the other procedure, false vocal folds are sutured together.

Laryngeal Suspension. A surgical procedure to promote laryngeal elevation in patients whose larynx does not raise up and move forward to help close the airway during swallow; the procedure raises the larynx and tilts it forward under the base of the tongue; a suture made from the middle of the mandible to the laryngeal cartilage helps accomplish this; head and neck cancer patients, not neurological patients, are candidates for this procedure.

Medialization Laryngoplasty (Thyroplasty). A surgical method now preferred to Teflon injection to the vocal folds; designed to help position a paralyzed vocal fold into a more medial position so the folds can approximate for phonation and swallowing without aspiration; a small silicon prosthesis is placed in a window surgically created in the thyroid cartilage at the level of the paralyzed fold; the prosthesis helps position the paralyzed fold in a more medial position; performed under local anesthesia; has been successful in achieving complete medialization of a paralyzed fold.

Medications. Medications are available for patients whose swallowing disorders are due to such neurological diseases as Parkinson's disease, myasthenia gravis, and multiple sclerosis; these patients

D

have esophageal swallowing disorders; note that patients with oral-pharyngeal swallowing problems typically are not treated with medications.

Nasogastric Feeding (NG Tube). A nonoral feeding method for dysphagic patients who cannot tolerate oral feeding; a tube inserted through the nose, pharynx, and esophagus into the stomach feeds the patient; recommended when this type of feeding is needed for a short duration (less than 30 days); less acceptable to patients than some of the other procedures because of constant nasal irritation and social appearance.

Pharyngostomy. A nonoral, surgical feeding method for dysphagic patients who cannot tolerate oral feeding; insertion of a feeding tube into the esophagus and stomach through a hole (stoma) surgically created through the pharynx; often more acceptable to patients than the nasogastric feeding.

Surgical Reduction of Cervical Osteophytes. A surgical procedure to remove the bony growth on the cervical vertebra that can narrow the pharyngeal area, displace the posterior pharyngeal wall anteriorly, and thus cause swallowing problems; the procedure poses risk of nerve damage and causing a more serious dysphagia.

Teflon Injection Into the Vocal Folds. A surgical implant method to improve airway closure during swallowing in dysphagic patients by adding implanted muscle mass that will help close the airway; Teflon may be injected into a normal or reconstructed vocal fold or any remaining tissue on top of the airway; other substances injected include glycerin and gel foam; often performed on patients who undergo partial laryngectomy; also performed on patients with such neurological disorders as Parkinson's disease; note that aspiration caused by lack of vocal fold closure may occur only in 10% of patients; its use is on the decline because of such complications as the formation of Teflon granuloma.

D

Total Laryngectomy. Total removal of the hyoid bone and the larynx to permanently separate the food and air passages; performed on patients who already have undergone partial laryngectomy and now cannot control aspiration; a last-resort procedure to control aspiration.

Tracheostomy. A surgical procedure to reduce or eliminate aspiration and improve pulmonary toilet; partially protects the lower respiratory tract from material that may pass the laryngeal sphincter; however, the procedure's effectiveness in reducing aspiration is limited.

Groher, M. E. (1997). *Dysphagia: Diagnosis and management* (3rd ed.). Boston: Butterworth-Heinemann.

Huckabee, M. L., & Pelletier, C. A. (1999). *Management of adult neurogenic dysphagia.* San Diego: Singular Publishing Group.

Logemann, J. (1998). *Evaluation and treatment of swallowing disorders* (2nd ed.). Austin, TX: Pro-Ed.

Pearlman, A. L., & Schulze-Delrieu, K. (1997). *Deglutition and its disorders.* San Diego: Singular Publishing Group.

Dysphonia. A general term that means disordered voice; any voice disorder with the exception of Aphonia.

Dystonia. Movements that are repetitive, slow, twisting, writhing, and flexing. Uncontrolled adductor and abductor laryngeal spasms occur; voice is breathy, strained, and hoarse.

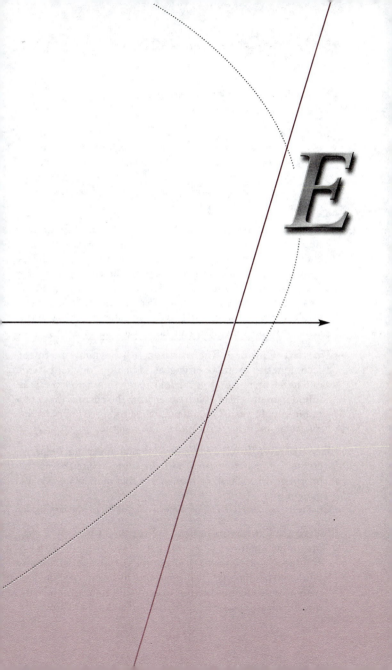

E

Echolalia. Parrot-like repetition of what others say; a major characteristic of autism.

Ear Training. Teaching a client to auditorily discriminate between speech sounds as against teaching production of those sounds; the same as Auditory Discrimination Training or Perceptual Training; see also, Traditional Approach under Treatment of Articulation and Phonological Disorders: Specific Techniques or Programs.

Effectiveness of Treatment. Assurance that treatment, not some other factor, was responsible for the positive changes documented in a client under treatment; requires controlled evidence gathered through clinical experimentation; data should show that treatment was better than no treatment; may use a group experimental design or a single-subject experimental design to establish this; not the same as Improvement or Functional Outcomes.

Effortful Closure Techniques. Behavioral treatment techniques to promote laryngeal adduction for clients with unilateral or bilateral vocal fold paralysis or weakness as found in many clients with dysarthria; the client is taught to grunt, cough, push, lift, and pull while trying to phonate; the muscular effort helps push the folds together.

Effortful Swallow. A swallowing maneuver that helps increase the posterior motion of the tongue base during the pharyngeal swallow; to implement this maneuver, ask the patient to:
- Squeeze hard with all of the muscles as he or she swallows

Electronic Communication Systems. Methods of augmentative communication for persons with limited or no oral speech; also known as electronic gestural-assisted communication strategies, these systems use electronic devices with a switching mechanism to activate a message and control the electronic system and use a display that shows the message; used in teaching Augmentative Communication, Gestural-Assisted (Aided).

Electronic Device for Alaryngeal Speech (Electrolarynx).   Hand-held electronic instruments that generate sound; used by persons who have undergone laryngectomy to produce alaryngeal speech; for rehabilitation procedures, see Laryngectomy; Treatment Procedures: Laryngectomy.

E

Electronic Gestural-Assisted Communication Strategies.   The same as Electronic Communication Systems.

Elicited Aggression.   Aggressive behavior directed against any object or person when an aversive stimulus (as in operant punishment procedures) is delivered; not necessarily directed against the person delivering the aversive stimulus; a potential undesirable side-effect of punishment.
- A child may kick the table when "No" is said to a wrong response
- A child may sweep the stimulus materials off the table when a token is taken away in a response cost procedure
- Note that to reduce elicited aggression in treatment, use punishment procedures sparingly and use more positive reinforcement and discriminative reinforcement that may indirectly control undesirable behaviors

Hegde, M. N. (1998). *Treatment procedures in communicative disorders* (3rd ed.). Austin, TX: Pro-Ed.

Empirical Validity.   Credibility or truthfulness of statements based on research data; assurance that treatment procedures have been shown to be effective through experimentation involving clients (as against logical arguments or scholarly speculation); a criterion for treatment selection.

Empiricism.   A philosophical position that statements must be supported by observational or experimental evidence; basis of modern science; contrasted with Nativism or Rationalism.

Environmental Contingency.   Interdependent relation between antecedents, responses, and the consequences the responses generate and thus help maintain those responses; environmental events that shape and sustain behaviors; reinforcers and punishers used in treatment in a manner that immediately follow the target behaviors; the treatment variable in behavioral approach; contrasted with Genetic/ Neurophysiological Contingency with which it interacts.

Escape.   A behavior that reduces or terminates an aversive event and hence increases in frequency; typically leads to avoidance; often maladaptive as in a stutterer's avoidance of speaking situations; reduction of avoidance may be a clinical goal.

* Work on eliminating the aversiveness of the event by teaching the needed, alternative skill (e.g., increased fluency in difficult speaking situations)
* In gradual steps, encourage the client to come in contact with the aversive event (avoided speaking situation)
* Reinforce the approach behavior (e.g., picking up the telephone instead of having someone else respond)

Escape Extinction.   A procedure to reduce negatively reinforced behaviors by blocking an escape and thus preventing negative reinforcement for it; a response reduction strategy; useful in treatment sessions in which children exhibit many undesirable behaviors to escape from treatment regimen (e.g., crawling under the table during treatment).

* Prevent the occurrence of an undesirable response (e.g., crawling under the table) exhibited to escape from aversiveness (e.g., training trials)
* Physically restrain the child every time an attempt is made to leave the chair to prevent reinforcement of escape behavior
* Measure the frequency of attempts to crawl; if there is no reduction, use a different technique

Ethnocultural Variables in Treatment.   Variables related to an individual's cultural, ethnic, and other personal variables that may affect treatment of communicative disorders; there is more written about assessment of ethnoculturally varied clients' disorders of communication; research on the effects of ethnocultural variables on treatment techniques is limited; see under each disorder entry (e.g., Aphasia, Articulation and Phonological Disorders, Language Disorders in Children) for specific and detailed guidelines on treating clients with varied ethnocultural backgrounds; a few major and general guidelines include the following:

- Select assessment procedures that are ethnoculturally relevant; see *PGASLP* for guidelines
- Note that many of these suggestions are relevant to any disadvantaged family, not just a minority family; many poor, less educated, rural, and working-class families of any race may face problems similar to those faced by families of ethnocultural minority communities
- Understand the cultural communication patterns of the client and the family
- Understand the families' views and beliefs about health, wellness, illness, specific diseases, disability, handicap, and impairment
- Find out the family members' beliefs about disorders of communication and the value they place on communicative skills
- Find out about the educational levels and sophistication about health care systems; without imposing a clinical recommendation, educate the client and the family about clinical resources available to them
- Understand the family environment, living conditions, financial resources to support treatment that needs to be paid for; help them find financial support from local, regional, state, federal, and private sources to help pay for clinical services
- Find out about a family's transportation needs; many do not receive help in speech and hearing clinics because they cannot afford to travel to clinical facilities that often are

E

located in distant areas from where disadvantaged people live

- Assess the time that is available for family members to get involved in clinical treatment, home treatment, and communication skill maintenance over time
- Understand the phonological, semantic, syntactic, and pragmatic rules of the client's dialect (e.g., African American English or an English dialect influenced by a primary language in a bilingual child)
- Place communication patterns in the larger cultural context; avoid the narrow view of differences in linguistic rules among the languages of different ethnic groups
- Achieve a larger understanding of culture, literature, history, and heritage of the people served; avoid the pitfalls of stereotypic and narrow linguistic descriptions of differences; note that this is an enriching experience to clinicians themselves
- Do not assume that clients of different ethnocultural background automatically reject the mainstream communication patterns or that they have not acculturated to mainstream values—many have; the only right thing to do is to find out in an objective and nonevaluative manner
- Do not accept cultural stereotypes about any group; for instance, do not assume that a boy from an Asian background does not maintain eye contact during conversation with his teacher *because of his cultural background*; he may have learned to avoid eye contact *because of his stuttering*
- Work with your colleagues to make sure that needed interdisciplinary services are made available to the clients and their families
- Receive family input in selecting treatment targets; recommend the targets you think are appropriate for the client, but discuss them with the client and his or her family members; make modifications in light of this discussion
- Serve as a resource to other professionals in helping them understand communication patterns of ethnoculturally

different clients and their families so that communication between service providers and receivers is more effective

- Treat communicative disorders that are diagnosed with ethnoculturally appropriate assessment; for instance, treat articulation disorders in African American children only when they have a disorder in African American English; in bilingual children, treat articulation disorders only if they have a disorder within the phonological system of their primary language or a disorder in English that is not due to the primary language's phonological patterns; treat a dialectal variation to induce standard English patterns only when the client, family, or both demand it

- Select treatment stimulus materials that are ethnoculturally appropriate; select materials that the clients are familiar with; in the case of children, find out their preferences in selecting toys, pictures, line drawings, objects, and other stimulus materials; seek family members' input and, if possible, select treatment stimuli from the client's home environment (e.g., ask the child to bring his or her favorite toys to treatment sessions and use them as stimuli for treatment tasks)

- Select treatment procedures that are known to have ethnocultural generality; evaluate treatment studies for their subject selection criteria; apply a given treatment procedure with caution if, in experimentally testing that procedure, an ethnoculturally diverse population has not been adequately sampled

- Select participants from varied ethnocultural backgrounds for your clinical treatment research

- In the absence of treatment research data on a particular disorder in a particular ethnic group (which is typically the case), assume tentatively that generally effective treatment procedures might work with clients of varied ethnocultural background; note that such treatment principles as modeling, demonstration, instructions, positive reinforcement, corrective feedback, extinction, differential reinforcement, shaping, and so forth have been researched with good generality; nonetheless, expect to modify them to suit individual clients

- Gather systematic client performance data on treatment procedures that are of unknown ethnocultural generality; if possible, publish your data as case studies to help other clinicians select treatment procedures appropriate for their varied clients

- Modify treatment procedures in light of the performance data and the client's ethnocultural background; publish information and data on such modifications that were found to be effective with certain clients

Kayser, H. (1995). *Bilingual speech-language pathology: An Hispanic focus.* San Diego: Singular Publishing Group.

Payne, J. C. (1997). *Adult neurogenic language disorders: Assessment and treatment.* San Diego: Singular Publishing Group.

Peña-Brooks, A., & Hegde, M. N. (2000). *Assessment and treatment of articulation and phonological disorders in children.* Austin, TX: Pro-Ed.

Roseberry-McKibbin, C. (1995). *Multicultural students with special needs.* Oceanside, CA: Academic Communication Associates.

Event Structures.   Sequentially organized, familiar events taken from daily life and routinized to teach language structures to children; for procedures, see <u>Language Disorders in Children</u>; <u>Treatment of Language Disorders: Specific Techniques or Programs</u>.

Evoked Trials.   Structured opportunities to produce a response when the clinician does not model; part of the discrete trial procedure; often used in the beginning stages of treatment; most useful in teaching articulation and language structures; contrasted with <u>Modeled Trials</u>; include <u>Baseline Evoked Trials</u> and <u>Treatment Evoked Trials</u>; in administering an evoked trial:

- Present a stimulus, such as a picture or an object, to the client by placing it on the table

E

- Ask a relevant question (e.g., "What is this?" "What do you see?" "What are these?" and so forth)
- Allow a few seconds for the client to respond
- Move the picture or object toward you
- Record the response as correct or incorrect; if no response, record this fact as well
- Represent the stimulus and begin another trial
- Note that this is the basic structure of a discrete trial used in establishing evoked baselines; if it is a treatment evoked trial, reinforce the client's correct responses and give corrective feedback for incorrect responses

Exemplar.   An example of something; in treatment, a response that illustrates a target behavior; these may be words, phrases, sentences, gestures, and so forth; for example, the word *soup* is an exemplar if used in teaching the /s/ or /p/; thus, all words, phrases, and sentences used in teaching correct production of phonemes are exemplars; the sentence *The boy is running* is an exemplar if used in teaching the noun phrase, the auxiliary, or the main verb plus *ing*; thus, all phrases and sentences used in teaching language structures are exemplars; pictures and objects used in treatment also may be considered exemplars; an individual stimulus item designed to evoke a specific target response:

- Select multiple exemplars for each target behavior to be taught (e.g., 20 words to teach the /p/ in initial positions; 20 sentences that contain the regular plural s)
- Teach multiple exemplars of each target behaviors to enhance the potential for generalized production
- Probe after teaching a few (4 to 6) exemplars to see if generalized productions emerge with untrained stimulus items
- Teach more exemplars if the client does not meet the probe criterion (e.g., 90% accuracy of the target phoneme production in a set of 10 untrained words)
- Note that generalized production often results with a few exemplar training items (typically less than 10 exemplars)

Expansions. A language treatment technique in which a client's incomplete or telegraphic utterances are expanded into grammatically more complete productions; for procedures, see Language Disorders in Children; Treatment of Language Disorders: Specific Techniques or Programs.

Experiment. A controlled condition in which an independent variable (such as treatment) is manipulated to produce changes in a dependent variable (production of speech or language); a means of establishing cause-effect relations; needed to establish treatment effects; may use the Group Design Strategy or the Single-Subject Design Strategy.

Experimental Group. In a clinical experiment, the group that receives treatment and hence shows changes in skills taught; part of the Group Design Strategy for establishing treatment effectiveness; contrasted with a Control Group.
- Select participants randomly (Random Selection)
- Assign participants into control and experimental groups randomly (Random Assignment)
- Alternatively, match subjects in the experimental and control groups (Matching)
- Assess the experimental and control groups to make sure they are equal
- Treat the experimental group while withholding treatment to the control group
- Demonstrate that the experimental group changed (improved), whereas the control group did not

Expiratory Board. A prosthetic devise used to improve respiratory muscle strength for speech; client pulls a board attached to wheelchair toward his or her abdomen and leans against it to stabilize the muscles; often used in treating breathing problems associated with Dysarthria.

Exclusion Time-Out. Response-contingent exclusion of a person from a reinforcing environment; a variety of Direct Methods of Response Reduction; a form of Time-Out.

- Contingent on an undesirable behavior, remove the child from the stream of activities (e.g., make the child sit outside the classroom or in a corner)
- Bring the child back to the stream of activities after a brief period of time
- Note that this procedure is generally not recommended because it takes time away from treatment
- Prefer nonexclusion time-out to exclusion time-out; in nonexclusion time-out, a brief period of silence (about 5 seconds) with no eye contact is imposed on an undesirable behavior; more efficient than removing the child from the stream of activities

Expressive Aphasia.   Aphasia whose main characteristic is difficulty in expressive language and speech; a general term that suggests difficulty talking with no significant impairment in auditory comprehension; often refers to Broca's aphasia.

Extension.   A language treatment method in which the clinician makes comments on the child's utterances to add additional meaning; for procedures, see Language Disorders in Children; Treatment of Language Disorders: Specific Techniques or Programs.

Extinction.   A procedure to reduce undesirable response by terminating reinforcement for that response; similar to ignoring in everyday life; one of the Direct Methods of Response Reduction; use the following guidelines in implementing an extinction procedure:

- Factors that affect extinction; note that whether and how fast a behavior will be extinguished depends on the:
  - amount of past reinforcement for that response; a heavily reinforced response is more difficult to extinguish than the one reinforced less heavily
  - duration of reinforcement; a response reinforced for a longer duration may be difficult to extinguish than the one reinforced for a short duration

Extinction

- previous exposure to reinforcement; a response that has been extinguished in the past will be more readily extinguished now than the one that is being extinguished for the first time
- Effective use of extinction in treatment session:
  - remove reinforcers for the response because this operation defines the procedure
  - educate the client's significant others about extinction because parents find it difficult to watch their child's behavior (e.g., crying) put to extinction; explain that other methods of temporarily stopping an undesirable behavior (e.g., picking up a child crying in a treatment session) may promote that behavior in future sessions
  - make an analysis of the reasons for the undesirable behavior you wish to extinguish; if it looks like it is maintained by attention, then withdraw attention; see Extinction of Positively Reinforced Behaviors; if it looks like the undesirable behavior helps the child avoid working hard in therapy (which is aversive to the child), then physically prevent such escape behaviors as crawling under the table when treatment trials are presented; see Extinction of Negatively Reinforced Behaviors; if it looks like the undesirable behavior is automatically reinforced (e.g., head banging), remove the sensory stimulation that results from such behaviors (e.g., make the child wear a padded helmet); see Extinction of Automatically Reinforced Behaviors
  - do not use extinction to control aggressive, self-destructive, and generally disruptive behaviors because extinction is a slow process and the response is allowed to be made with no reinforcers; allowing such responses to be made may result in injury to others and self; prevent the occurrence of such responses and use Differential Reinforcement to encourage alternative, desirable behaviors
- Note that extinguished responses recover sooner or later; when this happens, promptly extinguish again

Extinction of Reinforced Behaviors

- Note that some children may react very emotionally when you start extinction; for instance, a child's crying behavior may intensify when extinction is begun; do not give in at this point

- Combine extinction with positive reinforcement for a clearly stated alternative, desirable behavior (e.g., telling the child that "As soon as you stop crying, we can go out and see your mother" and following through)

Extinction of Automatically Reinforced Behaviors. The procedure of terminating automatic reinforcers for responses to be reduced; one of the Direct Methods of Response Reduction; especially useful in reducing self-stimulatory behaviors of clients who are autistic, profoundly mentally retarded, or brain injured because these behaviors are thought to be automatically reinforced by the sensory consequences they generate for those who exhibit them.

- Determine the sensory consequence of the undesirable behavior to be reduced (noise from banging on the table; stimulation from banging the head)
- Reduce or eliminate the sensory stimulation derived from the behavior to be reduced (cover the table with soft material or make the child wear a padded helmet)

Extinction of Negatively Reinforced Behaviors. The procedure of terminating negative reinforcers for responses to be reduced; one of the Direct Methods of Response Reduction; also known as Escape Extinction; appropriate to reduce such behaviors as crawling under the table during treatment, leaving the chair and walking around the treatment room, interrupting treatment trials by suddenly interjecting "You know what?" types of responses, and grabbing the clinician's pen or the stimulus material; such behaviors are exhibited because treatment trials are aversive to the child and the behavior provides escape from treatment work; the undesirable behavior is negatively reinforced because of such escape from aversive work; this escape needs to be prevented to stop reinforcement for it.

- Physically prevent the behavior; sit close to the child and physically restrain when you see an early sign of the child leaving the chair; sit immediately opposite the child and hold the child's chair between your legs; remove stimulus materials from the child's reach
- Continue to present treatment trials
- Note that by preventing the escape behavior, you stopped its reinforcement as well; this is escape extinction
- Note that negatively reinforced undesirable behaviors cannot be extinguished by simply withdrawing attention

Extinction of Positively Reinforced Behaviors. The procedure of terminating positive reinforcers for responses to be reduced; one of the <u>Direct Methods of Response Reduction</u>; appropriate to reduce such behaviors as crying maintained by reinforcement; should **not** be used to reduce aggressive, self-destructive, and generally disruptive behaviors, negatively reinforced behaviors, automatically reinforced behaviors, or behaviors that are due to physical pain and discomfort.

- At the very outset of extinction, tell the client that you will pay attention only when the undesirable behavior stops (e.g., say "As soon as you stop crying, I will take you out to see your mother.")
- Pay no more attention until the behavior stops; turn your back and sit motionless; do not try to use other means of stopping the behavior; do not peek at the child
- Do not be unnerved when the behavior initially intensifies (<u>Extinction Burst</u>); continue to ignore the behavior
- Pay immediate attention when the behavior subsides or stops (e.g., say "That is very good! You stopped crying; we can now go see your mother.")

Extinction Burst. A sudden, initial, and temporary increase in responses at the beginning of extinction; not a reason to abandon extinction when it is appropriately chosen.

Extraclinical Settings (Training In). Training given in such nonclinical settings as a playground, classroom, home, and other places; essential part of Maintenance Strategy; training is less formal, involving spontaneous, functional communication; often administered by such significant others as teachers, family members, and friends.

Extrapyramidal System. A neural pathway that carries motor impulses from the brain to various muscles via several relay stations; also called the indirect motor system; damage to this system may cause muscle tone problems and may affect voluntary movements of speech muscles; involved in Dysarthria; contrasted with the Pyramidal System.

Eye Contact. Looking at the listener's face during conversation; a pragmatic language intervention target; subject to ethnocultural variations, as in some cultures, eye contact between certain conversational partners (e.g., between a student and a teacher) may not be appropriate; for procedures, see Language Disorders in Children; Treatment of Language Disorders: Specific Techniques or Programs.

Eye Gaze. A method of nonverbal communication often taught to individuals with severe neuromuscular impairment; a method of Augmentative and Alternative Communication; the client is taught to gaze at a word, a phrase, a symbol, or an object to convey a message.

Eye Glass Hearing Aids. Amplification system built into the frames of eyeglasses; see Aural Rehabilitation.

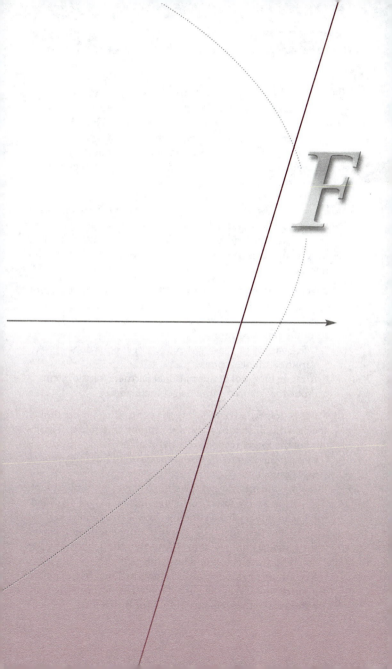

Facilitated Communication.   A once-popular technique of language treatment for children with autism and others with severe language impairment in which a facilitator maintains physical contact with the hand, wrist, or elbow of the client to facilitate writing, typing, or pointing on a message board; controlled studies have produced negative evidence; results suggest that the facilitator may be the source of the messages typed; the American-Speech-Language-Hearing Association is not convinced of its effectiveness and recommends additional research; the American Psychological Association and the Association for Behavior Analysis have concluded that the method is ineffective and invalid; not recommended.

Factorial Stimulus Generalization.   Generalized production of unreinforced responses given in relation to new stimuli, settings, and audience; the most complex form of stimulus generalization.
- Use a variety of stimuli to evoke target behaviors
- Vary treatment settings
- Arrange different conversational partners for the client
- Probe for factorial stimulus generalization

Fading.   A method of reducing the controlling power of such special stimuli as modeling and prompting while still maintaining the target responses the stimuli evoke.
- Reduce the frequency of the special stimulus (e.g., modeling) gradually
- Reduce the intensity of the stimulus (e.g., present <u>Prompts</u> in progressively softer voice until it is no longer provided)
- Present only a partial stimulus (as in <u>Partial Modeling</u>)
- Make the stimulus progressively more subtle (e.g., make the hand gesture given to slow down the speech of a person who stutters less and less conspicuous)
- Make a mechanical stimulus nonfunctional (e.g., turn off a microphone that the client still holds, or turn off a computer screen that remains in front of the client)

- Increase the distance from the client and the special stimulus in graded steps (move the microphone or the computer screen away from the client)

First Words. The first few words a child typically acquires; language treatment targets for young children who are nearly nonverbal.

- Select child-specific words
- Select the names of family members, child's favorite toys (car, doll), food items (milk, juice, candy), clothing items (sock, shoe), action verbs (come, go, walk), simple adjectives (big, small), animals (kitty, doggie), household objects (pen, book, spoon, chair, table), and words from similar categories
- Use the structured, Direct Language Treatment Approaches if the child is nearly nonverbal and has attention deficit:
  - use the Discrete Trials
- Use indirect language stimulation if the child interacts well and can concentrate on loosely structured treatment activities; use a play-oriented situation:
  - frequently model the target word productions
  - use the Mand-Model approach
  - use the Incidental Teaching Method
- Train parents to stimulate language at home; teach parents to:
  - have the child label an item before you hand it to him or her
  - read stories to the child and have the child name pictures
  - ask questions about the pictures (e.g., "How does the kitty go?")
- Give training in varied contexts and probe for generalized productions
- Move on to teaching Phrases (Word Combinations)

Fixed Interval Schedule (FI). An intermittent schedule of reinforcement in which an invariable time duration separates opportunities to earn reinforcers; the first response made after the interval is reinforced; responses made during the interval are not reinforced; limited use in treating communicative disorders.

Fixed Ratio Schedule (FR).   A schedule of reinforcement in which a certain number of responses are required to earn a reinforcer; an FR1 in which every response is reinforced is a continuous schedule; schedules greater than 1 are intermittent; frequently used in treatment sessions.
- Specify the schedule to the client ("I will give you a token every time you say it correctly.")
- Reinforce according to the specified schedule

Flaccid Dysarthria.   A type of motor speech disorder caused by damage to the motor units of cranial or spinal nerves that supply speech muscles (lower motor neuron involvement). See Treatment of Dysarthria: Specific Types under Dysarthria.

Fluency.   An aspect of speech and language production; quality or state of being fluent.

Fluency Disorders.   Speech disorders characterized by excessive amounts of dysfluencies, excessive duration of dysfluencies, or both; speech that is produced with excessive amounts of struggle and effort (Stuttering); speech that is characterized by excessively fast rate, indistinct articulation, and possibly language formulation problems (Cluttering); impaired fluency due to Neurogenic Fluency Disorders; Stuttering is the most researched and more frequently diagnosed and treated fluency disorder in the United States.

Fluency Reinforcement Techniques.   Reducing stuttering by increasing fluency through positive reinforcement; fluent intervals or fluent utterances may be reinforced through verbal praise or tokens that are exchanged for small gifts; can be effective in treating young children who stutter; for procedures see Stuttering, Treatment; Treatment of Stuttering: Specific Techniques or Programs.

Fluency Shaping Techniques. A collection of stuttering treatment techniques based on the assumption that normal-sounding fluency should be the intervention goal; include teaching such skills as airflow management, gentle onset of phonation, and reduced rate of speech through syllable prolongation; contrasted with Fluent Stuttering: Van Riper's Approach; described under Stuttering, Treatment; Treatment of Stuttering: Specific Techniques or Programs.

Fluent Aphasia. A type of aphasia characterized by fluent but mostly meaningless speech full of neologistic words and jargon compounded by auditory comprehension deficits; contrasted with Nonfluent Aphasia; includes Wernicke's aphasia, transcortical sensory aphasia, conduction aphasia, and anomic aphasia; see Aphasia and Treatment of Aphasia: Specific Types.

Fluent Speech. Speech that is smooth, flowing, effortless, and rapid within acceptable limits; negatively defined, it is speech that does not contain excessive amounts of pauses, repetitions, sound and silent prolongations, interjections, and other forms of dysfluencies; speech that is not produced with excessive effort and struggle; a treatment target for persons who stutter.

Fluent Stuttering: Van Riper's Approach. A stuttering treatment approach based on the assumption that reduced abnormality of stuttering, not fluent speech, is a realistic goal for most persons who stutter; includes teaching such skills as cancellation, pull-outs, and preparatory sets along with counseling, desensitization, and stabilization of fluent stuttering; for procedures see Stuttering, Treatment; Treatment of Stuttering: Specific Techniques or Programs.

Follow-Up. Assessment of response maintenance subsequent to dismissal from treatment; done according to a schedule (such as 3 months after dismissal or at 6-month intervals).

Frequency of English Consonants

- Set up a schedule with decreasing frequency (e.g., twice in the first 6 months of dismissal, the next follow-up after 1 year, the next after 2 years)
- Take a speech-language sample
- Measure the frequency of the target behaviors (production of clinically established speech sounds, language structures, fluency or dysfluency, vocal qualities, etc.)
- Calculate the percent correct use of the clinically established target behaviors
- Give Booster Treatment if the target behaviors are below the previously set criterion (such as 90% accuracy)

Frequency of Occurrence of English Consonants. Use the following frequency of occurrence information in selecting treatment targets for children who misarticulate; note that frequency of occurrence is not an absolute criterion of selection; consider other factors as well (described under Articulation and Phonological Disorder); note that frequency suggests ranking based on the relative frequency of 24 English consonants (e.g., 16th for /p/ means that it ranks 16 in occurrence among the consonants); the lower the ranking, the higher the frequency; two different rankings for the same sound suggest discrepancy among studies:

Sound	Frequency	Sound	Frequency	Sound	Frequency
/t/	1st or 2nd	/ð/	8th or 9th	/b/	18th
/n/	1st or 2nd	/k/	10th	/j/	18th
/r/	3rd or 4th	/w/	11th	/v/	19th or 21st
/s/	3rd or 5th	/h/	12th or 13th	/θ/	20th or 21st
/l/	4th or 9th	/f/	15th or 16th	/ʃ/	20th or 21st
/d/	5th or 6th	/g/	15th or 19th	/dʒ/	22nd
/m/	6th or 8th	/p/	16th	/tʃ/	23rd
/z/	7th	/ŋ/	17th	/ʒ/	24th

Functional Equivalence Training

Delattre, P. (1965). *Comparing the phonetic features of English, German, Spanish, and French.* Heidelberg, Germany: Verlog.

Shrieberg, L. D., & Kwiatowski, J. (1983). Computer assisted natural process analysis (NPA): Recent issues and data. *Seminars in Speech and Language, 4,* 397–406.

Functional Equivalence Training. An indirect method of reducing an undesirable behavior by reinforcing a desirable behavior that serves the same function as the undesirable behavior (e.g., teaching a verbal request to a nonverbal child who whines to get adult attention; the verbal request serves the same function as whining and thus is reduced in frequency); the same as the Differential Reinforcement of Alternative Behaviors (DRA); to implement this procedure:

- Find out the functions of an undesirable behavior that need to be reduced by analyzing:
  - the conditions under which an undesirable behavior occurs
  - the consequences it seeks (e.g., attention, reduction in needs, reduction in aversive stimulation, or sensory stimulation)
- teach a desirable, alternative behavior that is followed by the same consequence
- record the frequency of both the undesirable behavior (which should decrease) and the desirable (which should increase)

Functional Outcome Measures of Treatment. Measures that go beyond counting the correct production of specific target behaviors in treatment sessions; often involve qualitative measures of overall changes in the client's behaviors; measures of changes in the client's quality of life; measures of generalized production of communicative skills in natural environments; measured that are based on rating of communicative effectiveness of clients in everyday situations;

F

Functional Outcome of Treatment. Generalized, broader, and socially and personally more meaningful consequences of treatment; measured in more global terms than the effects measured in treatment sessions

- Document functional outcomes of treatment by measuring:
  - improvement in certain quality aspects of life of a client that may be due to treatment (e.g., improved social or academic performance of a child who has received language treatment; an adult's return to work after receiving rehabilitation services following traumatic brain injury; a stuttering male's improved dating skills or his enhanced communicative skills with his boss at work)
  - generalized and effective production of clinically established communicative skills in social, personal, family, educational, and occupational contexts; note that minimally, clients should produce at home and other settings what they have been taught to produce in the clinic
  - functional communication in natural settings (e.g., effective expressions of needs and wants by persons who have received treatment for aphasia; managing daily communication needs by a child who has received augmentative or alternative communication therapy; effective use of a hearing aid in social situations and documented benefits derived by a person who has received aural rehabilitation)
  - expansion of clinically established skills in natural settings (e.g., new and longer sentences produced in natural settings by a client who has received language treatment)
- Obtain information on functional outcomes from institutional caregivers and family members by:
  - interviewing them on different domains of skills and communicative behaviors
  - having them rate a client's communicative effectiveness in natural contexts
- Note that functional outcomes

Functional Outcome of Treatment

- are not the same as <u>Effectiveness of Treatment</u>; treatment effectiveness is established in controlled experimental research
- are simply measured changes in the client's communicative behaviors in natural settings; favorable outcomes, if documented, may be due to any factor including the family involvement, caregiver attention, and so forth; it cannot be claimed that treatment was effective
- outcomes research makes sense only after the effectiveness of a treatment is established

F

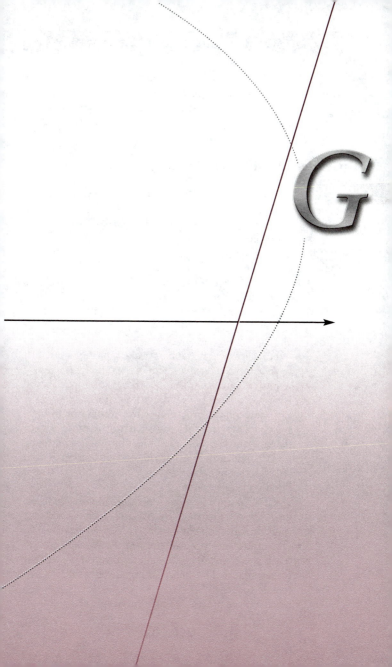

Gastroesophageal Reflux. Backward flow of stomach secretions into the esophagus; may lead to a reflux disorder in which the esophagus is irritated; can cause voice problems and other complications.

Gender Identification Therapy. Communication therapy with an emphasis on voice therapy designed for individuals who, at some point in their lives, assume a different gender; speech-language pathologist may be asked to help achieve proper gender identification after the change.

- Note that voice modification in a woman who has changed to a man may be achieved by hormone treatment that will thicken the vocal folds and lower the pitch
- Note that voice modification in a man who has changed to a woman may require extensive voice therapy, as the medical treatment to achieve an overall female pitch has met with limited success; also note that just a higher pitch may not be sufficient; the client may need to learn overall female speaking patterns
  - make a thorough assessment of the entire vocal range; identify a pitch that is appropriate, comfortable, and is not associated with laryngeal tension
  - use biofeedback or computerized programs to have the client practice the new pitch
  - teach stereotypically feminine intonation patterns (e.g., rising intonation at the end of sentences that characterize female speech)
  - discourage falsetto voice
  - teach the person to speak with more mouth openness, more air, and "placing" the voice in the head and face (presumably, men place their voice in the head)
  - teach the client to speak more softly than before
  - teach the client to speak slightly faster and with increased pause durations as these are characteristics of female speech
  - teach a more precise articulation of speech sounds

- teach the client to use more indirect speech and indirect requests (e.g., "Do you mind doing . . ." instead of "Do this" type of command)
- teach the client to emphasize feelings and relationships as against facts in speech
- teach female body language (more smiling, touching, eye contact)
- avoid such masculine habits of throat clearing and coughing

Andrews, M. L. (1999). *Manual of voice treatment* (2nd ed.). San Diego: Singular Publishing Group.

Gender Reassignment.   Sex change; someone who has been living as a man may now become a woman or vice versa through a sex-change operation; he or she may seek communication treatment to achieve the new and intended gender identity.

Generality of Treatment.   The applicability of a treatment procedure in a wide range of situations involving other clients and clinicians; demonstrated through Replication of treatment efficacy research; a Treatment Selection Criterion:

- Select treatment procedures that are known to have generality; consider the following kinds of generality in evaluating and selecting a treatment procedure:
  - applicability of a treatment procedure by a wide variety of clinicians; has the technique been effectively used by different clinicians?
  - applicability of a treatment procedure in a variety of clients; is the treatment procedure known to be effective with clients of different ages, socioeconomic conditions, educational levels, and ethnocultural backgrounds?
  - applicability of a treatment across clinical settings; is the treatment known to be effective in such varied clinical settings as a private clinic, hospitals, university speech and hearing clinics, extended care facilities, and rehabilitation facilities?

- applicability of treatment across geographic settings; is the treatment known o be effective in clinical facilities across the country?
- applicability of treatment across response classes; is the treatment known to be effective in treating a variety of disorders? (e.g., techniques such as modeling and reinforcement, known to be effective in speech and language treatment, may be equally effective in treating disorders of swallowing)
- Note that *effectiveness of treatment* implies experimental evaluation; existence of controlled data showing that treatment is better than no treatment; just because a technique is widely used in different clinics by different clinicians, in different geographic locations, and in treating different clients is no assurance that the technique is effective; no amount of expert advocacy in the absence of controlled data should convince clinicians to use a technique routinely

Generalization.   A declining rate of unreinforced responses in the presence of untrained stimuli; a temporary, intermediate goal of treatment; includes Verbal Stimulus Generalization, Physical Setting Generalization, Audience Generalization, Factorial Stimulus Generalization, and Response Generalization; each may be promoted with specific techniques; see Maintenance Strategy to promote lasting treatment effects.

Generalized Production.   Production of clinically established behaviors in relation to new stimuli, new audiences, and in new situations; measured through Probes.

Genetic/Neurophysiological Contingency.   The interdependent relation between genetic and neurophysiological variables that determine or influence behaviors; contingency that interacts with Environmental Contingency.

Gentle Phonatory Onset.   A stuttering treatment target; initiating voice in a gentle, soft, easy, relaxed manner; also a treatment target in treating hard glottal attack; for procedures see Stuttering, Treatment; Treatment of Stuttering: Specific Techniques or Programs; and Voice Disorders, Treatment of Voice Disorders.

Gestural Communication. Method of communication that supplements oral communication with smiles and a variety of other facial expressions, body movements including shoulder shrugging, hand movements, pantomime, pointing, and head nodding or shaking; part of normal oral communication; in gestural communication, expressions are important in communicating the speaker's messages; gestural communication may be unaided as in smiling or hand movements; or aided, as in gestures combined with a communication board; procedures described under Augmentative Communication, Gestural (Unaided) and Augmentative Communication, Gestural-Assisted (Aided).

Glossectomy. Partial or total surgical removal of a diseased or severely damaged tongue.

Glottal Fry. A normal voice register that may occur at the end of sentences; very low-pitched vocalization that may sound like the popping of popcorn; also called vocal fry.

Gradient of Generalization. Progressively decreasing, unreinforced response rate as a stimulus is varied on a given dimension, resulting in a curve that approximates the bell-shaped curve; the reason why generalization is not a final treatment goal.

Gradual Increase in Length and Complexity of Utterances (GILCU). A component of the Monterey Fluency Program; for procedures see Stuttering, Treatment; Treatment of Stuttering: Specific Techniques or Programs.

Granulovacuolar Degeneration. A build-up of fluid-filled vacuoles and granular remains within nerve cells; a basic neuropathology of Alzheimer's Disease and found in some normal elderly people.

Group Design Strategy. A research strategy in which the experimental treatment effect or efficacy is demonstrated by treating individuals in one group (the experimental group) and not treating individuals in another, comparable group (control group); helps demonstrate that treatment was better than no treatment; one of two strategies for treatment evaluation; contrasted with Single-Subject Design Strategy.

- In implementing a basic control-group/experimental-group treatment research in which a single treatment is evaluated:
  - identify a population (a large number of subjects with known characteristics) of participants with the disorder for which the treatment to be evaluated has been designed
  - select a sample of participants randomly from the population
  - randomly assign the participants to an experimental and a control group
  - match participants in the two groups on relevant variables if random selection and assignment are not possible,
  - administer pretests of the disorder (or measure specified skills) in the two groups
  - treat participants in the experimental group
  - withhold treatment from the control group
  - administer posttests of the disorder (or measure specified skills) in the two groups
  - compare the performance of the two groups on the pretest and the posttest
  - conclude that the treatment was effective if the experimental group improved while the control group did not
- In evaluating the absolute and relative effects of multiple treatments:
  - use multigroup experimental designs in which two or more groups receive treatment (each group receives only one treatment)

Group Design Strategy

- In evaluating interaction between treatments and personal characteristics of clients (e.g., Does age of the clients matter in the effectiveness of a given treatment?):
  - use factorial designs that help establish the relative effectiveness of treatments depending on such personal characteristics as age, socioeconomic factors, and the severity of the disorder

Hegde, M. N. (1994). *Clinical research in communicative disorders: Designs and strategies* (2nd ed.). Austin, TX: Pro-Ed.

G

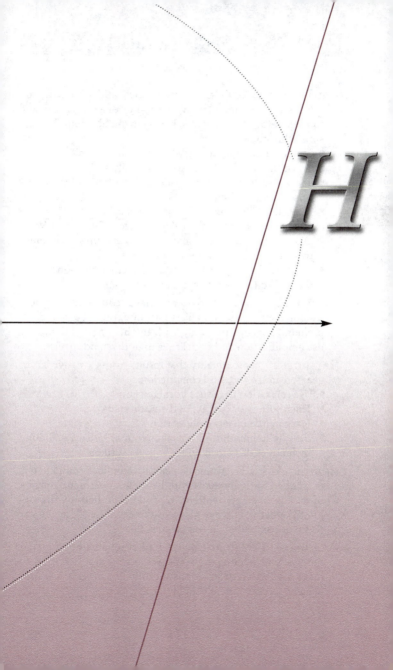

Hard Glottal Attack.   Abrupt voice initiation with too much stress on individual words; words of a sentence sound too separated; a vocally abusive behavior; also found in persons who stutter.
- Teach gentle, relaxed, easy onset of phonation
- Teach the client to blend words initially
- Teach gentle onset in persons with stuttering by instructions and modeling
- Use the Chewing technique, Whisper-Phonation, the Chant-Talk, and the Yawn-Sigh, all described under Voice Disorders, Specific Normal Voice Facilitating Techniques to treat hard glottal attacks in voice clients
- Contrast the easy-onset production with a hard-onset production to treat all clients with this problem

Hard of Hearing.   Persons who have reduced hearing acuity but nonetheless are able to acquire, produce, and comprehend language primarily with the help of audition; may use amplification and visual cues to understand speech.

Harshness.   Voice quality that results from excessive laryngeal tension, effort, and constriction.
- Use relaxation to reduce vocal tension
- Teach soft, easy contact of the vocal folds
- Teach gentle onset of phonation
- Use a combination of Specific Normal Voice Facilitating Techniques described under Voice Disorders

Hearing Aid.   Electronic device that amplifies sound and is prescribed for individuals with hearing impairment; may be of analog or digital variety; types include body-worn, behind-the-ear (BTE), eye glass, in-the-canal (ITC), in-the-ear (ITE), or completely in-the-canal (CIC).

Hearing Aid Evaluation.   An aural rehabilitation procedure in which different kinds of hearing aids are tried to make a selection of an aid that best fits the hearing loss profile and gives the most benefit to the client.

Hearing Aid Orientation.   An aural rehabilitation procedure in which the use and care of a hearing aid is taught to a person with hearing impairment.

Hearing Conservation.   A program designed to prevent or reduce the risk of hearing loss; includes procedures to monitor hearing over a period of time and to educate the client, family, employers, and employees about protecting their hearing.

Hearing Impairment.   Reduced hearing acuity; a hearing level that is greater than 25 dB HL for adults and 15 dB HL for young children in the process of language acquisition; includes the Hard of Hearing and the Deaf; classified as shown under Hearing Loss; oral speech and language disorders are a common concomitant of hearing impairment, especially deafness; mostly, the treatment procedures for Language Disorders in Children, Articulation and Phonological Disorders, and Voice Disorders are applicable with the following special considerations:

General Guidelines

* Begin speech and language stimulation training as early as possible
* Have the child under appropriate medical and audiological management
* Get the family involved from the beginning in speech and language stimulation activities
* Have the child fitted with an individual hearing aid
* Work closely with educators and special educators, especially the educator of the deaf
* Train family members to work with the child at home conducting sessions that parallel yours

   #### Teaching Oral Language
   * Begin oral language training as early as possible
   * Teach the basic words initially; select functional words
   * Teach phrases and sentence structures subsequently

- Pay special attention to teaching grammatic morphemes, as they are especially difficult for children with hearing impairment
- Pay special attention to pragmatic use of language, as it is especially difficult for children with hearing impairment; teach such skills as Topic Initiation, Topic Maintenance, and Turn Taking described under Language Disorders in Children; Treatment of Language Disorders: Specific Techniques or Programs.
- Pay special attention to teaching abstract terms, terms with dual meanings, and the meaning of proverbs, as they are especially difficult for children with hearing impairment
- Pay special attention to teaching synonyms and antonyms, as they are especially difficult for children with hearing impairment
- Use visual cues in all training sessions
- Refer to specialists who can teach such nonverbal communication systems as American Sign Language if the clients, families, or both prefer

Teaching Articulatory Skills

- Give ample visual cues in teaching speech sound production
- Use such procedures as the Phonetic Placement Method
- Pay special attention to fricatives, stops, and affricates, as these are especially difficult for children with hearing impairment
- Teach voiced and voiceless sound distinctions
- Use mechanical visual feedback

Treating Voice Disorders

- Use the standard techniques described under Voice Disorders
- Use mechanical, visual feedback with such instruments as VisiPitch
- Modify such abnormal voice qualities as harshness, hoarseness, stridency, and monotone

- Modify resonance disorders; modify both hypernasality and hyponasality

Treating Prosodic Problems

- Teach smooth flow of speech
- Reduce pauses that may be too frequent and placed inappropriately
- Teach normal intonation
- Teach appropriate breath control to improve phrasing
- Modify the pitch
- Modify loudness

Hearing Loss.   Roughly the same as Hearing Impairment; classified as follows:

- Mild hearing loss: 15–40 dB HL
  Moderate hearing loss: 41–70 dB HL
  Severe hearing loss: 71–90 dB HL
  Profound hearing loss: 90 dB and higher

High Probability Behaviors.   Behaviors of high frequency that can reinforce those of low frequency; an effective treatment method to increase low frequency treatment targets.

- Identify behaviors your client exhibits frequently (e.g., listening to music, watching television, or skiing)
- Design a method by which you in the treatment sessions and the family members at home can control opportunities for those behaviors
- Give tokens in treatment sessions for producing the low-frequency communicative skills
- Let the client accumulate the tokens and exchange them for opportunities to engage in the high-probability behaviors (brief periods of listening to music in treatment sessions, watching TV at home, or going on ski trips)

Hoarseness.   Voice quality that results from leakage of air and aperiodic vibration of the vocal folds; pitch may be too low; any condition that changes the mass and size of the vocal folds, including vocal nodules, may cause hoarseness of voice.

Huntington's Disease

- Obtain a medical evaluation and clearance before starting voice therapy
- Modify the vocally abusive behaviors
- Use a combination of Specific Normal Voice Facilitating Techniques, described under Voice Disorders.

Huntington's Disease.   An Autosomal Dominant, degenerative neurological disease; caused by neuronal loss in the caudate nucleus and putamen along with diffuse neuronal loss in the cortex; symptoms include Choreiform Movements and Dementia; associated with motor speech disorders and language impairment; general management procedures described under Dementia.

Hyperadduction.   Closure of vocal folds with excessive force and tension.
- Teach laryngeal relaxation
- Teach breathy onset of phonation
- Teach gentle, relaxed, easy phonatory onset
- Massage the larynx
- Use such other specific normal voice facilitation techniques as the Yawn-Sigh Method and the Chewing Technique described under Voice Disorders; Specific Normal Voice Facilitating Techniques.

Hyperkeratosis.   Keratotic lesions in the pharynx or larynx; a pinkish, rough lesion with horny growth; associated with Voice Disorders; nonmalignant in the initial states; may be a precursor to malignant lesion; due to continued irritation of tissue, including chronic smoking; treatment is to stop behaviors that result in continued irritation (e.g., cessation of smoking).

Hyperkinetic Dysarthria.   A type of motor speech disorder; its neuropathology is damage to basal ganglia (extrapyramidal system) resulting in rapid involuntary movements and variable muscle tone; may affect all aspects of speech, but a dominant symptom is prosodic disturbances; see Hyperkinetic Dysarthria, under Treatment of Dysarthria: Specific Types.

Hypernasality. Nasal resonance on nonnasal speech sounds; a resonance disorder; intervention described under Voice Disorders; Treatment of Disorders of Resonance.

Hypertonia. Excessive muscle tone or tension; a sign of neurological damage; a symptom in many clients with neurogenic communication disorders (e.g., cerebral palsy, dysarthria).

Hypoadduction. Inadequate approximation of vocal folds; results in breathiness and weak voice; often associated with neurological involvement; a symptom found in such neurogenic communication disorders as Dysarthria and Voice Disorders due to vocal fold paralysis.

- Elicit coughing, grunting, throat clearing, and laughing to improve Adduction
- Use Digital Manipulation of the Larynx described under Voice Disorders; Specific Normal Voice Facilitating Techniques; use this technique along with pressure applied to the abdominal muscles to increase subglottic pressure
- Teach pushing, pulling, and lifting exercises and combine them with phonation; see Dysarthria

Hypokinetic Dysarthria. A type of motor speech disorder; its neuropathology is damage to basal ganglia (extrapyramidal system) resulting in slow movement, limited range of movement, and rigidity; may affect all aspects of speech, but especially voice, articulation, and prosody; see Hypokinetic Dysarthria under Treatment of Dysarthria: Specific Types.

Hyponasality. Reduced or absent nasal resonance in the production of nasal sounds; the same as Denasality; intervention described under Voice Disorders; Treatment of Disorders of Resonance.

Hypotonia. Reduced tone or tension.

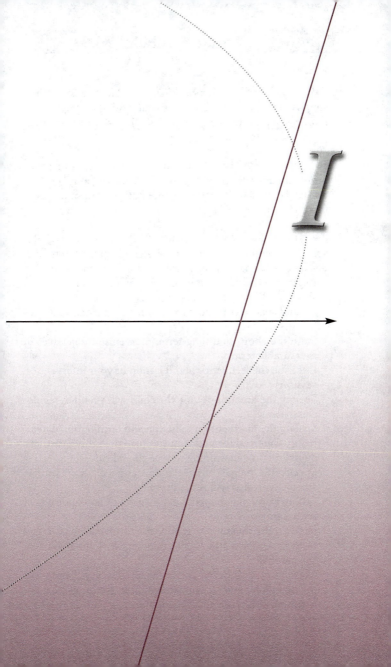

I

Iconic Symbols. A symbol that looks like the object it is supposed to represent; used in teaching Augmentative Communication, Gestural-Assisted (Aided); easier to learn than Noniconic Symbols.

Ideographic Symbols. Graphic representation of ideas; more abstract than pictographic symbols; may be line drawings; used in teaching Augmentative Communication, Gestural-Assisted (Aided).

I

IEPs (Individualized Education Programs). Child-specific intervention programs designed for children with disabilities or special needs served in public grade schools.
- Assess the child's communicative strengths and weakness
- Write an IEP for each child you serve; consult with teachers and special educators to include specific goals and objectives they suggest
- State the short- and long-term intervention objectives in measurable terms
- Describe the frequency and duration of your intervention sessions
- Specify the amount of time the child will spend in regular classroom
- Specify the intervention initiation and termination dates
- Justify the need for your services (use the school district's guidelines in determining service eligibility)
- Specify the names of special education or other professionals who also will serve the child
- Talk to family members to get their input and approval of treatment goals
- Hold an IEP meeting to finalize the intervention plan and to get the signatures of all attending, including those of the parents
- Make periodic assessment of the child to see if the goals are being met and to evaluate whether the goals or treatment procedures need to be modified

Individualized Family Service Plans

IFSPs (Individualized Family Service Plans). Special education programs designed for children with disabilities in the age range of birth through 2 years and their family members.

- Develop a plan similar to IEPs
- Include information on the family's needs and strengths
- Orient the plan toward family involvement

Imitation. A response that follows a modeled stimulus and takes the same or similar form of its stimulus; frequently used in the beginning states of treatment of most if not all communicative disorders; Modeling is the treatment technique to evoke imitation; to teach imitative responses:

- Model the correct response for the client; use instructions and demonstrations as found appropriate
- Place extra vocal emphasis on the specific target behavior in a modeled utterance (e.g., "Say *two cups*," with an emphasis on the grammatic morpheme in teaching the regular plural productions)
- Reinforce the client for imitating the modeled response
- Reinforce approximations initially, especially in the treatment of correct articulation of phonemes
- Require greater match to the modeled response in successive trials
- Fade modeling gradually to transition to evoked responses

Imitation of Aversive Control. Use of aversive methods to control others by persons who were subjected to aversive control themselves; a potential, undesirable side-effect of punishment procedures; a reason to limit punishment procedures in treatment by using strong positive reinforcement techniques for desirable target behaviors.

Imposition of Work. One of the Direct Methods of Response Reduction in which an undesirable behavior is reduced by immediately imposing work designed to reduce or eliminate the negative effects of that behavior; also known as overcorrection; has two components: restitution and positive practice.

Restitution

- Immediately following an undesirable behavior (e.g., throwing toys around), ask the child to neutralize the effects of that behavior (pick up the toys)
- Ask the child to go beyond neutralizing the effects of his or her behavior by improving the situation (ask the child to put the toys on a shelf and then clean up the mess created by another child)

Positive Practice

- Ask the child to practice an incompatible, appropriate behavior repeatedly without reinforcement (ask the child to organize your stimulus materials)

Improvement. Documented positive changes in the client's behaviors compared to initial assessment or baseline performance; needed to justify treatment; what a clinician can claim when routine treatment is offered; not the same as Effectiveness of Treatment, which requires controlled experimental evidence that demonstrates that treatment was better than no treatment.

Incidental Teaching Method. A naturalistic language treatment method that uses everyday verbal interactions to teach functional communication skills; procedure described under Language Disorders in Children; Treatment of Language Disorders: Specific Techniques or Programs.

Incompatible Behaviors. Behaviors that cannot be produced simultaneously, such as sitting and walking; used to reduce certain undesirable behaviors; targets in the Differential Reinforcement of Incompatible Behaviors (DRI).

Independent Variables. Hypothesized or demonstrated causes of events scientists investigate; treatment methods clinicians use; anything a clinician does that affects the client's behavior, including instructions, modeling, demonstration, positive reinforcement, and corrective feedback; contrasted with Dependent Variables.

Indirect Language Stimulation. A collection of somewhat varied, naturalistic, unstructured, or minimally structured language stimulation procedures based on play activities with no systematic reinforcement for specified target behaviors; for procedures, see Language Disorders in Children; Treatment of Language Disorders: Specific Techniques or Programs.

Indirect Methods of Response Reduction. Reducing certain behaviors by increasing other behaviors; indirect because no contingency is placed on behaviors to be decreased; in many cases, more desirable than the direct methods of response reduction because they avoid negative side effects of punishment; include Differential Reinforcement of Alternative Behavior, Differential Reinforcement of Incompatible Behavior, Differential Reinforcement of Low Rates of Responding, and Differential Reinforcement of Other Behavior.

Indirect Treatment for Swallowing Disorders. Treatment of swallowing disorders in which food is not presented to the patient; mostly involves various kinds of exercises; see Direct Treatment for Swallowing Disorders.

Informative Feedback. Information provided to the client on his or her performance levels that reinforces clinical target skills; may be verbal or mechanical; contrasted with Mechanical Corrective Feedback, Nonverbal Corrective Feedback, or Verbal Corrective Feedback in which the information provided is specific to the wrong responses to be decreased.

Verbal

- Periodically, tell the client how well he or she is doing (e.g., "You have improved to 85% today.")
- Show and describe charts and graphs that depict increases in target skills

Mechanical
- Display positive changes and improvement data on computer monitors and other display devices

Infrared Systems.   A variety of Assistive Listening Devices that includes a transmitter that transmits messages on light pulses to a receiver worn by a person with hearing impairment; useful in such large listening environments as concert halls and classrooms.

Inhalation Method.   A method of air intake to produce esophageal speech; for procedures, see Laryngectomy; *Treat Esophageal Speech*.

Inhalation Phonation.   A technique of voice therapy to evoke true vocal fold vibration in clients who are aphonic; for procedures, see Voice Disorders, Specific Normal Voice Facilitating Techniques.

Initial Response.   The first, simplified component of a target response used in Shaping.

Injection Method.   A method of air intake to produce esophageal speech; for procedures, see Laryngectomy; *Treat Esophageal Speech*.

Instructions.   Verbal stimuli that promote the production of target responses; often used in treatment sessions; combined with Demonstrations, Modeling, and Manual Guidance (as in Phonetic Placement Method)
- Design instructions that clarify the target behavior for the client
- Simplify your instructions and tailor them to the individual client
- Write your instructions and practice their delivery, but deliver them naturally; do not read them
- Repeat instructions until the client understands them
- Combine them with demonstrations, modeling, and manual guidance

Intelligibility.   The degree to which a speaker's speech is understandable to others; impaired for various reasons, but typically will be inadequate articulation of speech sounds; a treatment target in treating speech disorders in a variety of clients including children with articulation disorders and adults with dysarthria.

Intelligibility Drills.   A method to help improve intelligibility of speech in speakers who have Dysarthria.
- Prepare a list of words that contain many target sounds the client has difficulty with
- Ask the client to read the list aloud
- Turn back from the client to judge the accuracy of speech sound productions based only on phonatory cues
- If the production of a sound is unclear, ask the client to find out why and try again
- If this second attempt also fails, turn around, look at the printed word, and give corrective feedback to the client
- Ask the client to try saying the same word again

Yorkston, K. M., Beukelman, D. R., & Bell, K. (1988). *Clinical management of dysarthric speakers.* San Diego: College-Hill Press.

Intention Tremor.   Tremor that is absent during periods of rest, but manifests itself during voluntary movements.

Interdisciplinary Teams.   Teams of different specialists who assess and design treatment programs for clients; typically headed by one specialist; members finalize assessment and treatment plans after one or more meetings.

Interfering Behaviors.   Behaviors that interrupt the treatment process; includes such behaviors as leaving the chair, asking irrelevant questions during treatment, crying, wiggling in the chair, and inattentiveness; sometimes a priority focus for clinical intervention because speech-language behaviors cannot be trained unless such interfering behaviors are reduced or eliminated.

- Use one of the Differential Reinforcement procedures to increase the alternative desirable behaviors, which will then reduce the interfering behaviors

Intermediate Care.   A health care facility where persons with disability or chronic illness needing long-term care are admitted; facilities that persons enter after they have been discharged from a hospital and still need professional care.

Intermediate Response.   Responses other than the initial and the final responses used in Shaping a target skill.

Intermittent Reinforcement.   Several schedules of reinforcement in which only some responses or responses produced with specified delay are reinforced; produces stronger response rates than Continuous Reinforcement; includes the Fixed Ratio, Fixed Interval, Variable Ratio, and Variable Interval Schedules; useful in promoting response maintenance over time; to be used in the intermediate and final strategies of treatment, as it is not very effective in establishing the target responses.

Intermixed Probes.   Procedures used to assess generalized production of a trained skill by alternating trained and untrained stimulus items; alternating trained and untrained stimuli helps prevent extinction of trained responses because responses given to trained stimuli are reinforced (those given to untrained stimuli are not); see Articulation Disorders for an example.

- Have at least 10 items not trained (e.g., 10 words or phrases with the plural s when this grammatic morpheme is the treatment target; 10 words or phrases with /z/ in the medial position when this phoneme is the treatment target)
- Prepare a Probe Recording Sheet on which you have alternated trained and untrained exemplars; have at least 10 untrained exemplars that may be words, phrases, or sentences used in training phonemes or grammatic morphemes

- Present a trained exemplar on the first trial (e.g., the picture of two *cups* if this word has been trained); evoke the response by asking a question (e.g., "What are these?"); reinforce the correct production
- Present an untrained exemplar on the second trial (e.g., the picture of two *books,* a stimulus item not used in training); ask a question to evoke the response; provide no reinforcement or corrective feedback
- Alternate trained and untrained exemplars on the subsequent trials
- Calculate the percent correct probe responses based only on responses given to the untrained exemplars
- Give additional training when an adopted probe criterion is not met (e.g., 90% accuracy)
- Move on to next level of training or to new target behaviors when the criterion is met

Hegde, M. N. (1998). *Treatment procedures in communicative disorders* (3rd ed.). Austin, TX: Pro-Ed.

Intersystemic Reorganization.   Use of certain gestures, manual signs, or rhythmic and unusual movements (e.g., tapping, pantomiming, AMER-IND gestures or idiosyncratic gestures a patient invents) to facilitate speech production; often used in the treatment of patients with aphasia.

- Select a set of simple, easily recognizable gestures for the client (e.g., cupping the hand behind the ear to suggest "speak louder"; or select AMER-IND gestures to suggest specific meanings)
- Teach the client to produce the gesture and understand its meaning; use modeling and manual guidance of the gestural movements; educate the client about the meaning of the gesture if it is not clear; make sure the client can use them reliably and communicatively
- Combine the gesture with speaking; model both the gesture and the verbal expression that goes with it; have the client imitate both in combination; when the client is producing the combination, simultaneously model them or

the component on which the client falters; use manual guidance (molding the patient's hands to form the gesture)
- Teach the gesture-speech combination outside the clinical setting to promote its generalized productions in natural settings
- Fade the gestures if only the speech can be maintained
- Teach the client to self-cue verbal expression with the help of gestures (in which case, the gestures are not completely faded, but retained at a reduced form and rate to help get the verbal expressions going)
- Do not use this procedure with severely aphasic clients who cannot learn to gesture or to combine gestures with speech

Rosenbek, J. C., LaPointe, L. L., & Wertz, R. T. (1989). *Aphasia: A clinical approach.* Austin, TX: Pro-Ed.

Intervention.   Introduction and manipulation of external variables to affect the course of a disorder, disease, problem behavior, or condition with a view to eliminate the condition or effect positive changes; the same as treatment.

In-the-Ear Hearing Aid.   A small hearing aid that fits within the ear canal and concha.

Intonation.   Variations in pitch that give speech a pleasant melodic quality; a normal aspect of speech; a treatment target in many clients with communication disorders or when stutter-free speech is instated with slow speech that results in monotonous speech.

Intraverbal Generalization.   Stimulus and response generalization within forms of verbal behaviors; primarily includes expansions of language skills acquired under treatment.

Intubation Granuloma.   A lesion of the larynx that occurs at or near the vocal process of the arytenoid because of trauma caused by the insertion, positioning, or removal of an endotracheal tube; treatment is surgical; no voice therapy except for vocal rest.

Isolated Therapy Model. A special education service delivery model in which children are taken out of the classroom for special instruction, including speech-language instruction; the same as the Pull-Out Therapy Model.

Isolation Time-Out. Response-contingent removal of a person from a reinforcing environment and placing him or her in a nonreinforcing environment; a variation of Time-Out; involves physical isolation (such as placing the person in an isolation booth); may be considered only in reducing highly abusive, aggressive, or self-destructive behaviors; not especially useful in communication treatment sessions; misuse of this technique is common in educational settings; Nonexclusion Time-Out is preferred.

I

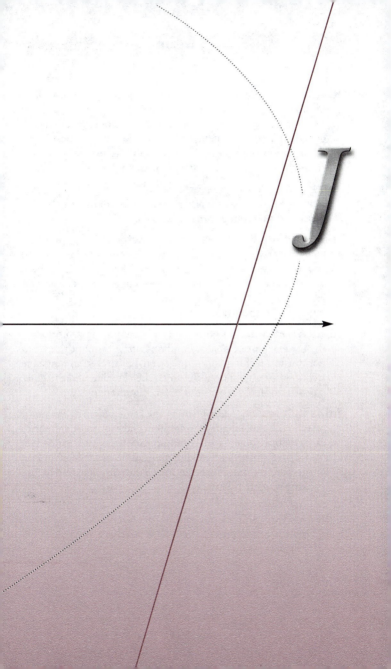

Jargon. A term with varied meanings in speech-language pathology; generally, it means technical or specialized terms of sciences, business, trade, and professions; in child language, it means syllable strings an infant produces with adult-like intonation patterns; in aphasia, it means expressions the patient invents yet are meaningless to the listener.

Jitter. A cycle-to-cycle variation in frequency of vocal fold vibrations that exceeds 1%; a voice disorder of pitch; also described as frequency perturbations.

Joint Action Routines or Interactions. A child language intervention method in which repetitive, routinized activities are used; similar to Script Therapy or may be a variation of it; for procedures, see Language Disorders in Children; Treatment of Language Disorders: Specific Techniques or Programs.

Joint Attention. Two or more people paying attention to the same event or object simultaneously; thought to be important in teaching communication skills; used in language treatment with children in which the clinician and the child pay attention to an event or object simultaneously.

Joint Reference. Establishing the same object as the point of reference in language treatment; lack of joint reference can create problems in communication, as two conversational partners will be talking about different things; in language therapy, drawing attention to the stimulus item before evoking speech or language.

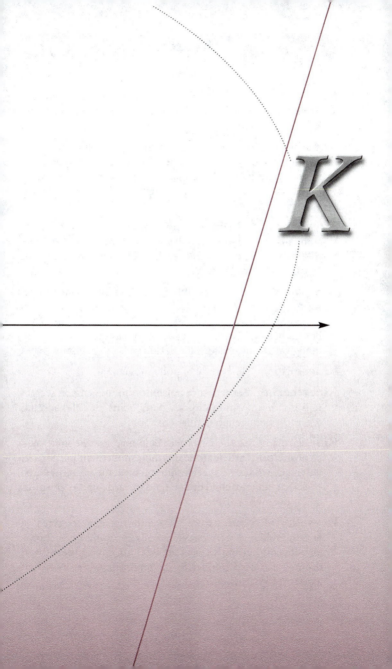

Keratosis. Horny growth (e.g., a wart or callous growth) on certain organs, including the mouth, pharynx, and larynx; see Hyperkeratosis.

Keyboard. A device that gives input to the computer with different layouts of letters, numbers, and other command inputs; may include key depression, touch membrane, or touch screen surfaces; used in Augmentative and Alternative Communication.

Keyguard. A plastic or Plexiglas material used to cover the standard keyboard; has holes for each key; the AAC user slides a pointer over the cover; helps prevent accidental hitting of irrelevant keys.

Key Word. A word in which a generally misarticulated sound is correctly produced; needed to implement the Paired-Stimuli Approach described under Articulation and Phonological Disorders; Treatment of Articulation and Phonological Disorders: Specific Techniques or Programs.

Kinesiology. The study of body movement.

Kinesthesia. Sensation or awareness of movement, weight, tension, and position of body parts; joint, muscle, and hair receptors help generate this sensation.

Kinesthetic Cues. Cues that help increase the awareness of positions of articulators and their movement patterns involved in producing speech sounds correctly; visual or verbal cues that help the child understand the articulatory positions and movement patterns.

Korsakoff's Syndrome. A syndrome characterized by anterograde and retrograde amnesia resulting from chronic alcoholism; currently, used to refer to any amnestic syndrome; also used to refer to the amnestic (memory deficit) aspects of Wernicke-Korsakoff syndrome.

K

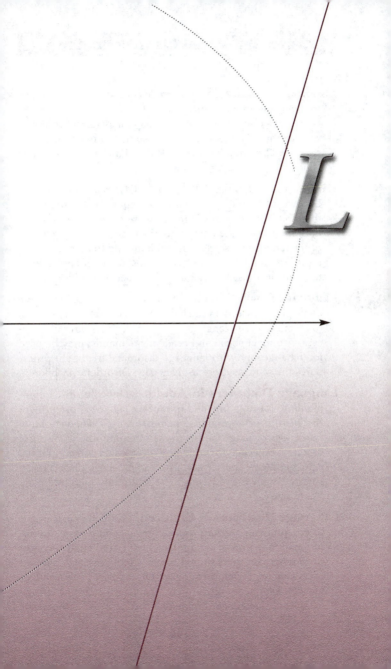

Language-Based Classroom Model. A model of service delivery in which the speech-language pathologist is in charge of a class organized especially for students with communication disorders, although some normally speaking children also may be involved; the clinician teaches these children all day or part of the day.

Language Delay in Children. Generally the same as Language Disorders in Children, except for the connotation that children with language delay are slow in learning and that they will catch up with their normally progressing peers; language disorders in children tend to persist; hence, disorders and delay are not synonyms; treatment procedures the same as those for Language Disorders in Children.

Language Disabilities in Children. Generally the same as language disorders; includes an acceptable connotation that children with language problems lack certain skills necessary to meet social and academic demands; may be used interchangeably with language disorders; treatment procedures the same as those for Language Disorders in Children.

Language Disorders in Adults. Difficulty in comprehending, formulating, and producing language; often there is a history of normally acquired and used language functions; loss of language functions often are due to physical diseases, especially neurological diseases; includes Aphasia, Apraxia, Dementia, Dysarthria, and language disorders associated with Right-Hemisphere Syndrome and Traumatic Brain Injury.

Language Disorders in Children. Difficulty in learning to comprehend and/or produce language in a varied group of children, some of whom have associated clinical conditions whereas others show no such conditions; also referred to as Language Delay, Language Disabilities, Language Deviance, Language Impairment, Language-Learning Disorders, and Language Problems; the term Childhood or

Congenital Aphasia is dated and controversial; the term Specific Language Impairment refers to a special group of children with language problems with no other difficulties, and is also controversial.

Ethnocultural Considerations in Treating Language Disorders in Children

- Language is not just a linguistic code, it is a part of cultural heritage
  - language should not be divorced from culture and society; excessive emphasis on language as a linguistic code with universal rules violates the true nature of language and communication
  - a child's language should be understood in the context of his or her culture
- Language may have some universal commonalities, but it is not spoken in a uniform manner
  - universal rules of language should not be overemphasized; diversity and variations in languages structure are closely related to diversity and variations in people who speak them
  - certain common linguistic rules of language should not be misinterpreted to mean certain standards all should follow
- A client's language performance should not be compared against norms established for another cultural community
  - each child's language should be evaluated against the cultural practices of the community to which the child belongs
  - the typical practice of routinely comparing a child's performance on some language measure to that of a typical group to which the child does not belong is inappropriate
  - the practice is even more objectionable when a standardized test that did not include members of the group to which the child belongs in its standardization

procedure is used to evaluate treatment effects or the child's progress in treatment

- Language differences go beyond just linguistic differences; cataloging linguistic differences is not sufficient; to understand it, you need to understand the culture of the client
  - multicultural literature in the past has often emphasized linguistic differences among languages; while these differences are important, the clinician needs to go beyond them
  - linguistic differences, after all, are a part of the larger cultural differences
- Defining language as a form of social behavior is immensely useful; such a definition implies that people's languages are as unique and different as their social behaviors are
  - viewing language as a form of social behavior deemphasizes the universal code notion of language promoted by structural linguists of the past
  - viewing language as a form of social behavior forces us to pay attention to cultural and social forces that shape patterns of communication
- Stereotyping ethnocultural groups is the same as not understanding them; individuals conform to their group norms to varying extents, and some do not conform at all; for instance, individuals of a particular ethnocultural group:
  - do not always dress like the traditional members of their group
  - do not always eat the foods of their group
  - do not always socialize among themselves
  - do not always share the religious beliefs of their traditional culture
  - do not necessarily reject the values of other ethnocultural groups

- Selecting language treatment targets for ethnoculturally diverse children; this requires a knowledge of the child's language characteristics and his or her cultural communication patterns; selected targets should be consistent with the child's dialectal variation; a feature that is a part of the child's language, but conflicts with another group norm should not be a target for modification; information on treating certain culturally diverse groups in the United States is now accumulating; see <u>Treatment of Language Disorders in African American Children</u> and <u>Treatment of Language Disorders in Bilingual Children</u> following the next major entry.

Treatment of Language Disorders in Children: General Guidelines

Several issues are relevant to the target behavior selection process. Consider the following:

- Selection of Target Behaviors
  - normative strategy, which requires clinicians to select target behaviors based on language development norms; a child with a language disorder does not meet the normative expectations; therefore, the skills that are missing from the standpoint of norms are considered the treatment targets
  - client-specific strategy, which emphasizes functional targets; accordingly, target behaviors should be child-specific; in selecting target behaviors for a child, his or her family and educational demands, family communication patterns, and the behaviors that, when taught, will make a difference, need to be considered; this view is more consistent with the functional view of language treatment and preserves the notion of uniqueness of each individual
- Sequencing the Language Targets for Treatment
  - normative strategy, which requires that selected target behaviors should be sequenced according to the

developmental norms; behaviors should be taught in the sequence in which children normally acquire them; although some behaviors may be more efficiently taught this way, there is no compelling evidence that this is always the best approach to sequencing target behaviors; rarely put to the test because of the strong assumption that this is the best

- experimental strategy, which encourages clinicians to experiment with different sequences of teaching the target behaviors and then using the one that produces the best results; the data may show that normative sequence is indeed the best or that other sequences are better or just as good

- Structure of Language Treatment Sessions
  - tightly structured sessions, which are preferred by some clinicians; tend to involve discrete trial teaching; the clinician controls the stimuli and response consequences; tend to have clearly defined target behaviors for teaching; measurement oriented
  - loosely structured sessions, which are preferred by some clinicians; tend to involve play-oriented sessions; the clinician does not directly control stimuli and consequences; tend not to have clearly specified target behaviors that are taught systematically; not very measurement oriented
  - the two options are perhaps not a matter of choice; the best approach might be to use them both but in different stages of treatment; the early stages of treatment are better structured to establish the target behaviors; the final stages of treatment should be less structured, more naturalistic, more conversation-oriented, and thus loosely structured; starting with good structure, clinicians should loosen the structure as behaviors become better established

- Treatment Efficacy
  - there are many language treatment procedures that have rarely been put to experimental test; techniques that are simply based on expert advocacy should be viewed critically
  - evidence-based practice requires that treatment procedures that have received experimental support should be selected; most behavioral treatment procedures have been experimentally tested; many suggestions that come from structural linguists and (some clinicians as well) are based on speculation and theoretical convictions; see <u>Treatment Selection Criteria</u>

Treatment of Language Disorders in Children

A Comprehensive, Integrated, Treatment Procedure for Language Disorders in Children

L

- Make a complete assessment based on an extended conversational speech and other culturally sensitive assessment tools; consult the cited sources and the *PGASLP*
- Determine what the child can and cannot do with language (comprehension and production; structures the child understands and uses and those that the child does not understand or use)
- Follow these steps in developing a language treatment plan for a child:
  - select target behaviors for training
  - plan a sequence of treatment
  - select stimulus materials
  - establish baselines
  - write a treatment and maintenance plan
  - implement the treatment plan
  - implement the maintenance plan
- Select language intervention targets that:
  - are child-specific and ethnoculturally appropriate
  - are useful in natural settings

- can make an immediate and socially significant difference in the child's communicative skills
- help meet the academic and social demands the child faces
- help expand communication skills into conversational speech in natural settings
- are within the child's reach as judged by current performance (words, phrases, sentences, conversational speech)

• Design a <u>Sequence of Treatment</u> that generally moves from:
  - words to phrases
  - phrases to controlled (less spontaneous) sentences
  - controlled sentences to spontaneous conversational speech
  - treatment in clinical settings to treatment in more naturalistic settings
  - more structured sessions to progressively less structured sessions
  - continuous reinforcement to intermittent reinforcement
  - primary reinforcers to social reinforcers
  - social reinforcers to natural consequences inherent in communication

• Prepare stimulus materials for treatment; select at least 20 exemplars to teach each selected target behavior (e.g., 20 phrases that contain the plural *s*)
  - select ethnoculturally appropriate, client- and target-specific stimuli that are colorful, attractive, and realistic; prefer objects to pictures
  - obtain stimuli from the child's home (the child's favorite books, toys, and objects)

• Prepare a <u>Response Recording Sheet</u> on which:
  - you can write target behaviors
  - record the occurrence of each behavior

• Establish <u>Baselines</u> of target behaviors through:

- repeated conversational language samples that help reliably document the occurrence of language targets
- a set of modeled discrete trials and a set of evoked discrete trials that (a) help capture the production of specific language targets that may not be adequately sampled in conversational speech; (b) are necessary in case of children with no or minimum conversational skills

- Administer <u>Modeled Baseline Trials</u> (note that on baseline trails, there is no reinforcement or corrective feedback for the child's responses):
  - place a stimulus picture or object in front of the child or demonstrate an action or enact an event (e.g., a picture of two books)
  - ask a question to evoke the target response ("Johnny, what do you see?")
  - model the response ("Johnny, say 'I see two books.'")
  - record the response on a recording sheet (note that there is no reinforcement or corrective feedback)
  - present the next picture (e.g., that of two cups); repeat the procedure until all the 20 exemplars or 30 or 50 basic words are baserated (basic words to teach a set of core vocabulary for a nonverbal child)

- Administer <u>Evoked Baseline Trials</u> (note that on baseline trails, there is no reinforcement or corrective feedback for the child's responses):
  - place a stimulus picture or object in front of the child or demonstrate an action or enact an event
  - ask a question to evoke the target response; do not model the response
  - record the response on the recording sheet
  - repeat the procedure for all the 20 or the total number of selected exemplars

L

Lang. Dis./Comprehensive Treatment

- Calculate the percent correct baseline response rate in conversational samples and on discrete modeled and evoked trials
- Write a treatment and maintenance plan

Word and Phrase Level of Training

- Begin treatment by teaching a set of **functional words** to a nonverbal or minimally verbal child; select at least 20 functional words, most of them may be among the First Words children acquire (e.g., such words as *mommy* and *daddy*; food items like *milk, candy, juice, apple, banana*; clothing and personal items like *socks, shirt, pants, shoe*; simple adjectives like *big, little*; animals like *kitty, doggie*; and household objects like *spoon, chair, book, pen*); select child-specific words (e.g., names of siblings and those of pets) after consulting with the parents; establish the target words with the discrete modeled trials:
  - place a stimulus picture or object in front of the child
  - ask a question to evoke the target response (e.g., "Johnny, what is this?")
  - model the response ("Johnny, say *sock*.")
  - positively reinforce the correctly imitated response; accept an approximation of the correct response
  - if the child gave a wrong response, give corrective feedback by saying "No, that is not correct; it is a *sock*, not a ___."
  - if the child did not say anything, just move on to the next trial
  - move the stimulus picture or item toward you to signal the end of a trial
  - record the child's response on the recording sheet (correct, incorrect, or no response)

- wait for a few seconds, draw the child's attention, and present the next trial
- when the child correctly imitates the target word on 5 consecutive trials, stop modeling and present evoked trials
- follow the same procedure as before: present the stimulus, ask the question ("What is this?"), but do not model the response
- reinforce the correct response and give corrective feedback for the wrong response
- if the child gave 3 or 4 wrong responses on the first introduction of evoked trails, reinstate modeling; again withdraw modeling or fade modeling with Partial Modeling when the child correctly imitates the word on 5 consecutive trails
- continue training in this manner until the child gives at least 9 correct responses out of 10 evoked (no modeling) trails (a 90% accuracy in producing the word without modeling)
- initially reinforce continuously; in gradual steps, reduce the amount of reinforcers by switching to intermittent schedules
- always use social reinforcers even when using tangible reinforcers
- fade tangible reinforcers if used

L

- Train 4 to 6 exemplars (words at this level) to a training criterion of 90% correct on a set of 10 trials before you probe
- Note that probes of words taught will involve presenting the same trained words, asking a question, and recording the response; probe trails do not involve modeling, reinforcement, or corrective feedback; just ask questions and record the response
- If the child can produce the words without modeling or reinforcement on at least 4 of the 5 consecutive

presentations, consider those words as tentatively trained

- Train 4 to 6 more (new) words; train the new words as you did the original 4 to 6 words; when they are produced correctly on probe trials (no modeling, no reinforcement, no corrective feedback)
- Continue to train the selected functional words (some 30 to 50); make sure that the words trained include nouns (*car, cup, sock, ball, kitty, candy, man, woman, baby*), adjectives (*big, small, blue, red, thin, thick, smooth, rough, happy, sad, hot, cold*), and main verbs (*walking, sleeping, eating, running, jumping, smiling*)
- When all of the initially selected words meet the probe criterion, form two-word phrases out of already trained words (e.g., *big car, red sock, small kitty; man sleeping, woman walking, doggie eating*)
- Begin training the phrases with the same modeled discrete trials; fade modeling and move on to evoked discrete trails
- Probe the phrase production without modeling, reinforcement, or corrective feedback when you have trained 4 to 6 phrases; if probe criterion (90% correct) is met, begin training on new phrases; if not, continue training on the original set of phrases
- When about 20 phrases are trained and have met the probe criterion, shift training to the level of grammatical morpheme and sentence training

Teaching Grammatical Morphemes and Syntactic Structures

- Note that one grammatic morpheme, the present progressive *ing,* may have been taught in the context of main verbs (e.g., walk*ing,* eat*ing*); similarly, irregular plural words (*men, women, children, teeth, feet*) also may have been trained as words; note also that some grammatical morphemes can be trained only in sentences (e.g., the auxiliary *is*; as in *The boy is running*) others could be trained in phrases (e.g., the regular plural *s* as in *Two books*); therefore, phrases and sentences are both involved at this level of training

- Initially, select grammatical morphemes that can be trained in phrases, as these are syntactically simpler and presumably easier for the child; select the regular plural inflections *s* (e.g., *two books, blue blocks, three cats, green plants*) and plural *z* (e.g., *four bags, two dogs, red balls, long trains*) for the initial training; other morphemes in phrases include the irregular plurals (*two women, big men, white teeth, big feet*); prepositions *on* (*on the table, on the bed*) and *in* (e.g., *in the hat, in the box*); possessive inflection (e.g., *mommy's hat, doggie's tail*) and so forth

- Use the discrete trial procedure to establish the morphemes; show a picture, ask a question, and model the phrases with an emphasis on the grammatical morpheme (e.g., "Johnny, What is this? Say two books."); fade modeling and train with evoked trails

- When 4 to 6 exemplars are trained to the training criterion of 90% correct on a set of 10 evoked trials, probe for generalized production of the morpheme; note that at this stage, probes are different than they were at the word level

- Use initially the <u>Intermixed Probe Procedure</u> in which you alternate trained and untrained exemplars to assess the generalized productions of the morpheme (such as the plural *s*) in *untrained* phrase; use at least 10 untrained stimulus items; administer intermixed probes as follows:

   1. first, present a stimulus, object, or event used in training; ask a question to evoke the response; reinforce or give corrective feedback; record the response on a <u>Probe Recording Sheet</u>; note that

the trained exemplar in an intermixed probe sequence is presented as it was during training

2. next, present a stimulus, object, or event not used in training (the *probe item*); ask a question; do **not** reinforce or give corrective feedback; record the response
3. present another stimulus used in training; use the same procedure as in #1
4. present another stimulus not used in training and use the same procedure as in #2

- Calculate the percent correct probe response rate; score responses given only to the untrained stimulus items (exemplars) for this calculation (e.g., if the child gave 5 correct responses out of 10 untrained stimulus presentations, the probe response rate is 50%)
- If the child does not meet the intermixed probe criterion of 90% correct production of the grammatic morpheme in phrases, train additional phrases with the same morpheme
- If the child meets the intermixed probe criterion, shift training to the sentence level; expand items already trained into short sentences (e.g., *I see three cats; I see big men*).
- Continue to train the grammatic morphemes in sentences; once again, use the same sequence as the modeled trials leading to evoked trials, intermixed probes, and additional training if the probe criterion is missed
- When the child meets the probe criterion for morphemes in sentences, move training to conversational speech
  - evoke speech in naturalistic contexts with pictures, toys, books, and so forth
  - engage the child in conversation

- reinforce the production of grammatic morphemes
- give corrective feedback for errors
- Select new grammatic features or syntactic structures for training; train each in an appropriate entry level (most of them in phrases or sentences; some in words); then move them through other levels (sentences, conversational speech) as described; for example, teach the production of
  - auxiliaries *is, are, was, were* and so forth (e.g., *girl is reading, boy is running; women are writing, dogs are chasing; he was sleeping, she was smiling; they were working, men were digging*)
  - copula *is, was, are,* and *were* (e.g., *girl is nice; boy was happy; turtles are slow; plants were green*)
  - regular past tense inflection (e.g., *he mailed; he mailed yesterday; he painted; he painted yesterday; she walked; she walked yesterday*)
  - irregular past words (e.g., *he came, she went; he came home; she went to store*)
  - articles *a* and *the* (e.g., *the girl, the boy; the girl is reading, the boy is running*); note that phrases that were trained earlier to induce the production of another phoneme may be used to add additional grammatic elements
  - pronouns *he, she,* and *it* (e.g., *he is playing, she is riding, it is hopping*)
  - conjunction *and* (e.g., *milk and cookies; I like milk and cookies; lions and tigers; I like lions and tigers*)
  - comparative *-er* and superlative *-est* (e.g., *dark; this is darker; this is the darkest; warm; this is warmer; this is the warmest*)
  - adjectives *big* and *small* (e.g., *big house, small house; this is a big house, that is a small house*)
  - tacts or simple active declarative sentences (e.g., *This is a nice house; that is a pretty flower.*)

L

- mands or requests (*Juice, please; Crayon, please; Please give me that ball; I want that book; I want that car.*)
- questions (e.g., *What is this? Where is it? Who is it? When do you eat breakfast?*)
- negation (e.g., *she is not sleeping, he is not eating, they are not walking*)

- When a target behavior meets the intermixed probe criterion of 90% correct on at least 10 exemplars taught in sentences, administer the pure probe; note that on a pure probe, you do not present trained exemplars; present only untrained exemplars to evaluate whether a trained grammatic morpheme or a feature is produced in untrained contexts:
  1. present a stimulus, object, or event not used in training (e.g., the picture of several elephants, not used in training)
  2. ask a question to evoke the response (e.g., "What do you see?")
  3. do **not** reinforce or give corrective feedback for the response; the child's response may be correct (e.g., "I see many elephant**s**.") or incorrect (e.g., "I see elephant.")
  4. record the response as correct or incorrect
  5. present another stimulus picture **not** used in training and follow the same procedure
  6. present at least 10 untrained stimulus events
  7. calculate the percent correct pure probe response rate

- If the pure probe response rate is less than 90% correct, give additional training using untrained stimulus items

- When a target behavior meets a pure probe criterion of 90% correct on at least 10 untrained exemplars produced in sentences:

L

- begin training on a more complex response level (e.g., longer sentences or conversational speech)
- select another behavior for training if the treatment time permits

Teaching Conversational Skills and Pragmatic Features

- Discard discrete trials when you reach the conversational speech level:
  - loosen the training structure
  - use more spontaneous speech
  - talk about events (e.g., build blocks and talk about it); stimulate speech about events and complex stimuli (such as pictured sequences in a story book)
  - tell or read aloud stories the child retells
  - use more natural consequences (instead of verbal praise for correct productions) including agreement (affirmation), negation, smile, handing requested objects, meaningful responses to questions, and so forth
- Integrate Pragmatic Structures into training at the spontaneous, natural, conversational speech training level:
  - teach maintenance of eye contact during conversation by prompting and reinforcing the child for doing so
  - teach Topic Maintenance (described later in this section under Treatment of Language Disorders: Specific Techniques or Programs) by progressively increasing the duration for which the child talks about a topic
  - teach Turn Taking (described later in this section under Treatment of Language Disorders: Specific Techniques or Programs) by reinforcing the child to alternately play the role of a listener and that of a speaker

L

- teach Conversational Repair (described later in this section under Treatment of Language Disorders: Specific Techniques or Programs) strategies including asking questions when statements are not understood

Decreasing Undesirable Behaviors

- Decrease undesirable behaviors through Response Reduction Strategies; note that these may be the wrong language responses or such interfering behaviors as leaving the chair, interrupting treatment trials with irrelevant questions, not looking at the stimulus materials, and so forth
  - give corrective verbal feedback ("No" or "Not correct") for incorrect language responses (e.g., omitting the plural *s* in words and phrases)
  - use Extinction for such behaviors as crying or asking irrelevant and interrupting questions
  - prevent responses that seem to be related to difficult demands you make and thus negatively reinforced (e.g., prevent the child from leaving the chair when difficult trials are presented; continue to present the trials)
  - heavily reinforce an alternative, desirable behavior that replaces an undesirable behavior (e.g., give extra tokens for sitting to reduce the off-seat behaviors)
  - see Differential Reinforcement for more details and other procedures

Implementing a Maintenance Program

- Implement a maintenance procedure
  - have family members, teachers, caretakers, peers, and others observe the treatment sessions
  - train the significant others, especially the family members and teachers, in evoking, prompting, and consequating target behaviors

- have family members conduct informal therapy sessions at home and bring recorded evidence to that effect
- ask the child's teacher to provide opportunities for communication in the classroom and to praise the child for producing targeted and other language skills
- hold informal training sessions outside the clinic room, outside the building, in other parts of the school or campus, and at other settings to the extent practical
- use intermittent reinforcement schedule and natural, social reinforcers
- delay reinforcement in later stages of treatment; increase the delay in gradual steps
- always take training to the natural conversational level
- teach Reinforcement Priming by training the child to draw attention to his or her newly acquired communicative skills
- teach Self-Control (Self-Monitoring) by training the child to recognize and measure his or her right and wrong responses
- continue treatment until the language skills stabilize in the natural environment
- ensure Follow-Up and provide Booster Treatment
- see Maintenance Strategy

Hegde, M. N. (1996). *A coursebook on language disorders in children.* San Diego: Singular Publishing Group.

Hegde, M. N. (1998a). *Treatment procedures in communicative disorders* (3rd ed.). Austin, TX: Pro-Ed.

Hegde, M. N. (1998b). *Treatment protocols in communicative disorders.* Austin, TX: Pro-Ed.

Shipley, K. G., & McAfee, J. (1998). *Assessment in speech-language pathology: A resource manual* (2nd ed.). San Diego: Singular Publishing Group.

L

Treatment of Language Disorders in African American Children. In treating language disorders of African American children, consider the following guidelines and the African American English characteristics; these characteristics, although different from standard English usage, are not indicative of language disorders; therefore, they are not targets of language treatment; acquiring standard English expressions may be a goal of some African American children and their families; in such cases, teaching standard English patterns of usage is acceptable.

- Make a thorough assessment of the child's African American English (AAE) and standard English usage; consult the cited sources and the *PGASLP*
- Make sure that the child and his or her family do use AAE; note that not all African Americans use AAE at home
- Consult with the child's family members about their goals for language treatment; ask whether they want to have the standard English language patterns taught as well
- Consult with an African American speech-language pathologist in your area or with one who specializes in AAE characteristics; develop resources on AAE and culture for future clinical use
- Select language treatment targets that are consistent with AAE and the goals of the family, are useful to the child, help meet the child's educational and social demands, and will quickly improve the child's communicative skills
- Work with the teachers and other special educators to have them appreciate the child's language patterns and not make negative evaluations
- Refer the child to other specialists as needed (e.g., to an audiologist); educate the family about needed and available services, resources, and support

- Consider the following AAE characteristics as summarized by Roseberry-McKibbin (1995); select treatment targets that are consistent with these characteristics; see also, <u>Treatment of Articulation and Phonological Disorders in African American Children</u>

AAE Characteristic	Mainstream American English	Sample AAE Utterances
Noun possessives may be omitted.	That's the woman's car. It's John's pencil.	That *the woman* car. It *John* pencil.
Noun plurals may be omitted.	He has 2 boxes of apples. She gives me 5 cents.	He got 2 *box of apple*. She give me 5 *cent*.
Third person singular may be omitted	She walks to school. The man works in his yard.	She *walk* to school. The man *work* in his yard.
Forms of *to be* (*is, are*) may be omitted.	She is a nice lady. They are going to a movie.	*She a* nice lady. *They going* to a movie.
Present tense *is* may be used regardless of person or number.	They are having fun. You are a smart man.	*They is* having fun. *You is* a smart man.
Person or number may not agree with past and present forms.	You are playing ball. They are having a picnic.	You *is* playing ball. They *is* having a picnic.
Present tense forms of auxiliary *have* may be omitted.	I have been here for 2 hours.	I been here for 2 hours. He done it again.
Past tense endings may be omitted.	He lived in California. She cracked the nut.	He *live* in California. She *crack* the nut.

L

Past tense *was* may be used regardless of number and person.	They were shopping. You were helping me.	They *was* shopping. You *was* helping me.
Multiple negatives may be used to add emphasis to the negative meaning.	We don't have any more. I don't want any cake. I don't like Broccoli.	We don't have no more. I don't never want no cake. I don't never like Broccoli.
None may be substituted for *any*.	She doesn't want any.	She don't want *none*.
In perfective constructions, *been* may be used to indicate that an action took place in the past.	I had the mumps when I was 5.	I *been had* the mumps when I was 5. I *been known* her.
Done may be combined with a past tense form to indicate that an action was started and completed	He fixed the stove. She tried to paint it.	He *done fixed* the stove. She *done tried* to paint it.
The form *be* may be used as the main verb.	Today she is working. We are singing.	Today *she be* working. *We be* singing.
Distributive *be* may be used to indicate actions and events over time.	He is often cheerful. She's kind sometimes.	*He be* cheerful. *She be* kind.
A pronoun may be used to restate the subject.	My brother surprised me. My dog has fleas.	My brother, *he* surprise me. My dog, *he* got fleas.

L

Them may be substituted for *those.*	Those cars are antiques. Where'd you get those books?	*Them cars,* they be antique. Where you get *them books*?
Future tense is and *are* may be replaced by *gonna.*	She is going to help us. They are going to be there.	She *gonna* help us. They *gonna* be there.
At may be used at the end of *where* questions.	Where is the house? Where is the store?	Where is the house *at*? Where is the store *at*?
Additional auxiliaries may be used.	I might have done it.	I *might could have* done it.
Does may replace *do.*	She does funny things. It does make sense.	*She do* funny things. *It do* make sense.

Roseberry-McKibbin, C. (1995). *Multicultural students with special needs.* Oceanside, CA: Academic Communication Associates.

Treatment of Language Disorders in Children of Asian Cultures. Children of Asian cultures are a heterogeneous group; very few generalized statements can be made abut these children; people of Asia speak a bewildering variety of languages, belonging to different languages, and each language may have many dialects; languages of China, the Indian subcontinent, and South East Asia differ widely; much of the available information described under the Asian heading pertains to the languages of China; some of the characteristics listed may apply to other Asian children; use the guidelines offered in this section with caution while treating children of Asian background.

- Make a thorough assessment of the child's primary language and English language skills; consult the cited sources and the *PGASLP*

- Make sure that the child and his or her family do use a primary language that is other than English at home; some Asian children may acquire English as their first language although the parents speak a different language at home

- Consult with the child's family members about their goals for language treatment; ask whether they want to have the standard English language patterns taught as well

- Consult with a bilingual speech-language pathologist in your area or with one who specializes in Asian languages in general or the child's primary language in particular; develop resources on the different Asian languages spoken in your service area for future clinical use

- Select language treatment targets that are consistent with the child's primary language and the goals of the family, are useful to the child, help meet the child's educational and social demands, and will quickly improve the child's communicative skills

- Work with the teachers and other special educators to have them appreciate the child's English language patterns that are due to his or her primary Asian language and not make negative evaluations

- Refer the child to other specialists as needed (e.g., to an audiologist); educate the family about needed and available services, resources, and support

- Consider the following characteristics of Asian communication patterns Roseberry-McKibbin (1995) summarizes; select treatment targets based on these characteristics for a child whose primary language is an Asian language; note that not all characteristics may apply to all Asian languages; see also, <u>Treatment of Articulation and Phonological Disorders in Bilingual Children</u>

Asian Language Characteristics	Sample English Utterances
Omission of plurals	Here are two piece of toast. I got 5 finger on each hand.
Omission of copula	He going home now. They eating.
Omission of possessive	I have Phuong pencil. Mom food is cold.
Omission of past tense morpheme	We cook dinner yesterday. Last night she walk home.
Past tense double marking	He didn't went by himself
Double negative	They don't have no books
Subject-verb-object relationship differences/omissions	I messed up it. He like.
Singular present tense omission or addition	You goes inside. He go to the store.
Wrong ordering of interrogatives	You are going now?
Misuse or omission of prepositions	She is in home. He goes to school 8:00.
Misuse of pronouns	She husband is coming She said her wife is here.
Omission and/or overgeneralization of articles	Boy is sick. He went the home.
Incorrect use of comparatives	This book is gooder than that book.

L

Omission of conjunctions	You _____ I going to the beach.
Omission, lack of inflection on auxiliary "do"	She _____ not take it. He do not have enough.
Omission, lack of inflection on forms of "have"	She have no money. We _____ been the store.
Omission of articles	I see little cat.

Roseberry-McKibbin, C. (1995). *Multicultural students with special needs*. Oceanside, CA: Academic Communication Associates.

Treatment of Language Disorders in Hispanic Children. Information on treating children whose primary language is Spanish is accumulating faster than information on other minority language groups in the United States; most guidelines offered here are relevant to all children whose primary language is other than English; adapt these guidelines to other groups by learning more about the primary language and communication patterns of your bilingual client in need of language treatment.

- Make a thorough assessment of the child's primary language and English language skills; consult the cited sources and the *PGASLP*
- Make sure that the child and his or her family do use a primary language that is other than English at home; some ethnoculturally diverse children may acquire English as their first language even though the parents speak a different language at home
- Consult with the child's family members about their goals for language treatment; ask whether they want to have the standard English language patterns taught as well

- Consult with a bilingual speech-language pathologist in your area or with one who specializes in the child's primary language characteristics; develop resources on the different languages spoken in your service area for future clinical use
- Select language treatment targets that are consistent with the child's primary language and the goals of the family, are useful to the child, help meet the child's educational and social demands, and will quickly improve the child's communicative skills
- Work with the teachers and other special educators to have them appreciate the child's English language patterns that are due to his or her primary language and not make negative evaluations
- Refer the child to other specialists as needed (e.g., to an audiologist); educate the family about needed and available services, resources, and support
- Consider the following characteristic of Spanish-influenced English as Roseberry-McKibbin (1995) summarizes; select treatment targets that are consistent with these characteristics; see also, Treatment of Articulation and Phonological Disorders in Bilingual Children

Spanish-Influenced Language Characteristics	Sample English Utterances
1. Adjective comes after the noun.	The house green.
2. s is often omitted in plurals and possessives.	The girl book is. . . .
3. Past tense -ed is often omitted.	We walk yesterday.
4. Double negatives are required.	I don't have no more.

5. Superiority is demonstrated by using *mas*.	This cake is more big.
6. The adverb often follows the verb.	He drives very fast his motorcycle.

Roseberry-McKibbin, C. (1995). *Multicultural students with special needs.* Oceanside, CA: Academic Communication Associates.

Treatment of Language Disorders in Native American Children. Children of Native Americans (American Indians) also speak a variety of languages belonging to different language families; however, it is likely that many children acquire English as their only language, as the American Indian languages are on the decline even within their own communities; follow the guidelines offered here with caution and try to develop information on the particular language and culture of the child being treated; if the child does speak one of the several Native American languages, he or she is then essentially a bilingual child with varying English proficiency.

- Make a thorough assessment of the child's primary language and English language skills; consult the cited sources and the *PGASLP*
- Make sure that the child and his or her family do use a Native American language at home and that English is a second language; many American Indian children do not learn their native language and English may be their only language
- Consult with the child's family members about their goals for language treatment; ask whether they want to have the standard English language patterns taught as well
- Consult with a speech-language pathologist who knows the child's Native American language or an

expert in that language; develop resources on the different Native American languages spoken in your service area for future clinical use

- Select language treatment targets that are consistent with the child's Native American language and the goals of the family, are useful to the child, help meet the child's educational and social demands, and will quickly improve the child's communicative skills

- Work with the teachers and other special educators to have them appreciate the child's English language patterns that are due to his or her primary language and not make negative evaluations

- Refer the child to other specialists as needed (e.g., to an audiologist); educate the family about needed and available services, resources, and support

- Consider the following characteristics of native American communication styles as Roseberry-McKibbin (1995) summarizes; select treatment targets that are consistent with these characteristics; note that the information is not specific to any one Native American language; you will have to get that language-specific information before you can plan an effective treatment program; see also, Treatment of Articulation and Phonological Disorders in Bilingual Children; among Native Americans:

  - mutual respect is a high cultural value; avoiding eye contact and looking down is a standard method of showing respect

  - children are especially taught not to maintain eye contact while talking to adults; maintaining eye contact during conversation with an adult is a sign of rudeness and defiance

  - Native American mothers, especially those in the Navajo population, may not talk much while caring for their infants

- children are taught to listen, observe, and learn thereby
- in the judgment of patents, their children may have better auditory comprehension skills than their expressive language skills
- some parents may not encourage their children to speak their native language until their articulation is acceptable; therefore, children in the early years may be deprived of language learning opportunities
- a long period of nonverbal communication (pointing and gesturing) may pass before children begin to use words
- talking too much or talking English may be viewed as imitating the White Man
- Native American etiquette requires that a speaker pause before answering a question; quick answers imply that the question did not require much thought
- if unsure of an answer, children may not respond to a question
- children may be reluctant to express their opinions until the adults indicate that they have earned their right express their own opinions
- public expression of strong feelings is generally discouraged
- expression of grief in the presence of outsiders may be acceptable only during official mourning ceremonies

Roseberry-McKibbin, C. (1995). *Multicultural students with special needs*. Oceanside, CA: Academic Communication Associates.

Treatment of Language Disorders: Specific Techniques or Programs. Several specific treatment programs are available; some are more comprehensive than others; some have better evidence than others; some have little or no evidence; clinicians need to check the evidence before selecting a technique.

Activity-Based Language Intervention. Treating language disorders with the help of various activities designed to promote language production; a classroom-based approach in which each child has an individualized educational plan; activities are part of classroom activities and use natural antecedents and consequences.

- Plan activities that promote the production of specific language structures in children
- Plan activities around a theme if appropriate (e.g., activities related to going on a camping trip)
- Read stories, narrate events, and sing songs about the theme; include the various language targets for the children in the class
- Ask questions about the presented information
- Forget to give needed objects during activities, leading the child to request them
- Give needed items one at a time so the child requests each one
- Put needed things out of reach so the child asks for them
- Put needed things in a clear jar that the child can see but cannot open to gain access and hence has to request help
- Hide the child's belongings to encourage requests
- Introduce novel items (e.g., wear a funny hat) and let those who talk about it wear it
- Pause during verbal or nonverbal actions so the child will request that you continue

Bricker, D., & Cripe, J. (1992). *An activity-based approach to early intervention*. Baltimore, MD: Paul H. Brookes.

Child-Centered Approaches to Language Intervention. Play-oriented, Indirect Language Stimulation in which the clinician does not target specific language structures to teach; the clinician may arrange stimuli that are more likely to evoke language structures; uses such techniques as Reversed Imitation (clinician's imitation of the child's utterance), Expansion, Extension, Parallel-Talk, Recast, and Self-Talk (all described later in this section); needs more evidence to document its effectiveness.

Conversational Repair. Skills of handling breakdown in communication; a pragmatic language structure and a treatment target during conversational skill training; refers to such skills as asking questions when messages are not clear and responding to requests for clarification; needs more evidence to support its widespread use.

Teach the Child to Request Clarifications From a Speaker. Play the role of a speaker who makes ambiguous or unclear statements:

- Make ambiguous statements (e.g., say "Give me the car" when you have displayed several toy cars)
- Wait for the child to request clarification
- If the child does not request clarification and responds anyway (such as picking one of the cars), say "No"
- Wait for the child to request clarification
- If the child does not request clarification, model a response for the child (e.g., "When you are not sure, I want you to ask me 'What do you mean?' OK?")
- Make another ambiguous statement
- Immediately model the request for clarification for the child
- Reinforce the child for imitating the request for clarification (e.g., "What do you mean?")
- Make another ambiguous statement
- Prompt (not model) a request for clarification (e.g., "What do you ask me?")
- Reinforce the child for asking for clarification (e.g., "What do you mean?")
- Introduce varied ambiguous statements

- Fade modeling and prompting
- Train parents in teaching the child to request for clarification
- Probe the generalized repair skill by presenting untrained messages
- Continue training until a set probe criterion (such as 90% accuracy in responding with the target skill) is met

Teach the Child to Vary the Expressions When Requested by a Listener Who Does Not Understand. Play the role of a listener who does not fully understand the expressions of the child:

- Ask the child to repeat
- Ask the child "What do you mean?"
- Tell the child "I do not understand"
- Negate a child's utterance so the child will clarify by assertion ("You did not go on the roller coaster 20 times did you?"; the child might say "No, I went on it two times.")
- Model the clarified statement by modifying what the child said ("You mean you went on the roller coaster two times, right?")
- Rephrase the child's utterance into a question and say it with a rising intonation ("You went on the roller coaster 20 times?")
- Model different ways of saying the same thing
- Ask the child to say it differently; reinforce varied phrases or sentences
- Periodically stop responding (e.g., to the child's request) to prompt the child to rephrase
- Train parents to prompt the child to vary expressions and to reinforce the child for compliance
- Probe the generalized repair skill by presenting untrained messages
- Continue training until a set probe criterion (such as 90% accuracy in responding with the target skill) is met

Conversational Skill. A language skill in maintaining a dialogue with one or more partners; an intervention goal for all clients with language disorders; collection of skills that include <u>Topic Initiation,</u> <u>Topic Maintenance,</u> and <u>Turn Taking</u> (all described later in this section).

- Use <u>Peer Modeling</u> (described later in this section); recruit peers who have good conversational skills to model those skills to the client
- Train the peers to model and have the client participate in conversation
- Closely monitor the behaviors of the peer models and the client
- Train peer models to be the hosts of a mock talk show
- Ask open-ended questions (you or the peer model)
- Ask follow-up questions (you or the peer model)
- Prompt the peer and the client for appropriate behaviors
- Train the client to ask questions
- Reinforce the client for new topic initiations, appropriate turn taking, and topic maintenance; if necessary, train these skills separately
- Show videotaped model interactions between adults, between children, and between children and adults
- Let the children analyze the tapes
- Let the children recreate what they saw on the tapes
- Train parents to conduct informal conversational skills training sessions at home

Delayed Stimulus Presentation. A child language intervention procedure in which the clinician delays providing such special stimuli as modeling for about 15 seconds to see if the child responds without such stimuli; provides the stimuli only when the child does not respond within the time limit.

- Establish joint attention regarding a stimulus (e.g., hold an object; establish eye contact with the child; look questioningly or expectantly)
- Do not speak for 15 seconds when the child approaches you or looks at you
- Model a mand or a name after the 15-second delay
- Give the object when the child imitates your modeling
- Give the object anyway when you have modeled 3 times and the child has not yet imitated

Direct Language Treatment Approaches. Intervention approaches in which the clinician selects specific language targets, designs a treatment environment and implements the treatment; uses specific stimuli including modeling, prompting, and manual guidance; uses explicit reinforcement contingencies; expects the child to imitate or produce specific targets upon stimulation; moves through a planned sequence of treatment stages.

Environmental Language Intervention Strategy (ELIS). A language intervention method for preschool children; developed and researched by J. D. McDonald and associates; a structured, direct treatment strategy; takes a semantic approach to teaching grammar; emphasizes generalized production at home; especially useful in training parents to conduct language stimulation sessions at home.

- Establish baselines of selected target language structures
- Structure treatment in three phases: imitation, conversation, and play
- Introduce the three procedures in the first three individual training sessions
- Train parents to record responses and administer the treatment program at home; train them in the Management of Behavioral Contingencies

- After the first three training sessions, integrate imitation, conversation, and play into a single session
- Spend the first 15 minutes on imitative productions
  - present a nonlinguistic stimuli (throw a ball)
  - present a linguistic stimuli (e.g., "Say, throw ball.")
- Spend the next 15 minutes on conversational speech
  - present the same nonlinguistic stimuli
  - ask a question (e.g., "What am I doing?")
  - model if necessary (e.g., "Say throw ball. What am I doing?")
- Spend the final 15 minutes on play activity during which the production of the target behavior is reinforced
  - let the child play with the material used in imitation and conversation
  - evoke responses from the child that are relevant to the child's actions (e.g., if the child throws the ball, ask, "What are you doing?")
- Give such positive reinforcers as tokens and verbal praise for correct responses
- Give such corrective feedback as Time-Out for incorrect productions
- Ask parents to conduct at home three weekly sessions similar to yours
- In each session, review the records of home training and suggest modifications

MacDonald, J. D., Blott, J. P., Gordon, K., Spiegel, B., & Hartman, M. (1974). An experimental parent-assisted treatment program for preschool language-delayed children. *Journal of Speech and Hearing Disorders, 39,* 395–415.

Event Structures in Language Treatment. Use of repetitive, sequentially organized, familiar events from daily life to teach language structures to children; an event structure may be the same as a Script used in Script Therapy (described later in this section); the two may be used in conjunction; also similar to Joint Action Routines or Interactions (described later in this section); needs more evidence to support its practice.

- Select a common event the child has repeatedly experienced (e.g., shopping for a toy, eating in a restaurant, taking part in a birthday party)
- Describe the event verbally
- Assign roles to yourself and the child (e.g., customer and the store clerk)
- Use props to act out the event
- Reverse roles and act out the events; repeat until the various language structures of interest are rehearsed
- Evoke words and phrases as you act out the event by using pauses at junctures (using the Cloze Procedure)
- Evoke increasingly complex or longer description of events
- Vary the sequence and event elements (e.g., after having worked with the event shopping for a toy, have the child work with the event shopping for clothing)
- Violate expected events or sequences and let the child question you or correct you (e.g., go to the sales clerk without trying the clothes)

Expansions. Expanding a child's incomplete or telegraphic statements into grammatically more complete productions; part of Indirect Language Stimulation.

- Arrange a play situation that provides opportunities for language production
- Engage in parallel play with the child or take part in the child's activities
- Expand the child's structurally incomplete productions into more complete sentences (e.g., a boy says "baby cry" as he looks at a picture; you expand it into "The baby is crying.")
- Do not ask the child to imitate your expansions

Expatiations. The same as Extensions.

333

Extensions. Comments on the child's utterances to add additional meaning; part of Indirect Language Stimulation; also known as Expatiations.

- Arrange a play situation that provides opportunities for language production
- Engage in parallel play with the child or take part in the child's activities
- Extend the child's semantically limited productions into semantically richer, structurally complete sentences through comments, (e.g., a girl says "play ball" as she plays with a ball; you extend it to include additional meaning: "Yes, you are playing with a big ball"; "You are playing with a blue ball.")
- Do not ask the child to imitate your extensions

Eye Contact. A potential pragmatic communication target behavior for certain children who do not look at the listener while speaking or at the speaker while talking; potentially culturally determined; need culturally sensitive assessment and treatment.

- Target eye contact from the beginning and especially during conversational speech training
- Use simple instruction and verbal praise
- Prompt the child by saying "Look at me" before you present stimuli, when you begin to talk, and when the child begins to talk
- Hold the stimulus parallel to your face so the child looks at the face and the stimulus simultaneously
- Praise the child for maintaining eye contact
- To track progress, measure the duration for which eye contact was maintained at the beginning (baseline) and throughout the treatment phase
- Fade the prompts or other cues used

Focused Stimulation. A technique of language intervention in which the clinician repeatedly models a target structure to stimulate the child to use that structure; usually a part of play activity.

- Design a play activity to focus on a particular language structure (e.g., the plural morpheme *s*)
- Collect various stimulus materials (books, cups, hats)
- Talk about the materials and repeatedly model the plural constructions (e.g., "I see two *books* here. The books have pictures. Here are two red *cups*. You can drink out of these *cups*. There are some *hats*. The *hats* are big.")
- Do not correct the child's wrong productions
- Respond to the child's nontarget responses without insisting on the correct response (e.g., the child says "The *book* is nice"; the clinician says "Yes, the books are nice.")
- Continue until the child begins to produce the target structure

Imitation of Child's Utterances. Reversed Imitation in which the clinician imitates a child's utterance during Indirect Language Stimulation; need more controlled clinical data to support its use.

Incidental Teaching Method. A Naturalistic Child Language Teaching Method (described later in this section) that uses typical, everyday verbal interactions to teach functional communication skills; the child often initiates an interactional episode; the clinician turns such episodes into opportunities to teach language; emphasis is on communication; effective when the child and the teacher interact for extended periods of time and in natural settings (e.g., in special education classrooms, institutions for the retarded and the autistic); excellent method for parents to learn and use at home)

- Select certain functional communicative skills for teaching (e.g., requests)
- Arrange therapy situations such that the child is likely to initiate a conversational exchange (e.g., place attractive toys on a shelf the child can see but

cannot reach; arrange a child's clothing items or some desirable food items)

- Stay close to the arranged materials and give nonverbal cues to speak (focused attention on the child and a questioning look)
- Give a verbal cue (e.g., ask "What do you want?") only if the nonverbal prompts fail to evoke a response from the child
- Give cues that evoke more complex responses (e.g., "Ask me in a sentence" if the child gives only single-word responses)
- Reinforce the child with natural consequences (e.g., "Good, here is the car"; "Very good, here is your sock"; "Fine, have some juice.")
- Arrange as many such teaching episodes as possible in a day

Hart, B. B., & Risley, T. R. (1982). *How to use incidental teaching for elaborating language.* Lawrence, KS: H & H Enterprises.

Indirect Language Stimulation. A collection of language stimulation procedures that are a part of play-oriented approach to teaching language disorders; also called Child-Centered Approach (described earlier in this section); less structured and more naturalistic; thought to be especially suitable for children who are passive, reluctant, or unmotivated to communicate; based on the assumption that variables observed in normally developing children are effective clinical treatment strategies; needs more controlled evidence to support this approach.

- Arrange a play situation that provides opportunities for language production
- Choose the play materials that are relevant for the targeted response
- Let the child lead the interaction
- Engage in parallel play with the child or take part in the child's activities

- Talk about what the child is doing, looking, playing, or talking
- Describe what you do (e.g., "See, I am drawing a face; I am drawing"; Self-Talk) (described later in this section)
- Describe or comment on what the child is doing (Parallel-Talk, described later in this section) (e.g., you say "You are drawing; you are drawing a face; you are making a nose.")
- Imitate the child's production (do *not* ask the child to imitate)
- Use Expansions (described earlier in this section); expand the child's telegraphic speech into grammatically more complete sentences (e.g., the child says "Mommy hat"; you expand this to "That is Mommy's hat.")
- Use Extensions (described earlier in this section); comment on the child's utterances to add additional meaning (e.g., the child says "Mommy hat," and you say "Yes, it is a big blue hat.")
- Recast (described later in this section) the child's utterances (expand the child's utterance type into a different kind of sentence (e.g., the child says "Mommy hat"; you ask a question, "Is this Mommy's hat?" or make a statement "This is not Mommy's hat.")
- Do not ask the child to imitate; do not target specific language structures; do not explicitly reinforce correct productions

Integrated Functional Intervention. Approach to language treatment that emphasizes natural contexts for training, conversational speech as the main mode of training, and increased involvement of parents and significant others in promoting and maintaining language skills.

Interactive Language Development Teaching. One of Directed Language Treatment Approaches to teach syntactic structures; the clinician reads a story to the child and then asks a series of questions designed to evoke specific language structures from the child.

- Select a story that targets language concepts (e.g., camping, cooking) and specific language responses (e.g., the auxiliary *is* or preposition *on*)
- Read the story to the child
- Ask questions frequently as you tell the story to evoke specific responses (e.g., "Daddy said a bear is coming [part of the story]. What did Daddy say?" [question to evoke the response "bear is coming"])

Lee, L., Koeningsknecht, R., & Mulhens, S. (1975). *Interactive language development teaching.* Evanston, IL: Northwestern University Press.

Joint Action Routines or Interactions. Use of repetitive, routinized activities in early language stimulation; an Indirect Language Stimulation method; similar to Script Therapy (described later in this section) or may be a variation of it.

- Use such established routines as "peek-a-boo"
- Design your own routines of action (e.g., always start treatment with telling the same short story that contains certain target language structures)
- Encourage the child to use the repetitive words, phrases, and sentences
- Reverse roles and let the child practice other language structures
- Violate a routine and let the child question you (e.g., skip the story and let the child ask "Story?" or "What about the story?")

Joint Book Reading. Systematic use of storybook reading to teach or stimulate language in children; allows for repetitive use and practice of the same phrases and concepts; helpful in establishing joint attention as well.

- Select story books that are linguistically and culturally appropriate for children under treatment
- Select books with colorful pictures
- Read the same story several times during a few sessions so that children memorize it
- Use prosodic features frequently to draw attention to specific language structures
- When the children know the story well, pause at points containing target language structures and prompt the children to supply the words, phrases, or sentences
- During different readings, pause at different junctures so the children produce different language structures
- Manipulate and vary pause locations that prompt progressively longer utterances from the children
- Ask a child to "read" (recite from memory, but looking at the text and the pictures) and pause
- Let the other children supply the words, phrases, and sentence

Kirchner, D. (1991). Reciprocal book reading. A discourse-based intervention strategy for the child with atypical language development. In T. Gallagher (Ed.), *Pragmatics of language: Clinical practice issues* (pp. 307–332). San Diego: Singular Publishing Group.

Whitehurst, G., Falco, F., Lonigan, C., Fischel, J., DeBrayshe, B., Valdez-Menchaea, M., & Caulfield, M. (1988). Accelerating language development through picture-book reading. *Developmental Psychology, 24,* 552–558.

Mand-Model. A variation of the Incidental Teaching Method (described earlier in this section); uses typical adult-child interactions in a play-oriented setting to teach language; supported by controlled evidence.

- Select a variety of attractive toys, pictures, and other stimulus materials
- Design a naturalistic interactive situation

- Establish a joint clinician-child attention to a particular material (such as a toy); if necessary, direct the child's attention to a stimulus
- <u>Mand</u> a response from the child (e.g., say "Tell me what you want" or "Tell me what this is.")
- Model the correct, complete response if the child fails to respond or gives a limited (e.g., single word) response
- Prompt if the child does not imitate the whole sentence you modeled (e.g., "Tell me the whole sentence.")
- Praise the child for imitating or for responding correctly without modeling
- Give the material the child wants as you praise

Rogers-Warren, A., & Warren, S. (1980). Mands for verbalization. *Behavior Modification, 4,* 230–245

Matching-to-Sample. A language teaching strategy; a child's response is reinforced only if it matches a sample; helps generate rule-based responding based on physical or functional similarity; supported by some evidence.

Teaching Matching-to-Sample on the Basis of Physical Similarity

- Display an array of stimuli in front of the child (e.g., a book, a ball, and a pencil)
- Hold a sample and show it to the child (e.g., a different book than the one displayed in front of the child)
- Ask the child to match it to the one displayed
- Reinforce the correct matching (e.g., pointing to the book)

Teaching Matching-to-Sample on the Basis of Functional Similarity

- Display an array of stimuli in front of the child (e.g., a large blue sneaker, a small brown ball)
- Hold a sample that matches the function of one of the objects but the physical property of the

other object displayed (e.g., a small brown shoe) and show it to the child
- Ask the child to match it to the one displayed
- Reinforce the correct matching (e.g., the blue sneaker)

Milieu Teaching. A collection of child language intervention procedures that emphasize natural, functional, conversational communicative contexts for teaching language; a naturalistic child language teaching method; uses natural consequences as reinforcers; includes the Mand-Model and Incidental Teaching Method (described earlier in this section); supported by controlled evidence.

Narrative Skills Training. A speaker's description of events (stories, episodes) and experiences in a logically consistent, cohesive, temporally sequenced manner; analyzed in terms of a Story Grammar (described later in this section); an advanced language skill targeted during the final stages of intervention.

- Use the Event Structure (described earlier in this section) approach to give children experience in establishing Scripts (schemes of events)
  - play such scripts as grocery shopping, eating in a restaurant, birthday parties, camping trips, vacations, playing certain games, and so forth
  - play daily routine scripts (get children involved in daily activities)
  - repeatedly read or tell the same stories so the children memorize the words, temporal sequences, characters, and events
  - let the children act out the stories
  - let the children switch the roles on repeated scripts
- Ask children to narrate experiences as they play out scripts and assume different roles
- As you retell stories, pause before important phrases or critical descriptions so the children supply them

- Prompt the phrases and descriptions as the children hesitate; fade the prompts
- Ask the children to tell the stories or narrate events without enacting the scripts but with the help of pictures or slides
- Ask the children to tell stories or narrate events without scripts, pictures, or slides
- Ask the children to narrate new events or experiences (not rehearsed or scripted)

Nelson, N. W. (1993). *Childhood language disorders in context.* New York: Merrill.

Paul, R. (1995). *Language disorders from infancy through adolescence.* St. Louis, MO: C. V. Mosby.

Ripich, D. N., & Creaghead, N. A. (1994). *School discourse problems* (2nd ed.). San Diego: Singular Publishing Group.

Naturalistic Child Language Teaching Method. An approach that emphasizes natural, functional, conversational communicative contexts for teaching language to children; uses loose training structure; uses natural consequences as reinforcers; includes Incidental Teaching Method, Joint Action Routines or Interactions, Mand-Model, and Script Therapy (all described in this section).

Parallel-Talk. Describing or commenting on what the child is doing during play activities; part of Indirect Language Stimulation.

- Arrange play activities designed to enhance opportunities for language production
- Play with the child
- Describe the child's actions (e.g., "You are playing with the ball; you are bouncing the ball.")

Peer Modeling. A child language intervention method in which the peers are trained to model the target skills for the child.

- Select a peer who agrees to help and is acceptable to the client

- Have the peer observe your treatment sessions
- Describe the target behaviors, modeling and imitation sequence, and reinforcement procedures
- Let the peer model and reinforce the child's productions in your presence
- Refine the peer's skills in modeling the target behaviors
- Ask the peer to submit recorded language samples that document appropriate modeling outside the clinic
- Periodically assess the results of peer modeling and provide additional training to the peer

Reauditorization. Clinician's repetition of what a child says during language stimulation; often combined with such other techniques as modeling (often without requiring imitation); need more evidence to show its usefulness or effectiveness.

- Repeatedly model a target language feature in varied linguistic contexts (e.g., you say "The book is *on* the table; the cat is *on* the tree; the dog is *on* the house.")
- Point to a target stimulus or ask a question (point to a bird on a tree; or ask "Where is the bird?")
- Repeat the child's production "in tree" or "bird is in the tree"

Recast. Expansion of a child's utterance type (sometimes presumed) into a different type of sentence; a method of play-oriented, unstructured, Indirect Language Stimulation.

- Arrange play activity designed to enhance opportunities for language production
- Play with the child
- Expand the child's utterance into a sentence type that may be different from the child's presumably intended sentence type (e.g., the child says "Big ball"; you expand it into a negative sentence, "No,

it is not a big ball"; or expand it into a question form, "Is this a big ball?")

- Do not ask the child to imitate your recast sentences

Request for Repair. A listener's (clinician's in intervention sessions) use of various devices to let the client know that his or her expression was not clear and that the message needs to be altered.

- Ask the speaker (the child) to repeat
- Ask a question ("What do you mean?")
- Use negation to prompt the child to clarify a statement ("You did not have seventy friends at your birthday party, did you?")
- Model the correct response by saying what the child meant ("You mean you had seven friends at your birthday party.")
- Turn a child's utterance into a question with a rising intonation ("You had seventy friends?")

Scaffolding. A collection of procedures to make it easier for a child to produce specific language behaviors or perform academic tasks; communicative assistance or support given to the child by peers and adults; a shared learning environment that promotes communication between the child and adults; ways to simplify communicative and academic tasks for the child; needs experimental support.

To Teach Language Use

- Support the child in his or her attempts to speak
- Direct the child's attention to important aspects of learning and communication
- Give feedback to the child's questions and comments
- Give semantically contingent feedback
- Provide prompts and models
- Let peers help the child
- Encourage the child to ask questions
- Let the child take part in problem-solving activities

- Expand and elaborate the child's utterances
- Fade the degree of support

To Promote Academic Learning in a Collaborative Model

- Ask the teacher to reduce academic demands that the child cannot meet or give more time for assignments
- Highlight important terms, issues, questions, definitions in a child's textbook; ask the child to find the meanings of terms in a dictionary
- Work on listening, reading, writing, and other skills that are required in the classroom

Kirchner, D. (1991). Reciprocal book reading. A discourse-based intervention strategy for the child with atypical language development. In T. Gallagher (Ed.), *Pragmatics of language: Clinical practice issues* (pp. 307–332). San Diego: Singular Publishing Group.

Paul, R. (1995). *Language disorders from infancy through adolescence.* St. Louis, MO: C. V. Mosby.

Ripich, D. N., & Creaghead, N. A. (1994). *School discourse problems* (2nd ed.). San Diego: Singular Publishing Group.

Script Therapy. Language intervention procedure in which events and routines known to the child or made familiar by the clinician (Scripts) are used; procedures are similar to those under Event Structures and Joint Action Routines or Interactions (described earlier in this section); used in teaching advanced language skills including narrative skills; a script is usually not a written document although it may be in treatment; refers mostly to presumed ideas or a mental scheme a child may have about such common experiences as eating in a restaurant or grocery shopping; needs experimental support.

- Select language targets appropriate for the children to be taught (e.g., such action-object-locative constructions as "Put the doll in the box")
- Select routinized scripts for each target (e.g., scattered toys that the mother and the child sort and put away before bedtime)

- Assign different roles to the participants; assign one to yourself (e.g., one plays the role of the mother of a child being taught)
- Scatter several toys and have a box, a shelf, a table, and other objects for storing the toys
- Begin by saying something to initiate the script (routine activity) (e.g., "OK, it is bedtime! Let us pick up these toys and put them away.")
- Model target responses ("I am putting the doll in the box") and if the child imitates, reinforce
- Ask questions (e.g., "What are you doing?") and reinforce correct responses ("I am putting the car on the shelf.")
- Complete the script and reenact the same or similar scripts
- Probe for generalized production (probe the same target responses with different scripts)

Paul, R. (1995). *Language disorders from infancy through adolescence.* St. Louis, MO: C. V. Mosby.

Young, K. T., & Lombardino, L. J. (1991). The efficacy of script contexts in language comprehension intervention with children who have mental retardation. *Journal of Speech and Hearing Research, 34,* 845–857.

Self-Talk. Clinician's description of her own activity as she plays with the child; a method of play-oriented, more or less structured, Indirect Language Stimulation.

- Arrange play activities designed to enhance opportunities for language production
- Play with the child
- Describe your own actions using language structures appropriate for the child (e.g., "I'm squeezing the rubber ducky here; see I'm squeezing.")

Story Grammar. The structure of narratives that may be treatment targets for children with language disorders; a story grammar includes the following elements:

- Setting statements (e.g., introduction to the story, the characters, the physical setting, the temporal context)
- Initiating events (e.g., episodes that begin a story)
- Internal response (e.g., the characters' emotions, reactions, thoughts)
- Internal plans (e.g., the characters' strategies for achieving their objectives)
- Attempts (e.g., actions the characters take to achieve their objectives)
- Direct consequences (e.g., results of actions)
- Reactions (e.g., the characters' response to the results)

Stein, N., & Glenn, C. (1979). An analysis of story comprehension in elementary school children. In R. Freedle (Ed.), *New directions in discourse processing* (Vol. 2, pp. 53–120). Norwood, NJ: Ablex.

Topic Initiation (Treatment for). The skill to start conversation with a new topic; a conversational skill; a pragmatic feature of language; a language treatment target; children with language disorders either fail to initiate topics or introduce inappropriate topics.

- Arrange a variety of stimuli that could trigger a new topic: objects, pictures, storybooks, topic cards (for children who can read), toys, structured play situations such as a kitchen and so forth
- Introduce one of the stimulus items or situations and draw the child's attention to it (e.g., a picture of a family setting up a tent in a park)
- Wait for the child to initiate conversation about the picture and the story
- If the child does not initiate a topic, instruct the child to say something about the picture
- If the child does not initiate, prompt by beginning the story ("They are setting up a. . . .")

- Lavishly praise the child for saying anything related to the topic depicted
- Accept statements that are remotely connected to the topic at hand; gradually, demand more relevant responses
- Do not interrupt the child or overly correct the forms of responses
- Ask the child to use the topic cards to initiate new topics
- Ask the child to think of new topics to talk about
- Prompt new topics
- Withdraw or fade such prompts, cues, cards, pictures and other special stimuli to make topic initiation more spontaneous
- Train parents to use your techniques so they can continue intervention at home

Topic Maintenance (Treatment for). A pragmatic language skill and treatment target; talking about a single general topic for extended duration; frequent and abrupt switching of conversational topics suggests lack of this skill.

- Target topic maintenance when training has moved to the conversational speech stage or sooner if the session structures allow it
- Let the child select topics of interest for talking
- Set a realistic duration for which you want the child to talk on a single topic; or set a target number of words to be produced on a topic
- Increase the duration or the number of target words in gradual steps
- Use such devices as *Tell me more. What about that? What happened next? Who said what? Where was it? When did that happen?* and so forth to stimulate more speech on the same topic
- Reinforce the child for maintaining the topic

- Stop the child when he or she abruptly switches the topic
- Move the child back to the target topic
- Train on a few topics and then probe with untrained topics to see if the skills have generalized
- Train on additional topic exemplars if the skills have not generalized

Turn Taking (Treatment for). Appropriate exchange of speaker and listener roles during conversation; a pragmatic language skill; an advanced treatment target; interrupting a speaker and not responding to cues to talk are indicators of deficient turn taking.

- Select turn taking as a target when treatment has advanced to conversational speech or sooner if the child can handle it
- Baserate the number of interruptions and failure to take cues to talk
- Design a signal for the child to talk (e.g., such verbal cues as "Your turn" or nonverbal cues as a hand gesture to suggest *you speak*)
- Design a signal that says *do not interrupt* or *do not talk* because it is your (clinician's) turn to talk (e.g., finger on your lips)
- Use such other discriminative stimuli as a real or toy microphone that you exchange with the child; the one holding the microphone talks and the other listens
- Reinforce the child for talking only when signaled or while holding the microphone
- Follow the same rule that you impose on the child (e.g., talk only when you hold the microphone)
- Teach the child to say "It is your turn"
- Reinforce the child for yielding the floor
- Teach turn taking until the child meets a performance criterion (e.g., no errors of turn taking in two consecutive conversational exchanges)

- Fade the signals or other special discriminative stimuli used to prompt the child
- Probe without signals or special discriminative stimuli
- Train until a probe criterion is met (at least 90% accuracy in turn taking while not receiving reinforcers)

Whole Language Approach. A philosophical approach to language, especially reading and writing, that has implications for oral language teaching; does not strictly refer to a method of teaching oral language; advocates that in teaching, language should not be broken down into components; believes that all aspects of literacy including reading, writing, listening, and talking should be simultaneously taught as an integrated whole; considers the Language-Based Classroom Model of intervention to be the best to teach language because all aspects of literacy can be effectively addressed; suggests that academic programs should be the basis of language teaching; advocates a naturalistic approach to language teaching; the approach has not been supported by efficacy research and many educational specialists now reject this approach; its use in teaching language to children with language disorders is questionable; there are better, experimentally supported alternatives.

Language Deviance in Children. Somewhat similar to the term Language Disorders in Children; includes a connotation of some abnormality in the acquisition or use of language for which there is little empirical support; not strictly a synonym for language disorders; treatment procedures the same as those for Language Disorders in Children.

Language Impairment. Generally the same as language disorders; includes an acceptable connotation of a disturbed function; may be used interchangeably with language disorder; treatment procedures the same as those for Language Disorders in Children.

Language-Learning Disorders. Generally the same as language disorders; links language disorder to a general learning disorder that negatively affects academic learning; often used in special educational contexts; treatment procedures the same as those for <u>Language Disorders in Children</u>.

Language Problems. Generally the same as language disorders; a more general term that may be used interchangeably with language disorders; treatment procedures the same as those for <u>Language Disorders in Children</u>.

Language Stimulation by Parents. Activities parents implement at home to stimulate language in infants and toddlers; may be the only recommendation for a child; may supplement or parallel clinicians' treatment; supported by some evidence; more needed

- Assess the child and his or her family
- Assess the parents' education, sophistication, time commitment, and motivation to conduct regular activities at home
- Design a language stimulation program for the child
- Test the program in the clinic for a few sessions to make sure it works
- Have parents observe your sessions
- Train parents in the effective methods; model the methods frequently
- Have parents conduct a session or two in the clinic
- Give feedback and refine their skills
- Train them to keep records of therapy that you can evaluate
- Give parents simple, clear written instructions
- Give parents video taped samples of treatment techniques
- Periodically assess the child and the parents' sessions at home
- Suggest needed modifications and movement to higher levels of training
- Initiate formal treatment when your assessment indicates a need for it

Laryngeal Cleft.   A cleft between the larynx (cricoid cartilage) and the esophagus; caused by a failure of dorsal fusion of the cricoid lamina; may be accompanied by other congenital anomalies, including feeding and respiratory problems soon after birth.
- Treatment is surgical closure of the cleft

Laryngeal Cysts.   Formation of small, fluid-filled sacs on the larynx, especially in the ventricle; often congenital; caused by accumulation of glandular secretion in submucosal; symptoms include swollen false (ventricular) folds; if enlarged, can result in hoarseness.
- Treatment is surgical removal of the cyst
- Follow-up voice therapy may be needed in some cases

Laryngeal Hyperkeratosis.   A thickening of the laryngeal mucosa resulting from an abnormal growth of the epithelium; causes may include cigarette smoking, heavy alcohol use, environmental pollutants, dust, noxious gases, and strained and tense speaking habits; usually occurs on the true vocal folds; may sometimes be premalignant.
- Modify the client behavior to reduce exposure to the listed causal factors

Laryngeal Leukoplakia.   Appearance of white patches on the laryngeal mucosa; voice may be hoarse; may be premalignant.
- Modify client behavior to reduce or eliminate smoking
- Do not offer voice therapy for hoarseness as it is not effective

Laryngeal Stoma.   An opening made into the trachea between the thyroid glands to allow for breathing in patients with laryngectomy.

Laryngeal Web.   Growth of a thin membrane across portions of the vocal folds; may be congenital or induced by trauma later in life; negatively affects respiration.
- Treatment is surgical removal of the web

Laryngectomee. A person who has had a partial or total Laryngectomy.

Laryngectomy. Surgical removal of all or part of the larynx because of disease or trauma.

Treatment Procedures, Laryngectomy
Preoperative Evaluation and Counseling
- Work as a member of the rehabilitation team
- In consultation with the surgeon, counsel the patient and the family about the effects of medical treatment on communication
- Invite and answer all questions from the patient and the family members; give answers that are consistent with advice from other professionals on the team
- Do not withhold information if the patient would like to hear it
- Obtain a sample of the patient's speech and writing; make an assessment of client's communication skills
- Describe various methods of speaking without a larynx; discuss communication options that may be preferable to the client; be consistent with the surgeon's preferences and recommendations
- Reassure the patient that he or she will talk again by using new techniques
- Have the patient meet and speak with a rehabilitated Laryngectomee who has mastered Alaryngeal Speech

Postoperative Management
- If no prior counseling, discuss the current condition of the patient and the prospects for new methods of communication
- Review the information provided during the preoperative counseling
- Discuss methods of Alaryngeal Speech (described later in this section)
- Demonstrate how electronic speech aids work

L

- Teach the patient to use a <u>Pneumatic Device for Alaryngeal Speech</u> (described later in this section), if appropriate, to support immediate communication
- Discuss the patient's rehabilitation plan; be cautious in making prognostic statements
- Give written information on rehabilitation plans and possibilities for the patient to read later
- Arrange a visit from a rehabilitated <u>Laryngectomee</u> to encourage the patient

Teaching New Methods of Communication
General Principles

- Select an appropriate method of communication that the client prefers, judged to be efficient, and is practical
- Teach the client to use the new method of communication
- Select either a <u>Pneumatic Device for Alaryngeal Speech</u> or an <u>Electronic Device for Alaryngeal Speech</u> (both described later in this section) for permanent communication
- Let the client use a pneumatic device during the early postsurgical period as it is easier to use within days after surgery; let the client switch to an electronic device if that is preferred
- Begin to teach the use of an electronic device only after the neck and throat areas recover from swelling and tenderness and the surgical suture lines heal
- Teach tracheoesophageal speech if the patient is surgically prepared for it
- Consider both individual and group therapy sessions
- Determine the frequency of treatment sessions based on the patient's physical condition
- Consider daily sessions in the beginning if the patient's physical stamina permits them
- Hold at least one weekly session
- Get family members involved in training sessions

Laryngectomy

- Let the patient's performance and progress dictate the pace of therapy
- Ask the client to practice the new method of communication at home

Teach Alaryngeal Speech With Electronic Devices

- Select a neck-held electronic larynx after discussing various models with the patient
- Demonstrate first what the instrument sounds like and then how speech produced with its help sounds like
- Experiment with the best position on the neck (usually under the jaw); let the head of the device a good contact with the skin without pressing it
- Manipulate the button for sound production and ask the patient to count aloud
- Ask the patient to clearly shape the words with the mouth
- Ask the patient not to exhale forcefully
- Teach the patient to handle the device
- Instruct the patient to coordinate sound and speech and to turn off the sound when not talking
- Reduce the patient's rate of speech to increase intelligibility
- Teach the patient to increase articulatory precision by practicing words that begin with voiceless consonants
- Shape progressively longer utterances
- Teach the client to maintain eye contact with the listener

Teach Alaryngeal Speech With Pneumatic Devices

- Use pneumatic devices during the early phase of rehabilitation
- Select a pneumatic device after discussing various options
- Teach the patient to place the cup end of the device firmly over the Laryngeal Stoma so that there is no air leak

- Ask the patient to hold the cup end over the stoma and produce a sound by blowing out
- Ask the patient to blow out two and three sounds for every breath
- Ask the patient to change the pitch by increasing the air pressure
- Ask the patient to place the mouth piece on top of the tongue, while keeping the cup end over the Laryngeal Stoma
- Ask the patient to say vowels and then words
- Shape progressively longer utterances
- Give appropriate positive and corrective feedback

Teach Esophageal Speech

- Begin esophageal speech training soon after patient starts eating food orally
- Describe the anatomy and the physiology of esophageal speech production
- Describe esophageal sound production to the patient
- Use diagrams to explain esophageal speech
- Teach the client the production of esophageal sound
- Try various procedures and settle on the one most effective with the client
- Teach the patient to use the injection method of taking air into the esophagus
  - ask the patient to press the tongue tip against the alveolar ridge to push the air back toward esophagus without the tongue making contact with the pharyngeal wall (glossal press)
  - ask the client to press the tongue tip against the alveolar ridge and to move the tongue back to make contact with the pharyngeal wall; thus push air back into the esophagus (glossopharyngeal press)
  - ask the patient to keep the velopharyngeal port closed
  - ask the client to inject the air in an audible manner, producing the sound called the "klunk"

L

- Teach the patient to use the inhalation method of taking air into the esophagus if necessary; be aware that some experts use only the injection method for most of their patients
  - teach the patient to synchronize the air intake through the stoma with air intake through the mouth into the upper esophagus; relaxed PE segment and the resulting negative pressure there will help air movement into upper esophagus
- Ask the patient to produce plosive consonants to stimulate esophageal sound
- Instruct the patient to say ta-ta-ta
- Ask the patient to use easy injection of air and say a series of ta-ta-ta
- Reinforce a likely emergence of esophageal sound
- Teach the patient to puff the cheeks out and move the air trapped in the mouth from one side to another; instruct the patient to move this trapped air quickly into the esophagus
- Ask the patient to produce words that typically trigger sound production: *church, stop, skate, scotch,* and *scratch*
- Use single phonemes initially
- Move on to single syllable words
- Increase response complexity
- Ask the patient to slow down the rate of speech

Teach Tracheoesophageal Speech

- Select a Voice Prosthesis for a patient who has undergone Tracheoesophageal Fistulization/Puncture)
- Insert the voice prosthesis into the fistula; make sure the fistula is properly healed; also make sure that there is no leakage of fluid around or through the prosthesis
- Ask the patient to inhale, occlude the stoma with a finger, and exhale
- Ask the client to produce sound as the air from the lungs enters the P-E Segment through the voice prostheses

L

357

Laryngitis

- Have the patient practice sound production
- Shape the sound into speech
- Increase the length of utterances
- Give appropriate feedback

Andrews, M. L. (1999). *Manual of voice treatment: Pediatrics to geriatrics* (2nd ed.). San Diego: Singular Publishing Group.

Casper, J. K., & Colton, R. H. (1993). *Clinical manual for laryngectomy and head and neck cancer rehabilitation.* San Diego: Singular Publishing Group.

Deem, J. F., & Miller, L. (2000). *Manual of voice therapy* (2nd ed.). Austin, TX: Pro-Ed.

Laryngitis.   Irritated and swollen vocal folds; causes include vocally abusive behaviors and infection; see the following three entries.

Laryngitis, Chronic.   Irritated and swollen vocal folds of long history; <u>Hoarseness</u> is the primary result; lowered vocal pitch and vocal tiredness also may result; may lead to vocal nodules or polyps.

- Impose vocal rest without whispering
- Reduce vocally abusive behaviors

Laryngitis Sicca.   Dryness and atrophy of the laryngeal mucosa, including the glandular structures with a rough, dry, and glazed look to the mucosa; causes include untreated chronic laryngitis, laryngeal radiation, and prolonged use of antihistamine drugs; also often described as dry voice; hoarseness, persistent cough, dry and tickly throat are common symptoms

- Treatment mostly medical (increased environmental humidity and use of lubricating agents)
- Do not recommend voice therapy

Laryngitis, Traumatic.   Irritated and swollen vocal folds; result of such vocally abusive behaviors as shouting, screaming, and loud cheering; hoarseness is the primary result.

- Do not recommend voice treatment for such temporary laryngitis as that following enthusiastic participation in ball games; natural period rest (one night's sleep) may be adequate

- Reduce vocally abusive behaviors if they persist

Laryngocele.   Air-filled or fluid-filled sacs that appear on the space between the true and false vocal folds; internal sacs remain within the thyroid cartilage; external sacs protrude above the thyroid cartilage; a combination has both the varieties; the basic condition is a congenital enlargement of the laryngeal ventricle, which may be worsened by straining, coughing, vocal abuse, playing wind instruments, and glassblowing; asymptomatic in infancy; such symptoms as hoarseness of voice, a bulge in the neck (with external laryngocele), and dysphagia may appear during adulthood.

- Treatment is medical and surgical
- Do not recommend voice therapy

Laryngomalacia.   A common laryngeal anomaly characterized by excessive flaccidity of the supralaglottic larynx resulting in an epiglottis that is collapsed over the glottis during inspiration; the main symptom is inspiratory Stridor (noisy inspiration); voice is typically not affected.

Laryngopharyngeal Reflux.   An upward flow of gastric juices into the laryngeal and pharyngeal structures; irritation caused by such flow; may cause such voice disorders as hoarseness, frequent throat clearing, and granulomas

- Treatment is medical (diet and medications)
- Do not recommend voice therapy

Laryngoplasty.   Surgical treatment to improve phonation in people with vocal fold paralysis or weakness; involves medial displacement of vocal folds with the help of implant materials to promote better approximation.

Left-Hand Manual Alphabet.   A manual communication method developed by L. Chen for clients with right-hand paralysis; appropriate for some clients with aphasia;

the signs closely approximate the letters; used in teaching Augmentative Communication-Gestural (Unaided).

Chen, L. Y. (1971). Manual communication by combined alphabet and gestures. *Archives of Physical Medicine and Rehabilitation, 52,* 381–384.

Lesson Plan.   A brief treatment plan which describes short-term goals and procedures; in case of student clinicians, approved by the clinical supervisor; in preparing lesson plans:
- Use Operational Definitions in writing treatment goals
- Give clear and brief description of procedures to be used

Lipreading.   Understanding speech by watching the mouth of the speaker; gaining cues from the movement of the articulators (e.g., the movements of the lips, the tongue, the jaw) and facial expressions; a skill that may supplement limited comprehension of speech through residual hearing; a skill that many children who are deaf learn without much effort; taught to children who are deaf by educators of the deaf.

Liquid Crystal Display (LCD).   Flat panel display systems used in computers and other electronic devices (e.g., calculators); used in many devices of Augmentative and Alternative Communication (AAC); contrasted with Cathode-ray Tube Display (CRT); backlit displays that have a light source behind the screen are easier to read under varied lighting conditions; contrasted with Cathode-ray Display (CRD).

Lobectomy.   Surgical excision of a lobe of an organ; removal of a lobe of lung, brain, thyroid, or liver.

Lobotomy.   Surgical incision of the fibers of a lobe of brain.

Logical Validity.   Consistency of statements that do not violate rules of logic; treatment procedures that may be logically consistent; no assurance that the procedures have experimental support; contrasted with Empirical Validity.

Lombard Effect.   Increase in vocal intensity under noisy environmental conditions or under induced masking with white noise; typically reflexive, but can be brought under voluntary control by instructions and reinforcement; a concomitant effect when masking noise is used to treat stuttering or voice disorders.

Loudness.   A sensation listeners experience as a function of physical intensity of sound; a vocal quality; an aspect of voice that may be disordered; a treatment target in clients with loudness disorders; see under Voice Disorders.

L

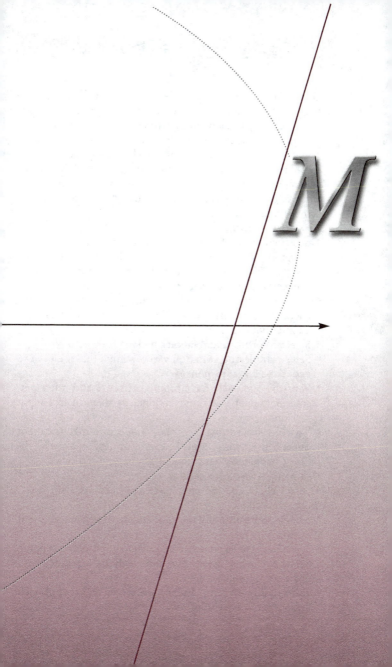

Maintenance Strategy. Methods designed to promote the production of treated communicative skills in natural environments and sustained over time; to be planned from the beginning of treatment; requires the extension of treatment to natural settings and training the client's significant others to help evoke and reinforce the target skills; all aspects of treatment including stimulus variables, response characteristics, and response consequences should be manipulated to achieve maintenance.

Stimulus Manipulations

- Select common, functional, client-specific stimulus items, preferably objects; let the client bring stimuli from home (e.g., a girl could bring her toys to serve as stimuli in speech or language training)
- Select stimuli that are ethnoculturally appropriate for the client; consult with parents in selecting culturally relevant stimuli that the child is familiar with
- Select colorful, unambiguous, and realistic pictures
- Select simple and common verbal stimuli that are used to evoke the target responses
- Vary the audience; have family members and other persons participate as conversational partners in treatment sessions
- Vary physical setting controls; conduct informal treatment outside the clinic room, in cafeterias, campus walks, library, bookstore, home, and other natural settings

Response Considerations

- Select client-specific and functional responses for treatment targets
- Select ethnoculturally relevant and appropriate treatment targets
- Select target behaviors that are likely to be produced at home
- Select target behaviors that can easily be expanded into more complex communicative behaviors
- Train multiple exemplars of each target skill and at each level of response complexity

M

- Take training to complex levels of target skills: always end treatment with sufficient training at the conversational level

Contingency Manipulation

- Use intermittent reinforcement schedules in the latter stages of training
- Use conditioned reinforcers (tokens with back-up reinforcers)
- Delay reinforcement in the latter stages of training
- Let the family members and others watch treatment sessions so they can better understand the treatment targets and teaching methods
- Train significant others in evoking and prompting the target behaviors at home and in other nonclinical settings
- Train significant others in reinforcing the production of target behaviors at home and in other nonclinical settings
- Reinforce generalized responses; have parents and others reinforce generalized productions at home
- Teach Reinforcement Priming to the client (e.g., teach the client to draw attention to his or her production of target behaviors at home so the ignoring parents can pay attention and reinforce the client)
- Hold informal Training Sessions in Natural Environments
- Teach Self-Control (Self-Monitoring) Procedures (e.g., counting one's target behaviors)
- Give treatment for a sufficient duration
- Ensure Follow-Up and arrange for Booster Treatment

Hegde, M. N. (1998). *Treatment procedure in communicative disorders* (3rd ed.). Austin, TX: Pro-Ed.

Management of Behavioral Contingencies. A clinician's or a parent's skill in arranging effective stimuli for target communication skills, requiring the production of specified skills, and in promptly and effectively providing differential feedback for the correct and incorrect productions; inherent to all behavioral intervention techniques; controlled evidence of significant amounts of generality supports the use of behavioral contingencies in the treatment of communicative disorders.

- Provide effective stimuli for target behaviors; use pictures, objects, enacted events, instructions, demonstrations, models, prompts, manual guidance, visual and tactile cues, and other stimuli for the target behavior
- Specify the response form; demonstrate what the client is expected to produce
- Give feedback promptly, clearly, naturally, and as frequently as needed
- Positively reinforce imitated or evoked target behaviors with Verbal Praise, Tokens that are exchanged for backup reinforcers, Informational Feedback, Biofeedback, and High Probability Behaviors
- Use Corrective Feedback, Response Cost, Time-Out and Extinction to reduce undesirable behaviors
- Use Differential Reinforcement to teach desirable behaviors that replace undesirable behaviors

Hegde, M. N. (1998). *Treatment procedures in communicative disorders* (3rd ed.). Austin, TX: Pro-Ed.

Mand-Model.   A child language intervention method that uses components of Incidental Teaching Method; uses typical adult-child interactions in a play-oriented setting to teach functional communication skills; for procedures, see Language Disorders in Children; Treatment of Language Disorders: Specific Techniques or Programs.

Mands.   A class of verbal behaviors that are triggered by a state of motivation; includes requests, commands, and demands; need to create a state of motivation to teach mands; often reinforced with primary reinforcers.

- Create a state of motivation:
  - arrange treatment around lunch or breakfast time so food may be used as a reinforcer (hunger is the state of motivation)
  - hold food in front of the child until the child asks for it

- place attractive toys on a high shelf and give them to the child only when requested
- offer a food item the child does not like (the child should verbally refuse it)
- eat something the child is fond of without offering it (the child should request it)
- give a tightly closed jar with candy in it (the child should ask you to open it)
- Reinforce promptly with the displayed or held back item; remove promptly an aversive item presented when the child makes an appropriate response

Manual Approach.   A deaf educational approach that promotes the use of sign language and other manual modes of communication for young deaf children.

Manual Communication.   A mode of nonverbal communication that may include sign language, finger spelling, gestures, and other forms of nonoral communication.

Manual Guidance.   Physical guidance provided to shape a response; the Phonetic Placement Method is similar to manual guidance; needed when the client cannot imitate a response; used in treating practically all types of communicative disorders.

- Use your fingers to shape articulators
- Take the client's hand and make it touch the target picture while training comprehension of commands
- Use tongue depressors to move the tongue to desired positions
- Apply slight digital pressure to the laryngeal area to lower a client's pitch
- Apply slight pressure on the chin of a child who does not readily open the mouth
- Fade manual guidance to promote the production of target responses without it

Manual Pointing.   A method of Augmentative and Alternative Communication in which the client points to a correct message among the several displayed on a screen or on a board; may or may not use a pointing device.

Manual Shorthand.   A method of communication that combines the Left-Hand Manual Alphabet with gestures; expressed by left-hand gestures; appropriate for clients with right-hand paralysis; used in teaching Augmentative Communication-Gestural (Unaided).

Chen, L. Y. (1971). Manual communication by combined alphabet and gestures. *Archives of Physical Medicine and Rehabilitation, 52,* 381–384.

Masking Noise.   Delivery of noise through headphones to mask auditory perception of pure tones or speech during auditory assessment; normally induces the Lombard Effect; used to induce stutter-free speech in stutterers and to induce higher vocal intensity in certain voice clients.

Matching.   A method in which subjects of similar characteristics are placed in the experimental and control groups used to evaluate treatment effects; part of the Group Design Strategy.

- Find pairs of subjects with the same or similar characteristics (age, gender, severity of the disorder, socioeconomic status)
- Assign one of the pair to the experimental group and the other to the control group
- Match groups on the basis of group means if pair-wise matching is not possible (the two groups with the same average IQ, for instance)

Maximal Contrast Method.   An articulation training method in which word pairs that contrast the most are used to train target phonemes; contrasted with Minimal Contrast Method in which word pairs that differ by one phoneme (e.g., *pat, bat*); in maximal contrast pair, the words may differ by several features or phonemic contrasts; treatment proce-

M

dure the same as those described under <u>Minimal Contrast Method</u>.

Mechanical Corrective Feedback.   A method to reduce incorrect responses in treatment; also known as <u>Biofeedback;</u> feedback is presented soon after an incorrect response is made; includes such feedback as provided on a computer monitor for incorrect responses (e.g., undesirable vocal pitch or intensity) and electromyographic feedback on muscle tension.

Melodic Intonation Therapy.   An aphasia treatment program that uses musical intonation, continuous voicing, and rhythmic tapping to teach verbal expressions to patients with severe nonfluent aphasia with good auditory comprehension; see <u>Aphasia; Treatment of Aphasia: Specific Technique or Programs</u> for procedures.

Memory Impairments.   Impairments in remembering, recalling, or acting on the basis of remote or recent experiences; impairment in learning or retaining current events or recently experienced events; typically described in such mentalistic or mechanistic terms as storage and retrieval and a variety of presumed mental or neurological processes; nonetheless, almost always it is the presence or absence of actions and behaviors that lead to such presumptions, theoretical speculations, and analogical reasoning; found in many persons with a variety of neurologic and psychiatric disorders; of interest to speech-language pathologists is the memory impairments found in patients of <u>Dementia</u> and <u>Traumatic Brain Injury</u> and to some extent in patients with <u>Aphasia</u>.

Treatment of Memory Impairments: Guidelines and Strategies
- Note that treating memory impairments as behavioral deficits (instead of presumed cognitive deficits) with

external stimulus manipulation (instead of trying to improve some presumed internal and underlying process) and response contingent consequences is effective

- See Aphasia, Dementia, and Traumatic Brain Injury for symptoms and their association with other communication and related deficits

- Note that a related skill, attention, if impaired, will result in further deterioration in recent or short-term memory

- As a speech-language pathologist, integrate memory improvement work with communication training; leave pure, abstract, and process-oriented work on memory to other professionals (e.g., neuropsychologists)

- Improve patient's awareness of memory problems by giving contingent feedback on responses that indicate memory lapses (e.g., point out misnaming, failure to recall required experiences, and missed appointments or scheduled activities)

- Select memory impairments that reduce the patient's communicative effectiveness; identify functional memory tasks (e.g., remembering names of children or grandchildren) instead of abstract and nonfunctional tasks (e.g., remembering just shown circles or squares drawn on a piece of paper)

- Improve patient's orientation before starting a more formal memory management program; note that efforts to improve memory skills may be ineffective with disoriented patients; see Alzheimer's Disease for suggestions on improving orientation

- Improve patient's attention; note that efforts to treat memory skills in inattentive patients is ineffective; alternatively, integrate attentional skills management to memory skill management; consider treatment suggestions offered under Attention Disorders

- Let the patient help select memory improvement strategies that he or she has used in the past

Memory Impairments

- Teach only a small amount of information at any one time; use language that is consistent with the patient's education and current level of functioning
- Always review what was done in the previous session, give an overview of information about to be offered, frequently review information just offered during treatment sessions, and review again at the end of the session
- Note if the client learns better by doing things instead of listening to instructions on how to do the same things; if so, schedule activities instead of passive listening to repeated instructions
- Improving memory skills requires repeated practice of skills and learning; impress on the patient and the family that there is no substitute for repeated practice
- Conduct frequent but short sessions, instead of long and infrequent sessions
- In both conversation and treatment sessions, present small amounts of information at a time; test comprehension before moving on to say more
- Always describe and explain the memory skills targeted for training; be specific and explicit in your description of targeted skills; note that it helps if the patient agrees with your goals and thus better cooperates with your treatment plan
- Work with health care staff and family to make sure that the goals and procedures are uniformly applied
- Start with few and the most important functional skills and add additional skills only when the client has mastered the initial skills
- Speak slowly to the patient and in simple language; train other staff and family members to do the same
- Highlight important information and alert the patient to crucial information soon to be offered (e.g., "I am going to tell you something very important"; "What I told you is very important"; "You should not forget this"; or "Listen carefully; this is important for you.")

Memory Log Books

- Teach the client to develop a <u>Memory Log Book</u> that helps keep track of activities and appointments
- Teach compensatory skills including written instructions on daily activities (e.g., cooking, shopping, household chores); write prompts on index cards the patient frequently consults or follows during the execution of an activity
- Teach the client to use electronic memory devices, calendars, wristwatches with alarms, and so forth that help keep appointments and remind him or her of scheduled activities
- Teach the client to maintain a pocket notebook on events and activities and train him or her to use it regularly
- Teach family members and health care staff to remind and prompt activities; to help the patient make use of written instructions, memory logs, lists, electronic devices, and so forth; have the family members reinforce the client's actual use of memory aids and the resulting improvement in behaviors

Memory Log Books. A memory aid for patients with memory impairments; consists of written material that helps sustain skills or prompt actions; recommended for patients who have retained at least a basic level of reading and writing skills; not useful for patients who are confused, have left-sided neglect, or have severe uncorrected visual defect

- Design a simple log book that will contain only essential information
- Design a colorful cover for the book so it is easy to locate
- Designate a regular place where book will always be kept; let the health care staff or family members know the place
- Select functional information to be included in the log book; consult with the patient, staff, and the family members in making this selection
- Include the patient's biographical information (name, age, address, phone number, family members' names); the current moth, year, and the name of the hospital; names of

main health care workers and individual clinicians treating the patient
- Train the patient to take the book to all appointments, including treatment sessions
- Include in the book pictures and names of therapists and family members; train the client to frequently consult this information to facilitate memory for their names and faces
- Designate a single health care worker who will help maintain, update, and modify the book as found appropriate
- Divide the book into easily identifiable sections, preferably of different color; organize information in the sections for easy consultation (e.g., a section on treatment session appointments, a section on daily activities, a section on medications and their schedules, a section on recreational activities, etc.)
- Train the client to consolidate all written forms of memory aids into the log book and not have multiple and odd pieces of information strewn around
- Teach the patient to write down information and then to periodically review the written information to act on it

Mendelsohn Maneuver. A swallowing maneuver that helps elevate the larynx more and for longer duration, resulting in an increased width and duration of cricopharyngeal opening; see Dysarthria; in implementing this maneuver:
- Educate the patient about the elevation of larynx (tell him or her about the Adam's apple or voice box going up)
- Have the patient palpate the elevation of the larynx when he or she swallows saliva several times
- Instruct the patient to hold the larynx up for a longer duration (several seconds) as he or she swallows; give such instructions as "Swallow long and strong" or "Stretch out the swallow"

Meninges. Membranes that cover the brain.

Mental Retardation. Intellectual, social, and adaptive behaviors that are significantly below normal during the developmental period, which extends up to age 18; communicative problems are a significant aspect of retardation; mostly, the treatment procedures for Language Disorders in Children are applicable with the following special considerations:

- Recommend or initiate treatment as early as possible
- Get the family involved in early Language Stimulation
- Get the help of other specialists including special educators and psychologists
- Make a comprehensive evaluation of the client's skills and deficiencies
- Consider the academic or occupational demands made on the client; select targets that help meet those demands; in the case of children, work closely with teachers in selecting target behaviors for treatment
- Select target behaviors that are functional (useful) to the client in educational, occupational, family, and social situations

- Design a comprehensive treatment plan that is most likely to include articulation and language and perhaps voice and fluency as well
- Select for initial training communicative behaviors that will produce the most effect in natural settings and in classrooms in case of children (e.g., select articulation training before language training if this leads to improved communication sooner; select language training if teaching a few functional words is the priority; teach a few functional signs before verbal expressions in the case of nonverbal and severely retarded children)
- Sequence the target behaviors carefully; use small step increments
- Model the target responses frequently; initially reinforce approximations of modeled responses; gradually require better approximations and finally require an exact match, if that is practical
- Fade modeling in gradual steps
- Shape responses whenever the client cannot imitate modeled responses

- Use objects and events more than pictures as treatment stimuli
- Establish target behaviors in structured treatment sessions but soon loosen the structure to resemble naturalistic situations
- Train in varied naturalistic settings to promote generalized production
- Use primary reinforcers initially and fade them; eventually use only verbal reinforcers
- Shape complex language behaviors in successive stages
- Train parents and teachers in prompting and reinforcing newly acquired communicative behaviors
- Implement a systematic maintenance program
- Consider nonverbal means of communication (e.g., American Sign Language) or Augmentative and Alternative Communication when appropriate
- Follow up and arrange for booster treatment

Metronome-Paced Speech. A method used to slow down the rate of speech; the client is asked to pace a syllable or a word to each beat of a metronome; used in the treatment of stuttering, cluttering, and certain forms of dysarthria; see also Stuttering, Treatment; Treatment of Stuttering: Specific Techniques or Programs and Treatment of Dysarthria.

- Begin treatment with a slow beat that reduces the rate of speech so that stuttering or cluttering is markedly reduced or speech intelligibility of dysarthric clients improves
- Have the client practice slow speech until fluency or improved speech intelligibility are stabilized
- Fade the metronome by gradually increasing the rate of its beat until the speech rate and prosody approximate the normal; note that this step is especially needed for persons who stutter or clutter.

Minimal Contrast Method. A method of treating articulation disorders in both children with developmental articulation disorder and adults with dysarthria; based on the

Minimal Contrast Method

assumption that it is necessary to teach the semantic differences between a child's (misarticulated) production and the correct adult production; involves the use of word pairs that differ only in one phoneme (hence the name, *minimal contrast*); also known as minimal-pair method or approach; see also <u>Maximal Contrast Method</u>.

- Select word pairs that differ by only one phonemic feature (e.g., *key-tea; pat-bat; four-pour*); note that for a given client, one of the phoneme is the erred one and the other is the target (e.g., in the case of /t/ substitution for /k/, a minimal pair will be *tea-key*)
- Select 8 to 10 word pairs for a phonemic contrast (e.g., to eliminate final consonant deletion, select such word pairs as *bow-boat, bee-beet, toe-toad,* and *pie-pine*)
- Select pictured stimulus items to represent both the words of all the pairs
- Place the pictures representing the word pairs in front of the child
- Model a given word pair (e.g., *bow-boat*) and ask the child to imitate; reinforce correctly imitated productions or approximations; give several trials
- Move to spontaneous naming task; ask the child to say a word, and point to it; then hand the child what he or she names (not what he or she points to if pointing and saying do not match, e.g., if the child points to *beet* but says *bee,* give the child *bee,* not *beet* that was pointed to)
- When the child does not accept the wrong picture (e.g., you handed *bee* when he or she pointed to *beet,* which was wanted), give corrective feedback; model *beet,* emphasizing /t/, and ask the child to imitate it
- Reinforce correct responses; train other pairs
- Arrange controlled play activities in which the target sounds and words are practiced in conversational speech (e.g., a toy *soap* used to pretend to wash hands, pots, dolls, and so forth while talking about the activity)

- Move on to more naturalistic conversational speech and reinforce correct productions of target speech sounds

Mixed Dysarthrias. A type of motor speech disorder that is a combination of two or more pure dysarthrias; the neuropathology is varied depending on the types of dysarthrias that are mixed; frequent causes include multiple strokes or multiple neurological diseases; speech disorders are varied and dependent on the types of pure dysarthrias that are mixed; see Treatment of Dysarthria: Specific Types.

Modeled Trials. Structured opportunities to imitate a response when the clinician models it; trials are separated by brief time interval; response accuracy scored for each trial; faded when imitation is established; applicable in the treatment of almost all communication disorders.

- Place stimulus item in front of the client; show an object, or demonstrate an action
- Ask the predetermined question (e.g., "What is this?")
- Immediately model correct response (e.g., "Johnny, say. . . .")
- Wait a few seconds for the client to respond
- Consequate the response if it is a modeled training trial
- Do not consequate the response if it is a modeled baseline trial
- Record the response on the recording sheet
- Remove stimulus item
- Wait 2–3 seconds to signify end of trial

Hegde, M. N. (1998). *Treatment procedures in communicative disorders* (3rd ed.). Austin, TX: Pro-Ed.

Modeling. Clinician's production of a target behavior for the client to imitate; needed when the clinician cannot evoke a response; used frequently in treating communicative disorders; much experimental evidence to support its use in treatment.

- Provide live or mechanically delivered model (audio or videotaped or computer presented)

- Use the client's own correct response as a model (presented mechanically)
- Model frequently in the beginning stages of treatment
- Ask the client to imitate as closely as possible
- Reinforce the client for correct imitations or approximations
- Withdraw or fade modeling in gradual steps as the client's imitative responses stabilize

Mode of Response.   Manner or method of a response; includes imitation, spontaneous production, conversational speech, and oral reading; useful in sequencing treatment targets:

- Teach a target behavior first in the imitative mode if necessary; model the target response
- Teach a target behavior in evoked mode, fading modeling
- Teach the target behavior in conversational mode
- Teach the target behaviors in oral reading if judged useful

Modification of Treatment Procedures.   See Treatment of Communicative Disorders: Procedural Modifications.

Monterey Fluency Program.   A treatment program for adults and children who stutter; behaviorally based; a fluency shaping program; for procedures see Stuttering, Treatment; Treatment of Stuttering: Specific Techniques or Programs.

Moto-Kinesthetic Method.   An articulation treatment method developed by Young and Stinchfield-Hawk; is similar to Phonetic Placement Method; emphasizes awareness of kinesthetic movement involved in articulation.

- Consider using the technique in the initial stages of treatment
- Manipulate the client's articulators with your fingers (Manual Guidance)
- Provide visual stimulation of the movements with the help of a mirror

Motor Speech Disorders.   A group of speech disorders associated with neuropathology affecting the motor control of speech muscles or motor programming of speech movements; includes Dysarthria and Apraxia of Speech.

Multi-infarct Dementia.   A form of dementia caused by multiple strokes resulting in extensive cortical damage; characterized by rapidly progressing and irreversible intellectual, behavioral, and memory impairments; see Dementia.

Multiple Baseline Designs.   A set of single-subject designs in which the effects of treatment are demonstrated by showing that untreated baselines did not change and that only the treated baselines did; practical designs to demonstrate treatment effects; has been extensively used in researching behavioral treatment procedures both in speech-language pathology and behavioral science; useful in integrating treatment research with service delivery; has three variations: across behaviors, settings, and subjects.

Multiple Baseline Across Behaviors Design.   A single subject design in which several behaviors are sequentially taught to show that a behavior changed only when brought under treatment and untreated behaviors remained unchanged; helps rule out extraneous variables leading to the conclusion that the treatment was effective.

- Select three or more target behaviors (e.g., three or more phonemes, grammatic morphemes)
- Establish baselines on all selected target behaviors on discrete trails and in conversational speech
- Teach the first behavior to a Training Criterion
- Repeat baselines on the remaining untreated behaviors
- Teach the next behavior and repeat the baselines on the remaining untreated behaviors
- Continue to alternate baselines and treatment until all the behaviors are trained
- Expect the untreated behaviors not to change; if changed, note that the experimental control is weakened and it is difficult to claim treatment effectiveness

Multiple Baseline Designs

- If all behaviors changed only when brought under treatment, conclude that treatment was effective and that no other factor is responsible for the changes

Multiple Baseline Across Settings Design. A single-subject design in which a behavior is sequentially taught in different settings to show that the behavior changed only in a treated setting and hence the treatment was effective.

- Baserate a target behavior in three or more settings (e.g., clinic, home, school, or office)
- Teach the behavior in one setting (e.g., fluency in the school clinician's office)
- Repeat the baserates in the remaining untreated settings
- Teach the behavior in another setting (e.g., fluency in the classroom)
- Continue to alternate baserates and teaching in different settings until the behavior is trained in all settings
- Conclude that the treatment was effective only if the repeated baserates show that the target behavior changed in a setting only when treatment was offered in that setting

Multiple Baselines Across Subjects Design. A single-subject research design in which several subjects are treated sequentially to show that only treated subjects changed and hence treatment was effective.

- Select a target behavior that needs to be taught to three or more clients
- Baserate the target behaviors in all subjects
- Treat one of the subjects
- Repeat the baserates on the untreated subjects
- Treat the second subject
- Repeat the baserates on untreated subjects
- Alternate treatment and baserates until all the clients are trained
- Conclude that the treatment was effective only if the repeated baserates show that clients showed positive

changes only when treated and that until the treatment was offered, no one changed

Hegde, M. N. (1994). *Clinical research in communicative disorders: Principles and strategies* (2nd ed.). Austin, TX: Pro-Ed.

Multiple Causation.   The philosophical position that most events, including communicative behaviors and their disorders, have several causes.

Multiple Phoneme Approach.   An articulation treatment program that is appropriate for children with multiple misarticulations; a highly structured behaviorally based method with an emphasis on production training in which all target phonemes are treated in all treatment sessions; includes extensively detailed steps; see Articulation and Phonological Disorders; Treatment of Articulation and Phonological Disorders: Specific Approaches for the procedures.

Multiple Sclerosis (MS).   A neurological diseases characterized by demyelination of cerebral white matter; symptoms include weakness, incoordination, and visual disturbances; associated with dysarthria.

Multisensory Approach.   A method of teaching deaf children with an emphasis on all available sensory modalities, including residual hearing, vision, and touch.

Mutational Falsetto.   Continuation of prepubertal voice after attaining puberty; voice is high-pitched.
- Have medical conformation of laryngeal maturation
- Establish a lower pitched voice; use techniques described under Voice Disorders; Treatment of Disorders of Loudness and Pitch.

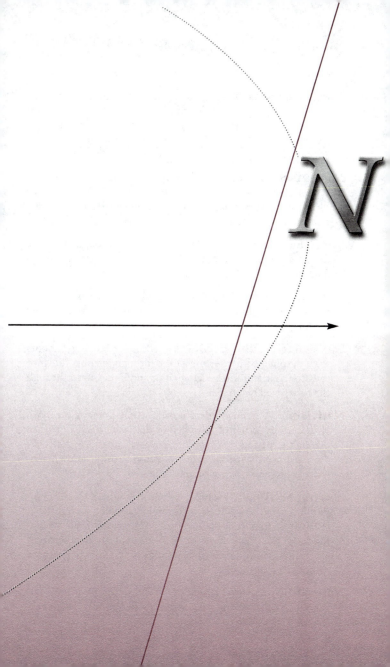

Narrative Skills. A language skill in describing events in a sequential, chronologically correct, and logically consistent manner; treatment procedures described under Language Disorders in Children; Treatment of Language Disorders: Specific Techniques or Programs; Narrative Skills Training.

Nasal Assimilation. A phonological process in which nasal consonants are substituted for oral consonants (e.g., /n/ for /d/); see Articulation and Phonological Disorders for treatment approaches.

Nasal Emission. Audible escape of air through the nose during speech; often found in children with cleft palate; reduction is a treatment target.

Nasendoscope. A mechanical device used to examine internal organs illuminated by a fiberoptic tube inserted through the nose.

N **Nasogastric Tube (NG).** A method of feeding patients with dysphagia by inserting a tube through the nose and into the stomach and introducing solid and liquid food through the tube; see Dysphagia.

Nativism. A philosophical position that humans are born with certain forms of knowledge that they need not learn through experience; basis for nativists' assertion that children are born with knowledge of universal grammar, sentence structure, or phonological rules.

Natural Settings. Nonclinical settings where clients communicate for the most part; communication in such settings is always a final treatment target; in the case of infants and toddlers, treatment may be implemented in such settings; extending treatment to such settings is essential to promote response maintenance.

Natural-Sounding Fluency. A stuttering treatment target when such techniques as Delayed Auditory Feedback,

Metronome-Paced Speech, and Rate Reduction are used; see Stuttering, Treatment; Treatment of Stuttering: Specific Techniques or Programs for additional information.

- Fade explicit management of airflow
- Fade the use of a metronome
- Fade the use of delayed auditory feedback
- Increase the rate of speech to near-normal levels
- Teach variations in intonation
- Teach normal rhythm of speech

Neck Brace. A brace around the neck used to stabilize the weakened neck muscles; often used in treating clients with dysarthrias.

Negative Reinforcers. Aversive events that are removed, reduced, postponed, or prevented; responses that accomplish these increase in frequency; less useful than positive reinforcers in teaching communicative skills.

Neglect. Often described as left-sided neglect, it is the tendency to ignore or be not aware of the left visual field in patients who have suffered right hemisphere brain damage; a major symptom and treatment target in patients with Right Hemisphere Syndrome; in reading, the patient may ignore the left side of printed pages; may neglect his or her own left side of the body; may neglect left-sided auditory stimuli as well.

Neologism. Creation of new but meaningless words by patients with Aphasia.

Neural Anastomosis. Connecting a branch of an undamaged nerve to a damaged nerve; a surgical treatment for certain dysarthric clients; a branch of the intact XIIth cranial nerve may be connected to the damaged VIIth cranial nerve to restore function and appearance.

Neuritic Plaques. Clumps of degenerating neurons; present in the brains of Alzheimer's patients and some normal elderly persons.

Neurofibrillary Tangles. Twisted and tangled neurofibrils; a basic neuropathology of <u>Alzheimer's Disease.</u>

Neurogenic Fluency Disorders. Somewhat varied problems of fluency that have a demonstrated neurological basis; also known as neurogenic stuttering; may follow a stroke, head trauma, extrapyramidal diseases, tumor, dementia, and drugs prescribed for asthma and depression; to be distinguished from stuttering, which is developmental with no gross neuropathology; may be persistent or transient; little or no research on treatment effects and efficacy; suggested techniques based on reported clinical experiences; evaluate the results of selected procedures carefully; abandon procedures that do not produce results with given clients.

- Make a thorough assessment and document neurological basis for the fluency disorder
- Reduce the speech rate to reduce or eliminate dysfluencies
- Use a <u>Pacing Board</u> to help the client reduce the speech rate
- Experiment with <u>Delayed Auditory Feedback (DAF)</u> to see if it is effective in slowing the speech rate
- Experiment with auditory masking to see if it is helpful
- Be aware that clients who exhibit stuttering along with slow and effortful speech may not benefit from pacing devices, DAF, and masking
- Consider relaxation and biofeedback to reduce speech muscle tension; evaluate the results carefully

Helm-Estabrooks, N. (1986). Diagnosis and management of neurogenic stuttering. In K. O. St. Louis (Ed.), *The atypical stutterer* (pp. 193–217). New York: Academic Press.

Rosenbek, J. C. (1984). Stuttering secondary to nervous damage. In R. F. Curlee & W. H. Perkins (Eds.), *Nature and treatment of stuttering* (pp. 31–48). Austin, TX: Pro-Ed.

Nonexclusion Time-Out. Response-contingent arrangement of a brief duration of time in which all interaction is terminated; the client is not removed from the setting; one of the Direct Methods of Response Reduction; often used in communication training.

- Give response contingent signal to start time-out (e.g., saying, "Stop" as soon as a dysfluency occurs); do not let the client talk during time-out
- Turn your face away from the client
- Stay motionless for 5 seconds
- Turn toward the client, and continue the interaction

Nonfluent Aphasia.   A type of aphasia characterized by nonfluent, agrammatic, halting speech with word retrieval problems; includes Broca's aphasia, transcortical motor aphasia, mixed transcortical aphasia, and global aphasia; contrasted with Fluent Aphasia; see Aphasia and Treatment of Aphasia: Specific Types.

Noniconic Symbols.   Abstract, geometric shapes that do not look like what they suggest; the meaning of such shapes to be established by training; more difficult to learn than Iconic Symbols, but more flexible; plastic chips or various shapes are an example; used in teaching Augmentative Communication, Gestural-Assisted (Aided).

Nonpenetrating (Closed-Head) Injury.   A head injury in which the skull may or may not be fractured or lacerated and the Meninges remain intact.

Non-SLIP (Non-Speech Language Initiation Program).   A nonspeech communication program that uses the Premack-type, color-coded plastic shapes each associated with a word; developed and researched by Joseph Carrier, Jr.; the client learns to communicate by arranging them in sequence to form sentences; also used to promote oral language acquisition in initially minimally verbal children; used in teaching Augmentative Communication, Gestural-Assisted (Aided).

Nonverbal Communication.   Modes of communication that do not involve spoken speech; use of gestures, signs, symbols, printed material, electronic display, communication boards, and so forth to communicate; also includes such fully developed nonoral languages as <u>American Sign Language</u>.

Nonverbal Corrective Feedback. A method used to reduce incorrect responses in treatment; feedback is presented soon after an incorrect response is made; includes various forms of gestures, hand signals, and facial expressions that suggest to the client that the response was wrong (e.g., the stereotypic sad face); a form of <u>Corrective Feedback;</u> often paired with <u>Verbal Corrective Feedback.</u>

Normal Prosody. Normal or socially acceptable rhythm, stress, intonation (pitch variation), intensity, transition between words and phrases, correct phrasing and pausing at appropriate junctures, and acceptable rate of speech; a target in treating various disorders of communication including apraxia of speech, cluttering and stuttering, dysarthria, foreign accent reduction, hearing impairment, voice disorders, and so forth.

- Select a particular aspect of prosody for treatment (e.g., pitch variations)
- Model the target behavior
- Demonstrate the target on a computer screen, if possible
- Tape-record the model and play it
- Ask the client to match the live or recorded model (imitate)
- Shape the target behavior in successive and progressively more complex steps
- Reinforce any movement in the direction of the model
- Set a higher level of response (e.g., sentences) when the target (a certain pitch or intensity) is achieved at a lower level (e.g., phrases)
- Give maximum feedback including auditory and visual feedback

Hargrove, P. M., & McGarr, N. S. (1994). *Prosody management of communication disorders.* San Diego: Singular Publishing Group.

Normative Strategy.   An approach to selecting target behaviors for clients based on age-based norms and developmental sequences; often used in selecting target speech sounds and language structures for children; some clinicians question its relevance and assumptions; contrasted with Client-Specific Strategy.

- Assess the communicative behaviors of the child to determine potential treatment targets
- Select behaviors that the child should already have acquired based on the age-based norms
- Teach the selected behaviors in the normative sequence in which they are acquired
- Note that this is by no means the only approach to target behavior selection and sequencing
- Do not hesitate to experiment with different sequences that may not conform to the normative sequence

Norms.   Average (mean) performance of a typical group of persons on a selected test in its standardization process; frequently established with the method of cross-sectional sampling of a group of children; most common problems are small sample size and limited sampling of behaviors measured; frequently used in selecting treatment targets, especially for children with speech and language disorders.

N

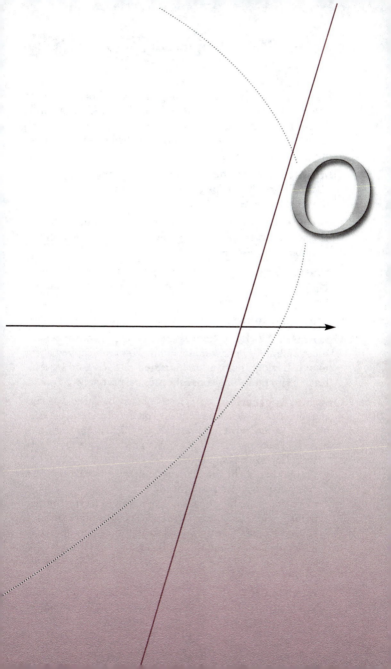

Objectivity

Objectivity.   Agreement among different observers who observe or measure the same event in the same manner; important in treatment research so that different observers agree that a treatment had an effect; helps replicate treatment procedures by other clinicians.

Obturator.   A structure that helps close an opening; a prosthetic device that helps close a cleft of the hard palate; the device has a plate that covers the cleft.

Omission.   A type of articulation disorder; not producing the sound in required word positions; see Articulation and Phonological Disorders.

Omission Training.   Reinforcing a person for not exhibiting a certain behavior; the same as Differential Reinforcement of Other Behavior.

Open-Head Injury.   The same as Penetrating Head Injury.

Operant.   A behavior that is affected by its consequences; most voluntary behaviors including communicative behaviors; behaviors that can be increased or decreased by reinforcing and punishing consequences, respectively.

Operant Aggression.   Aggressive behavior directed against the source of an aversive stimulus; a potential undesirable side-effect of punishment; contrasted with Elicited Aggression.
- A child may say "I hate you" when the clinician says "No" for an incorrect response
- A child may fight the clinician's attempt to take a token away in a response cost procedure
- Note that to reduce operant aggression in treatment, use punishment procedures sparingly and use more positive reinforcement and discriminative reinforcement that may indirectly control undesirable behaviors

Hegde, M. N. (1998). *Treatment procedures in communicative disorders* (3rd ed.). Austin, TX: Pro-Ed.

Operant Conditioning.   Skinnerian conditioning; method of selecting and strengthening behaviors of an individual by arranging reinforcing consequences; roughly the process and procedures by which most behaviors and skills are taught in treatment sessions.

Operant Level. The same as Baselines.

Operational Definitions. Definition of variables in measurable terms.
- Specify the topographic aspects of the target behavior (e.g., production of /s/ in word-initial positions, phrases, sentences)
- Specify the mode in which the response will be measured (e.g., reading, conversational speech)
- Specify the stimuli and settings (e.g., when shown pictures, in the clinic, or at home)
- Specify the accuracy criterion (e.g., 90% correct)

Oral Approach. A method of educating children who are deaf; the approach emphasizes oral language skills as against manual communication; uses auditory training, amplification, and speech reading to learn and sustain oral language skills; contrasted with Manual Approach.

Oral Apraxia. Deficits in making movements unrelated to oral speech; a motor programming disorder due to neurological damage in the absence of muscle weakness or paralysis; see Apraxia.

Oral Language. A form of communication based on articulated speech and language; the most common form of communication in most societies; most disorders of communication treated are the disorders of oral language.

Oral Phase. A swallowing disorder in which the patient has difficulty making the tongue movement to initiate the voluntary aspect of the swallow and in passing the food over the base of the tongue; see Dysphagia.

Oral Preparatory Phase of Swallow. A swallowing disorder in which the patient has difficulty collecting the masticated food to form a bolus as a preparation for swallow; see Dysphagia.

Organic Disorder. A disorder of communication or other behaviors for which there is a neurophysiological or anatomical basis; disorder due to some structural defect; examples include cleft palate speech, aphasia, dysarthria, and apraxia.

Orofacial Examination. An aspect of assessment done prior to initiating treatment; an examination of the structures of the face and mouth to detect their overall integrity and any deviations that may be present; see *PGASLP* for procedures.

Orthography. Study of alphabetic letters and their proper sequence in a given language; written representation of language.

Overarticulation. Exaggerated articulatory movements that may improve speech intelligibility; may be a treatment target in patients with Dysarthria.

Overcorrection. A procedure used to reduce behaviors by requiring the person to eliminate the effects of his or her misbehavior (Restitution) and practice its counterpart, a desirable behavior (Positive Practice); both described under Imposition of Work.

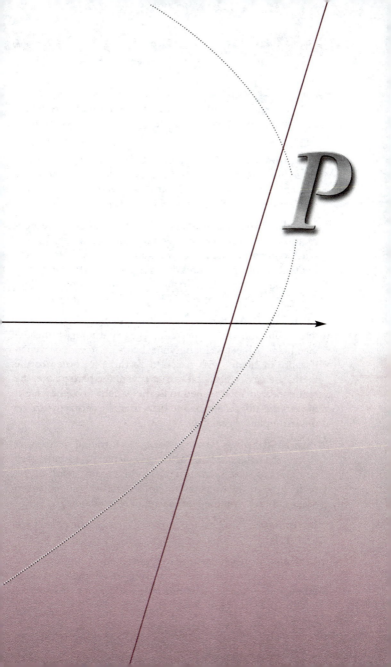

Pacing. A speech treatment procedure in which the rate of speech is reduced with rhythmic external stimulus to cue the production of syllables or words; used in the treatment of Aphasia and Dysarthria.

Pacing Board. A wooden board that has a series of colored slots that are separated by ridges; used in reducing the speech rate of clients with motor speech disorders; the speaker touches one slot for each word spoken.

Paired-Stimuli Approach. An articulation treatment method; uses correct production of sounds in a Key Word to teach correct production of the same sounds misarticulated in other words; procedures described under Articulation and Phonological Disorders; Treatment of Articulation and Phonological Disorders: Specific Techniques or Programs.

Palatal Lift Prosthesis. Constructed by a prosthodontist in consultation with a speech-language pathologist, this device helps achieve velopharyngeal closure to reduce hypernasality in clients with flaccid dysarthria; anchored to the teeth, the device has a plate that covers the hard palate; the rear end is custom-shaped to fit the patient's oropharynx; it pushes the soft palate up and back to make contact with the posterior pharyngeal wall.

Palate Reshaping Prosthesis. An intraoral device that lowers the palatal arch by artificially increasing its bulk; may be designed with teeth to replace the missing teeth of the patient; helps the tongue with limited vertical movement to make contact with the hard palate to chew food.

Palatoplasty. Surgical repair of the clefts in the palate; see Cleft Palate.

Palilalia. A speech disorder in which a word, a phrase, or a sentence is repeated with increasing speed and decreasing intelligibility; often a symptom of Parkinson's disease; reduction is a treatment target.

P

Palliative Treatment. Medical treatment that may reduce the intensity of some symptoms, increase the patient comfort level, but not cure the disease.

Palsy. Paralysis; see Cerebral Palsy.

Pantomime. A method of communication in which the speaker acts out a message by gestures and bodily movements; a target communication skills for some nonverbal or minimally verbal clients who can use gestures and bodily movements; unlike in other gestural systems, uses whole- as well as part-body movements; often more concrete and easier to understand than other gestures; used in teaching Augmentative Communication-Gestural (Unaided).

Papillomas. Wart-like growths on the larynx; thought to be of viral origin; may be life-threatening if they block the airway; may be a recurring condition; treatment is laser surgery, which also needs to be repeated; may need voice therapy to make the best possible use of the compromised larynx.

- Teach the client to achieve appropriate pitch and loudness; use techniques described under Voice Disorders; Treatment of Disorders of Loudness and Pitch.
- Teach proper respiration control; treat any other voice symptom with Specific Normal Voice Facilitation Techniques (described under Voice Disorders)

Paradigm of Treatment. An overall philosophy or viewpoint of treatment.

Paradoxical Effects. Increase in response rates when a known response reduction procedure (e.g., time-out or verbal "No") is used; potential side-effect of punishment.

- Always watch for undesirable side-effects when using response reduction (punishment) procedures
- Terminate the punishment procedure when paradoxical effects are evident
- Always reinforce desirable target behaviors and minimize the use of response reduction procedures

P

- Consider one of the Differential Reinforcement procedures in which an undesirable response is indirectly reduced by reinforcing alternative desirable behaviors

Parallel Talk. A child language treatment method; describing or commenting on what the child is doing during play
activities; procedure described under Language Disorders in
Children; Treatment of Language Disorders: Specific Techniques or Programs.

Paraphasias. Unintended word or sound substitutions; a
symptom of Aphasia; a treatment target for patients with
aphasia.

Paraplegia. Paralysis of the both the legs often due to spinal cord injury or disease.

Parent Training. Preparing parents (or other family members) to conduct informal treatment at home; to conduct
maintenance activities to sustain treatment gains at home
and other natural settings; see Language Stimulation by Parents; Maintenance Strategy; Peer Training.

Parkinson's Disease. A progressive neurological syndrome associated with depigmentation of the substantia ni-
gra, a midbrain structure functionally related to the basal
ganglia; there is loss of ability to produce or store dopamine;
symptoms include Tremor, Rigidity, depression, visuospatial
disturbances, and Bradykinesia; irregular and less legible
handwriting; soft, monotonous, and rapid speech; crowded
word productions without the usual pauses between phrases;
general management procedures described under Dementia;
in addition, consider the following suggestions:
- Reduce the rate of speech to increase intelligibility
- Use a Pacing Board to monitor the speech rate
- Decrease monotonous tone of voice
- Increase vocal intensity (subject to improvement of chest
musculature functioning)

Partial Assimilation

- Increase pauses between phrases
- Monitor the changes (if any) that occur with specific medication such as Levodopa (L-Dopa)

Partial Assimilation. A characteristic of speech articulation in which a sound takes on the properties of its neighboring sounds.

Partial Modeling. Withdrawing modeling of complete sentences in gradual steps; a method of Fading.

- Initially model complete sentences for the client to imitate (e.g., "The book is on the table.")
- Drop the last word when it is time to fade modeling (e.g., "The book is on the. . . .")
- Drop additional words, one word at a time, on subsequent trials ("The book is on. . . ."; "The book is. . . ."; "The book. . . ."; etc.)

Peer Modeling. A child language intervention method in which peers are trained to model the target skills for the child client; procedure described under Language Disorders in Children; Treatment of language Disorders: Specific Techniques or Programs.

- Select a peer who agrees to help and is acceptable to the client
- Have the peer observe your treatment sessions
- Describe the target behaviors, modeling and imitation sequence, and reinforcement procedures
- Let the peer model and reinforce the child's productions in your presence
- Refine the peer's skills in modeling the target behaviors
- Ask the peer to submit recorded language samples that document appropriate modeling outside the clinic
- Periodically assess the results of peer modeling and provide additional training to the peer

Peer Training. Training peers of clients to evoke and reinforce target behaviors in natural settings; a Maintenance Strategy.

- Ask the peers to initially observe your treatment sessions
- Describe the target skills the client is being taught
- Let the peers count the occurrence of the skill along with you
- Give them feedback on their counting
- Train the peers to prompt, evoke, model, and reinforce the target communication skill
- Have peers conduct a session in your presence
- Give peers feedback and refine their skills
- Give peers simple, clear written instructions
- Give peers a sample videotape of treatment procedures
- Ask peers to monitor the target skills in natural settings
- Ask peers to audio record a monitoring session outside the clinic or submit data recorded on paper
- Periodically review data submitted
- Periodically assess the client who is taught by the peers
- Initiate clinical treatment if peer training is not effective or their training cannot be improved

P-E Segment.   Pharyngeal-esophageal segment; a part of the pharynx and the esophagus; muscle fibers from the cricopharyngeus, esophagus, and inferior constrictor blend at this site to create a sphincter that can reduce the cross-sectional area of the esophagus.

Penetrating (Open-Head) Injury.   An injury where the skull is perforated or fractured and the Meninges are torn or lacerated.

Perceptual Training.   The same as Auditory Discrimination Training; in articulation treatment, it is assumed that clients should first learn to discriminate between speech sounds others produce before learning to produce them; in language treatment, it is assumed that clients should comprehend language structures before learning to produce them; both assumptions are questioned by some clinicians; the method needs more evidence.

In Articulation Treatment
- Present correct and incorrect productions of the target sounds alternatively
- Ask the child to judge each production as correct or incorrect
- Do not ask the child to produce the sounds
- Move to production training when the client can consistently discriminate your correct and incorrect presentations

In Language Treatment
- Teach nonverbal responses to verbal stimuli
- Ask the child to show objects or pictures you name
- Ask the child to follow directions and commands
- Do not ask the child to produce oral language
- Move to production training of a given language structure when the client can comprehend the meaning of that structure when spoken

Peristalsis.   Constricting and relaxing movements of a tubular structure (such as the pharynx) to move its contents (such as food in the pharynx); pharyngeal peristalsis may be disordered in patients with Dysphagia.

P

Perseveration.   Tendency to persist with the same response even though the stimulus has changed; often seen in patients with brain injury.

Pharyngeal Flap Operation.   A surgical procedure designed to reduce hypernasality in persons with repaired cleft or in those with weak or paralyzed soft palate (as in flaccid dysarthria); to improve velopharyngeal closure, the surgeon:
- Cuts a flap of tissue from the posterior pharyngeal wall
- Brings the flap down or raises it up (depending on how the flap is cut)
- Attaches the flap to the velum to provide extra muscular mass that helps achieve velopharyngeal closure
- Leaves an opening on either side of the flap to allow breathing, nasal drainage, and production of nasal sounds

Pharyngeal Phase of Swallowing

Pharyngeal Phase of Swallowing. A normal swallow stage in which the food is propelled through the pharynx and into the pharyngeal-esophageal (P-E) segment; may be disordered due to delayed or absent swallowing reflex; see Dysphagia.

Pharyngoplasty. A surgical procedure designed to reduce hypernasality in persons with repaired cleft or in those with weak or paralyzed soft palate (as in flaccid dysarthria); in this procedure, the surgeon
- Injects Teflon or other substance (e.g., Dacron wool or silicone gel bag) into the posterior pharyngeal wall
- Creates a bulge through such injection in the pharyngeal wall to help close the velopharyngeal port

Phonate. To produce vocal sound.

Phonatory Disorders. Disorders of phonation due to laryngeal structural problems or habitual patterns.

Phoneme. A group or family of closely related speech sounds whose individual productions may vary from production to production but nonetheless perceived as the same.

Phonemics. Study of the sound system and sound differences in a language.

Phonetic Derivation. The use of Shaping procedures (progressive approximation) to teach correct articulation to clients who do not imitate the clinician's productions; in using this procedure:
- Break the target sound production into its simpler components (e.g., teaching the production of /m/ by first having the client put the lips together, a simplified component of the total response)
- Teach the next component that will move the sequence in the right direction (e.g., add humming to the closed-lip posture)

- Teach other response components to achieve the total response (e.g., opening the mouth while humming through the nose, resulting in *ma*)
- Have the client practice the integrated response (e.g., *mommy*)

Phonetic Placement Method. An articulation treatment method; used when the client cannot imitate the modeled sound production; uses instruction, physical guidance, and visual feedback on how target sounds are produced; often used as a component of a comprehensive treatment program.

- Describe how the target sound is produced
- Demonstrate how the sound is produced
- Show the placement of articulators
- Give maximum visual feedback; use a mirror and a drawing of articulatory placements; use palatograms and breath indicators
- Show the differences between correct and incorrect productions of the same sound
- Help position the tongue of the client with tongue blades
- Use your fingers to manipulate and correctly position the client's articulators
- Let the client feel the presence and absence of laryngeal vibrations
- Reinforce correct responses

P

Phonetics. The study of speech sounds, their production, acoustic properties, and the written symbols that represent speech sounds.

Phonological Disorders. Multiple errors of articulation that form patterns based on Distinctive Features or Phonological Processes; the treatment target is to eliminate phonological processes.

Phonological Disorders (Treatment of). See Articulation and Phonological Disorders.

Phonological Processes

Phonological Processes.   Multiple ways in which children simplify adult production of speech sounds; these include such categories of processes as Deletion Processes, Substitution Processes, and Assimilation Processes; persistent processes in children are targets of intervention; treatment is directed against eliminating a phonological process; see Articulation and Phonological Disorders, Treatment of Articulation and Phonological Disorders: Specific Techniques or Programs.

Phonology.   The study of speech sounds, their patterns and sequences, and the rules that dictate sound combinations to create words.

Phrases (Word Combinations).   Productions that contain two or more words; grammatically incomplete, hence not sentences; treatment targets for language impaired children.
- Teach a few First Words
- Create two-word phrases out of words the child already has learned (e.g., such nouns and adjectives as *big man* or *small box*)
- Teach them with either Indirect Language Stimulation or Direct Language Treatment Approaches

Physical Prompts.   Visual signs or gestures given before a response is produced to demonstrate and prompt correct articulation (e.g., showing a lifted tongue tip just before the child attempts to produce a /t/; showing lip closure to prompt the production of a bilabial sound).

Physical Setting Generalization.   Production of trained responses in a setting not used in training; an important clinical goal; measured on a Probe; typically not reinforced.
- Select stimuli for treatment targets from the client's home
- Use common stimuli found in nonclinical settings
- Give training in varied physical settings such as outside the treatment room, outside the clinic building, and in

other places where target behaviors may be practiced in conversational speech in a relatively subtle manner

Physical Stimulus Generalization. Production of trained responses in the presence of untrained stimuli because of their similarity to trained stimuli; an important treatment goal; typically measured on a Probe; usually not reinforced.

* Use varied stimuli in training
* Use stimuli from the client's home
* Prefer objects to pictures
* Use multiple exemplars to train each target behavior
* Probe frequently with the help of untrained stimuli to evaluate physical stimulus generalization
* Provide additional training until the Probe Criterion is met

Pic Symbols. A set of Pictogram Ideogram Communication (Pic) symbols drawn in white on a black background; used in teaching Augmentative Communication, Gestural-Assisted (Aided).

Picture Communication Symbols. A large collection of pictures that represent words, phrases, sentences, social exchanges widely used in Augmentative and Alternative Communication; most symbols are transparent (meaning readily apparent).

Picture Exchange Communication System. A non-verbal communication system in which the client picks a picture and hands it to a caregiver or therapist who the gives what the picture implies or depicts; has been used in teaching communication to autistic children; children who cannot point to pictures to indicate what they want may nonetheless pick and hand a picture to someone to achieve the same effect; a transitional system eventually leading to verbal communication training.

Picsyms. A set of symbols containing line drawings that can be used to teach nonoral expression of nouns, verbs, prepositions, and so forth; each symbol also is associated with a printed English word; an open-ended system to which the clinician can add her or his own drawings; used in teaching Augmentative Communication, Gestural-Assisted (Aided).

Pictographic Symbols.   Pictorial representation of objects and events; easier to learn than abstract symbols; used in teaching Augmentative Communication, Gestural-Assisted (Aided).

Pneumatic Device for Alaryngeal Speech.   Sound source for patients with laryngectomy that uses the patient's exhaled air; a nonelectronic device, one end of which is placed in the mouth and the other end is placed over the stoma; a vibrating reed in between provides sound that the patient articulates into speech; contrasted with Electronic Devices for Alaryngeal Speech.

Polyps.   Protruding, soft, fluid-filled growths on the inner margin of the vocal folds; result of vocal abuse, often from a single abusive episode; often unilateral; may be *sessile* (broad-based) or *pedunculated* (the mass of the polyp is connected to the vocal fold by a stalk-like structure); associated with hoarseness and breathiness; surgically removed; see Voice Disorders; Treatment of Vocally Abusive Behaviors.
 • Identify the vocally abusive behaviors
 • Reduce vocally abusive behaviors
 • Teach appropriate vocal behaviors (e.g., gentle onset of phonation, soft speech)

Population.   A large, defined group with certain characteristics identified for the purposes of a study; part of the Group Design Strategy of research; a representative Sample is randomly drawn from the population.
 • Identify a large group of persons with defined characteristics (e.g., persons who stutter; people who have aphasia with additional defined characteristics relative to age, gender, severity, and so forth)
 • Randomly draw a sample of subjects needed for the study

- Assign them randomly to an experimental group and a control group in a treatment research study

Positive Practice. Required and unreinforced practice of a desirable behavior following Restitution for an undesirable behavior; a Direct Methods of Response Reduction; a part of Imposition of Work.

Positive Reinforcers. Events that, when presented immediately after a response is made, increase the future probability of that response; an effective method to increase the frequency of target communicative behaviors; extensively researched with a variety of clinical populations; commonly used in communication training.

- Select potential reinforcers after consulting with the client, the family, or both
- Present potential reinforcer immediately after the correct response is made
- Use a Continuous Reinforcement schedule in the beginning and an Intermittent Reinforcement schedule subsequently
- Prefer Conditioned Generalized Reinforcers, (e.g., Tokens) to Primary Reinforcers
- Always use verbal praise (even when you use other kinds)
- Use a different event when the one selected does not increase the response rate
- Call an event a reinforcer only when it increases a response rate

Postreinforcement Pause. A period of no responding after receiving a reinforcer; markedly evident in Fixed Interval Schedule of reinforcement.

Posttests. Measures of behaviors established after completing an experimental or routine teaching program; compared with Pretests; in a group design study, help rule-out the influence of extraneous variables.

Postural Strategies. Techniques of manipulating body positions, especially head and neck positions to prevent aspiration in patients with dysphagia; see Dysphagia.

P

Pragmatics

Pragmatics. The study of social use of language and the rules of such usage.

Pragmatic Structures. Aspects of appropriate language use in naturalistic communicative contexts; targets of language intervention; include such skills as Conversational Repair; Eye Contact; Narrative Skills, Topic Initiation, Topic Maintenance; and Turn Taking (all described under Language Disorders in Children; Treatment of Language Disorders: Specific Techniques or Programs).

Premack-Type Symbols. Plastic shapes or tokens designed by David Premack to teach communication to chimpanzees; Noniconic symbols that may be used to teach communicative skills to nonspeech clients; used in teaching Augmentative Communication Gestural-Assisted (Aided).

Prephonation Airflow. A target behavior for people who stutter and those who exhibit hard glottal attacks; includes a slight exhalation before initiating phonation; for procedures, see Stuttering Treatment, Treatment of Stuttering: Specific Techniques or Programs; Airflow Management; and Voice Disorders; Treatment of Voice Disorders; Specific Normal Voice Facilitating Techniques; Whisper-Phonation Method.

Pretests. Measures of behaviors established before starting an experimental or routine teaching program; compared with posttests; in a group design study, help rule out the influence of extraneous variables.

Primary Reinforcers. Reinforcers whose effects do not depend on past learning; often fulfill biological needs; contrasted with Conditioned, Secondary, or Social Reinforcers; also known as unconditioned reinforcers.

- Use primary reinforcers with infants, toddlers, and other children who do not respond well to Social Reinforcers

Principles (of Treatment)

- Use with children who are mentally retarded, those who are minimally verbal, and those who are autistic
- Use with persons who have brain injury in the initial stages of treatment
- Always combine with social reinforcers
- Gradually withdraw primary reinforcers and keep the clients on social reinforcers

Principles (of Treatment).   Empirical rules from which treatment procedures are derived.

Probes.   Procedures used to assess generalized production of clinically established responses; administered every time a few exemplars are trained to assess generalized productions; may be Intermixed Probes, Pure Probes, or Conversational Probes.

Probe Criterion.   A rule that specifies when to terminate training at a given topographic level of training or on a specified target behavior.

- A 90% correct Intermixed Probe response rate at each topographic level of training may suggest that the training may be moved to the next level (e.g., from the word to the phrase level)
- A 90% correct Pure Probe response rate for a behavior at the conversational level may suggest that the behavior is sufficiently trained and that the training may move on to another target behavior.

Probe Procedure.   Procedure to assess generalized production of target behaviors; see Intermixed Probes and Pure Probes for procedures.

Probe Recording Sheet.   A prepared sheet for recording probe response rates.

- Design and use a probe recording sheet similar to the following; modify as found necessary

P

Procedures of Treatment

Name of the Client	Treatment Target
Clinician	Date
Probe Recording Sheet	
Stimulus Items	Responses: + (Correct), − (Incorrect), 0 (No response)
1.	
2.	
3.	
4.	

Procedures of Treatment.   Technical operations the clinician performs to effect changes in client behaviors; actions of clinicians; contrasted with Treatment Targets; in describing treatment procedures:

- Specify what you ought to do to achieve the treatment target
- Specify the target communication skills
- Describe the stimulus conditions you need to arrange
- Specify the kinds of feedback you should give to the client under the differing conditions of correct, incorrect, and lack of responses
- Clarify how you measure the skills during treatment to document progress
- Describe how you plan to promote generalized productions and maintenance over time and across situations
- Specify the follow-up and booster treatment procedures

Production Training.   Treatment designed to teach a client to produce a specified speech or oral language target; contrasted with Perceptual Training or Auditory Discrimination Training; emphasis is on what the client ought to say rather than just listen or respond nonverbally.

- Model the target skills and ask the client to imitate your productions

410

- Fade modeling when imitation is established
- Evoke the target skills by appropriate questions and other devices

Prognosis.   A statement about the future course of a disorder under specified conditions, which typically include treatment or no treatment; good prognosis implies that the patient will recover from the clinical condition (with or without treatment, usually specified).

Programmed Learning.   A method of teaching skills in a systematic manner with immediate positive and corrective feedback using operant conditioning principles; used in the treatment of language and articulation disorders.

Program of Treatment.   An overall description of target behaviors, treatment variables, measurement procedures, generalization measures, maintenance strategies, follow-up, and so forth.

Progressive Assimilation.   A phonological process in which a sound takes on the properties of a preceding sound; elimination of such processes is a treatment goal in articulation and phonological treatment; see <u>Articulation and Phonological Disorders.</u>

Prolonged Speech.   A stuttering treatment target; syllables are prolonged to reduce the rate of speech; for procedures see <u>Stuttering, Treatment; Treatment of Stuttering: Specific Techniques or Programs.</u>

Prompts.   Special stimuli that increase the probability of a response; prompts may be verbal or nonverbal.
- Prompt promptly, as the client hesitates (e.g., in treating naming in a client with aphasia: "What is this?" "The word starts with a /t/.")
- Prompt more frequently in the beginning to reduce errors
- Prefer a subtle or short prompt to ones that are loud or long (e.g., in treating a person who stutters to speak slowly: "Slower" instead of "Speak at a slower rate.")

- Prefer a gesture to a verbal prompt (e.g., in treating a person who stutters to speak slowly: make a hand gesture to suggest a slower rate)
- Use <u>Partial Modeling</u> as a prompt
- Fade prompts as the responses become more consistent

Prosthesis.   A device fashioned for individual clients and fitted to compensate for deficient or deformed structure to improve their function.

Pseudobulbar Palsy.   Paralysis of the muscles of mastication, articulation, and swallowing caused by bilateral brain damage; so called because the symptoms mimic those caused by brainstem damage.

Pseudo Supraglottic Swallow.   A procedure to protect the airway during swallowing; used with patients who have dysphagia.
- Ask the patient to inhale, and hold the breath
- Swallow
- Cough

Public Law (P.L.) 94-142.   The Education of All Handicapped Children Act passed in 1975 by the U.S. Congress and signed into law; mandates appropriate special education, speech, language, and hearing services to all handicapped children in the age range of 3 and 18 years; extended to age range 3 to 21 in 1988; requires <u>Individualized Education Plans</u> for all handicapped children and education in least restrictive environment.

Public Law (P.L.) 99-457.   The 1986 Amendment to the Education of the Handicapped Act passed by the U.S. Congress and signed into law; mandates services to infants and toddlers required comprehensive state plans to educate handicapped youngsters.

Public Law (P.L.) 101-336.   The Americans With Disabilities Act passed by the U.S. Congress in 1990 and signed into law; prohibits discrimination against disabled individuals in employment settings; requires telephone relay services for the hearing impaired; requires handicapped access to public buildings.

Public Law (P.L.) 101-431. The Television Decoder Circuitry Act passed by the U.S. Congress in 1990 and signed into law; requires television manufacturers to include closed-caption circuitry in televisions (13 inch or larger screens).

Public Law (P.L.) 101-476. The Education of All Handicapped Children Act Amendments under the new title, Individuals With Disabilities Education Act passed by the U.S. Congress and signed into law in 1990; reauthorizes the original P.L. 94-142; additionally requires transition services to disabled students 16 years and older; also requires the use of assistive technology in educating children with disabilities.

Public Law (P.L.) 103-218. The Technology Related Assistance for Individuals With Disabilities Act Amendments passed by the U.S. Congress in 1994 and signed into law; encourages states to develop consumer access to assistive technology devices and services.

Public Law (P.L.) 105-17. The Individuals With Disabilities Act passed by the U.S. Congress and signed into law in 1997; promotes ethnocultural considerations in assessing and treating individuals with disabilities; requires parental involvement in the education of their disabled children.

Pull-Out Therapy Model. A special education service delivery model in which children are taken out of the classroom for special services, including speech-language services.

Punisher. A stimulus or a consequence that, when delivered soon after a response is made, is likely to reduce that response; a response-reducing consequence.

Punishment

Punishment. Procedures of reducing undesirable behaviors by response-contingent presentation or withdrawal of stimuli; includes <u>Direct Methods of Response Reduction</u> and <u>Indirect Methods of Response Reduction.</u>

- Minimize the use of response reduction procedures
- Simplify the target response and shape it to avoid or reduce the use of punishers
- Let the positive:corrective ratio be in favor of the positive (more reinforcers than punishers)
- Prefer indirect methods of response reduction in which you replace undesirable behaviors with desirable behaviors that you positively reinforce
- When the client's correct responses do not increase, change your treatment procedures
- Watch for potential undesirable <u>Side-Effects of Punishment</u>
- Note that <u>Time-Out</u> and <u>Response Cost</u> are especially effective procedures in reducing various disorders of communication and other undesirable behaviors children might exhibit during treatment sessions

Pure Probes. Procedures to assess generalized production with only untrained stimulus items; to be administered when the client has met the intermixed probe criterion, preferably toward the end of treatment: contrasted with <u>Intermixed Probes</u> in which trained and untrained items are alternated.

- Prepare a <u>Probe Recording Sheet</u> on which you have at least 10 untrained exemplars (untrained words, phrases, or sentences that contain the target sound or language feature)
- Present each exemplar on discrete trials
- Provide no reinforcement or corrective feedback
- Calculate the percent correct probe response rate
- Give additional training when an adopted probe criterion is not met (e.g., 90% accuracy)
- Move on to next level of training or to new target behaviors when the criterion is met

Pushing Approach.   A voice therapy procedure to promote better vocal fold approximations in clients who have
weakened or paralyzed; for procedures, see Voice Disorders,
Specific Normal Voice Facilitating Techniques.

Pyramidal System.   A bundle of nerve fibers that originate
in the motor cortex of the brain and travel to the brainstem;
upper motor neuron pathways; deliver motor impulses for
voluntary movements; has two tracts: corticobulbar and cor-
ticospinal; damage to the system can cause various neurogenic speech disorders; see Dysarthria.

P

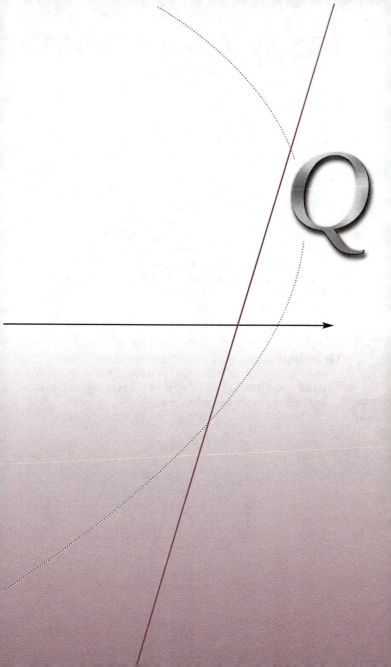

Quadriplegia.   Paralysis of all four limbs.

QWERTY.   The standard arrangement of letters on keyboards for typewriters and computers and certain Augmentative and Alternative Communication input devices.

Question.   Interrogative forms designed to request information; treatment targets for clients with language disorders; types of questions include:

- Intonation questions: Essentially declarative statements (not syntactically correct questions) that serve as questions because of their unique intonation
- Tag questions: Declarative expressions with an interrogative tag added at the end (e.g., You can do it, can't you?")
- Wh-questions: Question forms that begin with *who, what, which, when, where, whose, why,* and *how*
- Yes-No questions: Question forms that require either a *Yes* or a *No* as the response

Questionnaire.   Assessment instrument that asks a series of questions of relevance; respondent's answers are analyzed and often compared against the responses of a reference group; subjective measures.

Q

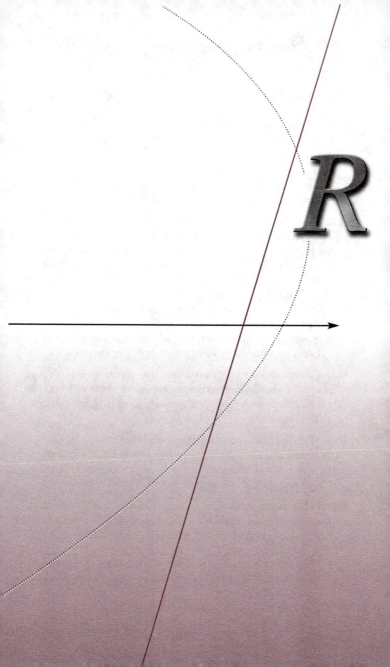

Random Assignment. A method of assigning participants selected for a study to either the experimental or the control group without the experimenter bias; used in treatment research; part of the Group Design Strategy.
- Select participants randomly
- Assign a number to each subject
- Assign every even-numbered subject to one group and every odd-numbered subject to the other group

Random Selection. A method of selecting subjects (clients) to evaluate treatment effects or efficacy; each potential subject has an equal chance of being selected for the study, hence no experimenter bias in subject selection; need a large number of potential subjects for the method to work; part of the Group Design Strategy.
- Identify a large number of potential subjects
- Assign a number to each subject
- Select the required number of subjects randomly (e.g., every second, every fourth, or every tenth person)

Range of Motion. The degree to which muscle movements can occur; limited range of speech muscle movements may cause speech disorders; problem found in some patients with Dysarthria.

Rate Reduction. A rate of speech slower than the normal or below a client-specific baserate; a target in the treatment of several communicative disorders including Stuttering, Cluttering, and Dysarthria.

Ratio Strain. Reduction in response rate due to a sudden thinning of reinforcement as when the clinician shifts from continuous reinforcement to a FR10 (every 10th response is reinforced) .
- Start with continuous reinforcement for target responses
- Move to a FR2 or FR3 (every second or third response is reinforced)
- Increase the ratio of reinforcement gradually

Rationalism.   A philosophical position that reason and intellect are the source of knowledge, not sensory experience; closely related to <u>Nativism;</u> contrasted with <u>Empiricism.</u>

Rebuses.   Pictures of objects and persons used in teaching <u>Augmentative Communication Gestural-Assisted (Aided);</u> different from just pictures in that words and grammatic morphemes are combined with rebuses; <u>Iconic</u> easier than <u>Noniconic</u> symbol systems to learn.

Recast.   A child language intervention procedure in which the clinician expands a child's utterance type into a different type of sentence; procedure described under <u>Language Disorders in Children; Treatment of Language Disorders: Specific Techniques or Programs.</u>

Recombinative Generalization.   A form of generalization of taught behaviors in which various combinations of new stimuli evoke differential responding; varied and novel sentences formed out of previously taught words exemplify recombinative generalization.

Recurrent Laryngeal Nerve Resection.   A surgical treatment procedure for adductor spasmodic dysphonia; the recurrent laryngeal nerve is unilaterally resectioned to paralyze one of the folds to prevent hyperadduction; voice therapy may be needed following this operation.

R

Reduced Modeling.   The same as <u>Partial Modeling.</u>

Regressive Assimilation.   An articulatory phenomenon in which a sound takes on the properties of a following sound.

Regulated Breathing.   A stuttering treatment target; includes inhalation, a slight exhalation before initiating phonation, and reduced rate of speech; for procedures see <u>Stuttering, Treatment; Treatment of Stuttering: Specific Techniques or Programs.</u>

Reinforce. Strengthen and increase behaviors by arranging immediate consequences for them; an important action clinicians perform in teaching target responses to children as well as adults; see <u>Reinforcers.</u>

Reinforcement. A method of selecting and strengthening behaviors of individuals by arranging consequences under specific stimulus conditions; widely used in the treatment of communicative disorders; see <u>Reinforcers.</u>

Reinforcement Priming. Seeking reinforcers for one's own behaviors; useful strategy for the client to learn in getting parents, teachers, peers, and others to notice the production of clinically established behaviors in natural settings and thus get reinforced; part of <u>Maintenance Strategy.</u>
- Teach others to reinforce the client for the production of target behaviors established in the clinic
- Teach the client to draw attention to his or her desirable communicative behaviors from others
- Verify that others are indeed reinforcing the client when attention is drawn to the production of target behaviors (e.g., have the client or the family members maintain and present records of reinforcement delivery)

Reinforcement Withdrawal. Taking away reinforcers to decrease a response; one of the <u>Direct Methods of Response Reduction;</u> includes <u>Response Cost</u> and <u>Time-Out.</u>

Reinforcers. Events that follow behaviors and thereby increase the future probability of those behaviors; widely used in treating communicative disorders.
- Select either the <u>Primary, Secondary, Conditioned Generalized, Informative Feedback,</u> or <u>High Probability Behaviors</u> to reinforce clinical targets
- Reinforce initially on a <u>Continuous Reinforcement</u> schedule
- Switch to an <u>Intermittent Reinforcement</u> schedule later
- Always use verbal (conditioned) reinforcers in conjunction with other types

Reinke's Edema

- Teach the client's significant others to reinforce the skills you establish

Reinke's Edema. Also known as polypoid degeneration; sausage-shaped, grayish-pink or red projection-like growth on vocal fold margins; typically bilateral; the floppy-appearing folds may be described as *elephant ears;* severe and persistent hoarseness is the vocal symptom; cause is excessive smoking and alcohol abuse.

- Treatment is surgical removal of the growth; performed on one fold at a time; if normal voice is restored, the second operation may be avoided
- Voice treatment involves modifying smoking and drinking behaviors

Reliability. Consistency with which the same event is repeatedly measured; important in clinical work and clinical research; includes inter- and intraobserver reliability.

Interobserver Reliability. The extent to which two (or more) observers agree in measuring an event.

- Measure a behavior of interest with its location identified for a unit-by-unit analysis (count not only the behaviors being measured, but also their locations in transcribed speech samples)
- Have another trained observer measure in the same manner (unit-by-unit analysis)
- Score the total number of locations for which both of you agreed for an Agreement count (A)
- Count the total number of locations for which only one of you, not both of you scored the behavior (stuttering, pitch breaks, articulatory error) for a Disagreement count (D)
- Calculate the unit-by-unit Agreement Index by using the following formula: $A/(A+D) \times 100$

Intraobserver Reliability. The extent to which the same observer repeatedly measures the same event consistently.

Replication

- Measure the behavior of interest using the unit-by-unit method
- Measure again by the same method
- Calculate the Agreement Index using the same formula as given under Interobserver Reliability

Hegde, M. N. (1994). *Clinical research in communicative disorders: Principles and strategies* (2nd ed.). Austin, TX: Pro-Ed.

Replication. Conducting repeated research to show that a given procedure works with different clients, in different settings, and for different clinicians; important in treatment efficacy research; includes direct replication and systematic replication; both designed to show treatment Generality; one of the Treatment Selection Criteria.

Direct Replication. The same investigator repeats the same treatment experiment in the same setting but with different subjects who have the same characteristics as the original subjects.

- Initially, show that a treatment works with some clients
- Select different clients who share the same personal (age, gender, health) and clinical characteristics (severity, age of onset) as the original subjects
- Repeat the treatment experiment
- Analyze the results to evaluate generality of the treatment method

Systematic Replication. The same or different investigators repeat a treatment experiment in different settings, with clients who have different characteristics than the original clients; may even include clients with totally different diagnoses.

- Initially, an investigator shows that a treatment is effective with a sample of clients
- The same or a different investigator repeats the treatment research with another sample, with different personal (gender, age, health) and clinical characteristics

R

(severity, age of onset) characteristics, and in a different setting than the original
• The investigator analyzes the results to evaluate the broader generality of the treatment method

Hegde, M. N. (1994). *Clinical research in communicative disorders: Principles and strategies* (2nd ed.). Austin, TX: Pro-Ed.

Response Class.

A group of responses created by the same or similar contingencies; functionally, but not necessarily structurally, similar responses; good treatment targets because there is generalized production within a class and discrimination between classes.

Response Complexity.

Different topographic levels of a target behavior; structural complexity of communicative behaviors typically create a sequence of treatment.
• Teach words before phrases
• Teach phrases before sentences
• Teach sentences before conversational speech

Response Cost.

A direct response reduction strategy in which the production of each response scheduled for reduction results in the loss of a reinforcer. In the **Earn and Lose** variety, clients earn a token for every correct response and lose one for every incorrect response. In the **Lose-Only** variety, the client who receives unearned tokens at the beginning of a session loses one for every incorrect response.

Earn and Lose
• Give a token, to be exchanged for back-up reinforcers, for correct responses
• Take a token away each time the client produces an incorrect response
• Exchange the tokens the client still possesses for back-up reinforcers at the end of the session

Lose-Only
• Give a certain number of tokens at the beginning of a session

R

Response Generalization

- Take a token away each time the client produces an incorrect response
- Exchange the tokens the client still possesses for back-up reinforcers at the end of the session

Response Generalization. Production of unreinforced (new, untrained) responses that are similar to trained responses; a goal of treatment; typically achieved through various strategies designed to promote Generalization because stimulus generalization in language training also involves response generalization.

Response Mode Generalization. Production of unreinforced responses in a mode not involved in training.

- Train skills in a certain mode (e.g., fluency in oral reading)
- Probe to assess generalized production (fluency in conversational speech)
- If there is no generalization, train the skills in that mode (fluency in conversational speech)

Response Recording Sheet. A prepared sheet for recording correct, incorrect, and no responses given in treatment sessions.

- Design and use a response recording sheet similar to the following; modify as necessary

Name of the Client	Treatment Target
Clinician	Date
Response Recording Sheet	
Stimulus Items	Responses: + (Correct), − (Incorrect), 0 (No response)
1.	
2.	
3.	
4.	

Hegde, M. N. (1998). *Treatment procedures in communicative disorders* (3rd ed.). Austin, TX: Pro-Ed.

Response Reduction Strategies

Response Reduction Strategies.   A collection of procedures that help decrease undesirable responses; include Direct Methods of Response Reduction and Indirect Methods of Response Reduction.

Response Substitution.   Increase in an undesirable behavior when another behavior is reduced; exemplified by increased frequency of wiggling in the chair when a child's disruptive hand movements are reduced by a response reduction method.
- Apply a response reduction strategy to the newly emerged undesirable behavior
- Apply such strategies sequentially if you have to

Response Unit.   A training target in the Paired Stimuli Approach to treating articulation disorders (described under Articulation and Phonological Disorders; Treatment of Articulation and Phonological Disorders: Specific Techniques or Programs); the client is asked to produce a key word and a target word as a single response unit (e.g., this-bus); the client earns one reinforcer only by correctly producing the target sound in both of the words.

Restitution.   An element of overcorrection in which the person eliminates the effects of his or her misbehavior and then improves the situation; described under Imposition of Work.
- Ask the child who disorganizes your stimulus materials to reorganize them
- Next, ask the child to organize the toys on the floor (the disorganized toys were not the child's making)

Reversed Imitation.   Clinician's imitation of a child's utterance during indirect language stimulation; in the operant Imitation, it is the client who imitates and the clinician who models.

Right Hemisphere Syndrome.   A syndrome of brain injury and its consequences sustained in the right cerebral hemisphere; may be caused by cerebrovascular accidents,

R

tumors, head trauma, or various neurological diseases; associated with perceptual, attentional, emotional, and communicative deficits; varying degrees of functional involvement depending on the site, nature, and extent of damage.

Treatment: General Considerations

- Note that treatment research on the techniques typically suggested is limited and in many cases, nonexistent; recommendations are based on clinical experience of several clinicians; use all suggestions with caution and with a view to collect data
- Counsel the family about communication treatment soon after the onset
- Note that some clinicians prefer to teach specific skills while others prefer to treat presumed underlying processes; process approach needs to demonstrate that skills improve when underlying processes are targeted for treatment; in practice, the two approaches may be integrated
- Begin treatment as soon as it is practical
- Select the client-specific treatment targets that:
  - will result in the most improvement in family, social, and vocational communication
  - help build other, more advanced communication skills
  - help focus on communicative treatment targets (e.g., attentional deficits may have to be treated before other language skills)
  - the clients can imitate
- Develop stimulus materials that:
  - range from simple to progressively more complex and from fewer to greater number of elements
  - are clear, unambiguous, and relatively concrete
  - are familiar, meaningful to the client, and attractive
- Establish baselines of target behaviors
- Provide extensive and intensive practice
- Be aware that there is no controlled clinical evidence to support the use of computerized cognitive rehabilitation programs

Right Hemisphere Syndrome

- Structure treatment sessions initially and loosen them as the client becomes more proficient in producing the target responses
- Use instructions, modeling, and prompts in all stages of treatment
- Fade the special antecedents used in early stages of treatment
- Shape the target behaviors
- Give prompt and effective feedback
- Work with the family members to promote generalization and maintenance

Treatment: Targets and Procedures

Treat Lack of Awareness of Problems Experienced

- Give immediate verbal feedback on errors
- Give visual feedback on errors
- Tape record and replay the speech to the client and discuss the errors
- Teach the client Self-Control (Self-Monitoring) skills

Treat Impaired Attention

- Shape sustained attending behaviors with changing criterion (Changing Criterion, Treatment Procedure)
- Reinforce the client for paying attention to the stimulus material and for maintaining eye contact
- Structure the initial treatment sessions and reduce distractions, including noise
- Give alerting stimuli before presenting the treatment stimuli (e.g., "Look at me" before modeling a response, "Get ready, here comes the next picture" before presenting the stimulus picture; touching the client before presenting a treatment stimulus)
- Draw attention before you speak to the client (e.g., "Listen, I am going to tell you something.")
- Vary the treatment stimuli, drop unattractive stimuli, use clear and forceful stimuli
- Give frequent, brief breaks in the initial phase of treatment; reduce the number and duration of the breaks gradually

R

- Introduce gradually some distracting stimuli while still reinforcing attention to treatment tasks

Treat Visual Neglect

- Note that the most commonly used strategy to treat neglect is to force attention to that side with a variety of cues and prompts
- Use printed material or any means that would force attention to the neglected side
- Teach the patient to keep a finger on the left margin while reading and track back to it before beginning a new line
- Color the left-side margins, draw a colored line through the margin, or use other discriminative stimuli to force attention to the left side of reading texts; fade such stimuli
- Tell the patient to "Look to the left" when the client reaches the end of sentences; fade such verbal cues
- Teach clients to recognize that what they read does not make sense; teach them to quiz themselves about what they read
- Design reading materials with large print and progressively smaller print and ask the client to read them aloud

Treat Impulsive Behaviors

- Teach the client to wait and withhold responses
- Give nonverbal signals to delay responses
- Fade the noverbal signals and introduce verbal signals to wait, withhold, and delay

Treat Pragmatic Language Skills

- Teach the client to initiate conversation; have the client discuss various topics in which you teach various skills by modeling them, ask the client to use them, and reinforce the client for using them; for instance:
  - teach the client to introduce the topic explicitly
  - teach the client to give background information on narratives and stories

- teach the client to periodically restate the topic of discussion
- prompt the client to maintain focus on the main topic
- teach the client to ask such questions as "Do you follow me?" or "Do you understand?"
- give corrective feedback

- Teach the client to request clarification when messages are not understood (e.g., "Please repeat that," or "I do not understand.")
- Teach the client to maintain eye contact during conversation; use such verbal stimuli as "Look at me"
- Reinforce progressively longer durations of topic of maintenance
- Teach the client to take turns in conversation; stop the client for inappropriate turn taking (e.g., interrupting you)
- Use the PACE program (Promoting Aphasics' Communicative Effectiveness; described under Aphasia; Treatment of Aphasia: Specific Techniques or Programs) for teaching social communication

Treat Impaired Reasoning Skills

- Teach the client to think and plan (e.g., discuss how the client might plan a vacation; help the client move in a logical manner)
- Pose different kinds of problems one might encounter in real life and ask the client to solve them (e.g., "How do you buy an airplane ticket?")

Treat Impaired Inference

- Tell stories and ask questions to evoke implied information
- Describe situations that require the client to draw logical conclusions

Treat Impaired Recognition of Absurdities

- Show pictures that depict logical and absurd events and ask the client to separate them (e.g., picture of a cat chasing a rat and picture of a rat chasing a cat)

R

- Present verbal or written statements that are logical or absurd and ask the client to separate them
- Ask the client to explain why a statement is absurd or logical

Treat Impaired Comprehension of Metaphors or Idioms

- Ask the client to select statements that give literal meanings
- Asking the client to sort out literal and figurative statements
- Set up hypothetical situations that require such judgments

Treat Comprehension of Figurative Meanings

- Begin with nonliteral meanings that the client presently uses and understands
- Provide multiple meanings for a single statement
- Discuss the difference between what the statement apparently says and what it means
- Use stimuli that the client was familiar with and used premorbidly

Treat Comprehension of Humor

- Associate captions with the cartoons
- Link the punch line with the body of the joke

Teach Compensatory Strategies

- Monitor the comprehension of the speaker's utterance
- Teach the use of such functional memory aids as lists of things do, writing down appointments, having a checklist of things to do before leaving the house, keeping related things together, and so forth
- Teach Self-Control (Self-Monitoring) skills including the generation of memory aids
- Teach the client to stop and self-correct when errors are made
- Make a few socially appropriate and inappropriate statements and ask the client to evaluate them
- Have the client evaluate social appropriateness of his or her own productions

- Teach the client to rephrase inappropriate comments to make them more appropriate

Brookshire, R. H. (1997). *An introduction to neurogenic communication disorders* (5th ed.). St. Louis, MO: Mosby Year Book.

Hegde, M. N. (1998). *A coursebook on aphasia and other neurogenic language disorders* (2nd ed.). San Diego: Singular Publishing Group.

Myers, P. S. (1999). *Right hemisphere damage.* San Diego: Singular Publishing Group.

Tompkins, C. A. (1995). *Right hemisphere communication disorders: Theory and management.* San Diego: Singular Publishing Group.

Rigidity.   Stiffness of muscles and joints.

Rochester Method.   A method of teaching communication skills to children who are deaf by combining speech with finger spelling.

R

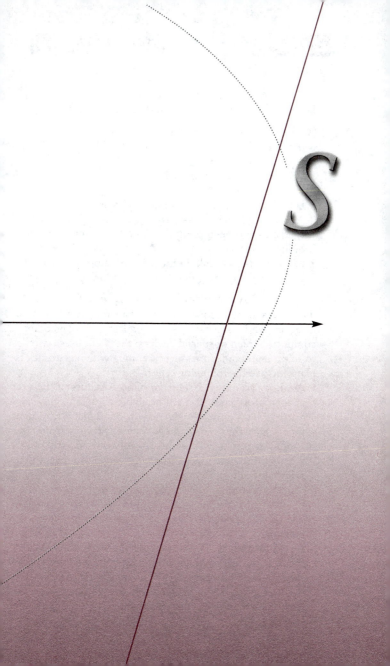

Sample.   A smaller number of individuals selected from a larger population for a research study.

Satiation.   Temporary termination of a drive or need because it has been satisfied; a potential problem with <u>Primary Reinforcers</u> (e.g., food).
- Give only small amounts of food or drink to reinforce individual responses
- Let the client accumulate food that he or she can eat later
- Arrange treatment sessions, especially with infants and toddlers who need primary reinforcers, around breakfast or lunchtime
- Ask parents to withhold the primary reinforcers you plan to use before coming to treatment sessions

Scanning in Augmentative Communication.   An indirect message-selection method in augmentative communication; various messages are typically displayed on a computer screen or special devices; the client uses switches to select an intended message; scanning with electronic displays include the following types:
- Auditory scanning: Useful for blind AAC users; the user gets auditory cues that tell available choices (e.g., *Things to eat, Things to wear* spoken with one voice); the client then selects the specific category among the presented categories; the items within the category selected are spoken with another voice (e.g., *hamburger, milk*); the client then selects the individual item
- Circular scanning: The screen displays message or symbol choices in a circular manner, and the client presses a switch to highlight the desired item or an intended message
- Direct scanning: The screen displays various message choices; the client holds a switch pressed down; consequently, the indicator (cursor) moves through the list; the client releases the switch as soon as the cursor is on the desired item, which is then highlighted

S

- Group item scanning: The screen displays messages or symbols in groups; the client first highlights a group (e.g., food items) and then an individual item in the group (a glass of juice)
- Multiple switch scanning: Highlighting messages or symbols with the help of two or more switches.
- Predictive scanning: Scanning based on previous selections; once a selection is made, the device presents only those choices that may be selected next; speeds up the selection process
- Row column scanning: Selecting a message of symbol by first highlighting an entire row and then an individual item within the row
- Step linear scanning: Scanning item-by-item with a switch that moves the cursor across choices; the user stops the cursor when it highlights the desired item

Schedules of Reinforcement. Different patterns of reinforcement that generate different patterns of responses; include <u>Continuous Reinforcement</u> schedules and <u>Intermittent Reinforcement</u> schedules.
- Use continuous reinforcement schedule in the beginning of treatment
- Shift to an intermittent schedule as learning becomes more stable

Script. A presumed mental representation of repeatedly occurring, sequenced events, episodes, or personal experiences; used in teaching advanced language skills including narrative skills; a description of baking cookies or running a hot dog stand is a script; it has a beginning and an end, actions people take, or roles people play; for procedures, see <u>Language Disorders in Children; Treatment of Language Disorders: Specific Techniques or Programs.</u>

Script Therapy. The use of <u>Scripts</u> in teaching language skills to children with language impairment; for procedures, see Language Disorders in Children; Treatment of Language Disorders: Specific Techniques or Programs.

Secondary Reinforcers. Conditioned reinforcers whose effects depend on past learning; appropriate reinforcers for all kinds of verbal responses except for certain kinds of mands that request food and drink; include Social Reinforcers, Conditioned Generalized Reinforcers, Informative Feedback, and High Probability Behaviors.

Self-Control. A behavior that monitors and modifies other behaviors of the same person; a necessary skill in maintaining clinically acquired communicative behaviors.

Self-Control (Self-Monitoring) Teaching Procedures.

Techniques of monitoring one's own behavior to effect significant and positive changes; useful to teach these techniques to clients within a Maintenance Strategy: take note of the examples and extend them to other disorders and other kinds of strategies:

- Teach clients to discriminate their own incorrect and undesirable responses; for instance:
  - model a child's misarticulated sound production and ask the child to listen to them
  - demonstrate a stuttering person's associated motor behaviors
  - model a child's phrases or sentences that do not contain required grammatic morphemes (e.g., "Two cup" or "Boy walking")
  - play back a taped sample of client's speech to point out undesirable voice quality
- Teach clients to contrast their desirable and undesirable responses; for instance:
  - contrast easy and hard glottal attacks of a voice client or a fluency client by modeling the two kinds of phonatory initiations
  - contrast incorrect and correct productions of phonemes by modeling them

Self-Control Teaching Procedures

- contrast correct and incorrect sentence forms (e.g., "Two cup" and "Two cups")
- contrast the desirable lower pitch with the client's excessively high pitch by modeling the two pitch levels or by tape-recording the client's voice that might catch both the levels
- Teach clients to measure their behaviors reliably; for instance:
  - ask a client to measure his or her dysfluencies in selected situations outside the clinic and submit the data
  - ask a client to measure the frequency of his or her vocally abusive behaviors for 3 days and submit the data
  - ask a client to measure his or her misarticulations in certain specific situations and submit the data
  - have clients tape-record a home speech sample and play it as you give feedback on the target behaviors to be measured
- Let clients measure their behaviors along with you in treatment sessions; note that children, too, can learn to make a tally mark to measure correct productions of sounds, grammatic morphemes, voice qualities, and so forth; for instance:
  - in the treatment sessions, ask the client to chart his or her own correct and incorrect productions of target phonemes along with you
  - ask a fluency client in therapy to chart his or her own dysfluencies, hard and abrupt voice onset, excessively fast speech, easy onset, and appropriate rate
  - ask an apraxic client to chart correct and incorrect articulatory movements
  - ask a child in language therapy to chart sentences with and without the target grammatic features
  - ask a voice client in therapy to chart his or her desirable vocal qualities
- Give clients frequent feedback on their measurement to improve their skill; for instance:

S

Self-Control Teaching Procedures

- give all clients feedback when they fail to record their correct and incorrect responses; point out the characteristics of those responses, model them if necessary, and ask them to resume their charting
- throughout the session give them informative feedback ("You and I agreed on three of the five instances" and "This time, you and I agreed on four of the five instances.")
- monitor the progress and make sure the clients' skill in measuring their behaviors improves over the sessions
- Teach clients to monitor their newly acquired skills by measuring them outside the clinic; for instance:
  - ask the fluency client to keep a pocket record of his or her use of slower rate or gentle phonatory onset; minimally, ask the client to gain a clear impression of the frequency of their use
  - ask a voice client with excessively soft voice to keep a record of the number of social situations in which he or she spoke with adequate loudness
  - ask a client with aphasia to keep a record of the number of times he successfully recalled his wife's name in a given day
- Teach clients to generate signals and prompts for their own actions in the natural environment; for instance:
  - ask a patient with aphasia to write down the names of family members and frequently consult the list before engaging in conversational speech
  - ask a client to wear electronic devices that remind him or her of appointments, to slow down the speech, to speak more softly or loudly, and so forth
- Teach clients to pause after they produce a wrong response both in the clinic and outside the clinic; for instance:
  - teach a stuttering client to pause briefly after each dysfluency and say the same word fluently without your help

Self-Control Teaching Procedures

- teach a voice client to pause soon after a hard glottal attack is produced and start again with a softer attack without your help
- teach a child in articulation therapy to stop as soon as he or she produces a target sound incorrectly without your help
- teach a client in apraxia therapy to stop as soon as a wrong articulatory gesture is initiated and then initiate the correct gesture without your help
- Teach clients to correct their own mistakes or nontarget responses
  - initially, give corrective feedback for every incorrect response
  - tell the client that you will on occasion not give correct feedback and the client should catch himself or herself making a wrong response and immediately correct the mistake without help
  - withhold corrective feedback on certain occasions
  - if the client does not immediately self-correct, give corrective feedback; remind the client that he or she should self-correct without your help
  - continue the procedure until the client reliably self-corrects; reduce the frequency of corrective feedback further while maintaining self-corrections
- Teach clients to anticipate problems and take corrective actions
  - teach a person who stutters to practice saying "Hello" with appropriate airflow when the telephone starts ringing
  - teach an aphasic client to practice names of people who are expected to visit shortly
  - teach a voice client with vocal abuse to reduce talking before a scheduled and unavoidable speech to be given to a group
  - teach another voice client to drink more water to ward off vocal problems related to vocal dryness

S

- In group therapy, teach clients to correct other participants' errors
  - in a group therapy involving children who have received treatment for stuttering, teach each child to monitor other children's speech rates and to give appropriate feedback
  - in group therapy involving aphasic clients, teach each to remind the other to practice specified skills (e.g., self-cueing words with the first word phoneme)
  - in language group therapy, teach each child to monitor the use of a specific grammatic feature in other children and give appropriate feedback

Self-Talk. A child language intervention procedure in which the clinician describes his or her own activity while playing with a child; procedure described under Language Disorders in Children; Treatment of Language Disorders: Specific Techniques or Programs.

Sequence of Treatment. Movement within a treatment program from the beginning to the end; a description of steps involved in implementing a treatment plan; progression of treatment from a simple to a more complex level; see Treatment in Communicative Disorders, General Sequence.

Service Delivery Models. Different arrangements of providing assessment and treatment services to children with communication disorders, include the Collaborative Model, the Consultant Model, the Language-Based Classroom Model, and the Pull-Out Therapy Model.

Shaping. A method of teaching nonexistent responses that are not even imitated; also known as successive approximation; supported by experimental evidence; highly useful in teaching a variety of skills.

- Select a terminal target response (e.g., the production of /m/ in word initial positions)
- Identify an initial component of that target response the client can imitate (e.g., putting the two lips together)

Side-Effects of Punishment

- Identify intermediate responses (e.g., humming or other kinds of vocalizations, opening the mouth as humming is continued)
- Teach the initial response by modeling and immediate positive reinforcement (e.g., putting the lips together on several trials)
- In successive stages, teach the intermediate responses (e.g., adding humming when the lips are closed; opening the mouth when the humming is continued; adding other sounds to form words)
- Continue until the terminal response is taught

Side-Effects of Punishment. Undesirable effects of punishment procedures; include emotional reactions, aggressive reactions, unexpected increase in the punished response, increase in a different response than the one punished, and so forth; to be eliminated or minimized by prudent use of response reduction methods.

- Always use positive reinforcers for desirable behaviors
- Keep reinforcement:punishment ratio in favor of reinforcement
- Shape a difficult response to avoid using response reduction methods
- Consistently apply response reduction methods to all undesirable behaviors
- Remove or reduce reinforcement for undesirable behaviors
- Never associate response reduction methods with positive reinforcement

Significant Others. People who typically interact with a client on a daily basis; include family members, teachers, friends, colleagues, baby sitters, and health care workers; important in helping the client learn and maintain communicative behaviors; recipients of training within a Maintenance Strategy.

Sig Symbols. A set of pictographic or ideographic symbols based on American Sign Language; used on communication boards; used in teaching Augmentative Communication Gestural-Assisted (Aided).

Single-Subject Design Strategy. Methods of demonstrating treatment effects by showing contrasts between conditions of no treatment, treatment, withdrawal of treatment, and other control procedures; typically, all subjects selected receive treatment (no control group); includes, among others, ABA Design, ABAB Design, and Multiple Baseline Design; contrasted with Group Design Strategy.

Social Reinforcers. A variety of conditioned reinforcers frequently used in treatment sessions; include verbal praise, attention, touch, eye contact, and facial expressions; resistant to satiation effect; may not work with nonverbal clients.

- With children who are nonverbal, profoundly retarded, and very young (infants and toddlers), pair social reinforcers with primary reinforcers
- Eventually, fade the primary reinforcers and maintain the responses on social reinforcers only

Soft Articulatory Contacts. A stuttering treatment target; includes relaxed, easy, and soft contact of articulators in speech production; used in conjunction with such other techniques as Airflow Management and Rate Reduction; for procedures see Stuttering, Treatment; Treatment of Stuttering: Specific Techniques or Programs.

Spasmodic Dysphonia. A voice disorder characterized in most cases by severe overadduction of vocal folds and strained or choked-off voice quality; in some cases, phonation may be impossible; in other cases, characterized by sudden abduction of folds and resulting aphonia; of unknown etiology; possible neuropathology; voice therapy is not particularly helpful although several techniques, including relaxed, easy, and less effortful phonation; the yawn-sigh method; auditory masking; amplified voice feedback, laryngeal massage, and other kinds of digital manipulations; none has produced lasting treatment effects; some clinicians combine voice therapy with medical management in a team effort; current medical management includes:

- Injection of Botox (botulinum toxin A) into one or both of the vocal folds to induce paralysis of the folds; some data suggest the best results are with unilateral injection
  - initially, the voice is weak and breathy, which improves with voice therapy
  - voice therapy is designed to eliminate habitual over adduction and effortful phonation by teaching more relaxed phonation
  - reinjection may be needed as the effects last only a few months
- Recurrent laryngeal nerve sectioning; a surgical procedure in which the recurrent laryngeal nerve is cut.
  - procedure has not produced long-term favorable effects and, in some cases, the symptoms worsen; the laryngeal nerve also may regenerate, resulting in the symptoms return
  - need to be combined with voice therapy; procedures to raise the pitch, head position changes, and digital manipulation of the larynx have all been clinically tried and found to be helpful to varying degrees

Spastic Dysarthria.   A type of motor speech disorder; its neuropathology is bilateral damage to the upper motor neuron (direct and indirect motor pathways) resulting in weakness, spastic paralysis, limited range of movement, and slowness of movement; may affect all aspects of speech; major speech problems include strained-strangled-harsh voice, hypernasality, slow rate, consonant imprecision, and monopitch and monoloudness; select appropriate treatment targets and procedures described under Treatment of Dysarthria; see Dysarthria: Specific Types.

Specific Language Impairment (SLI).   Language disorders in children who are otherwise normal although some may have subtle cognitive deficits; different language skills may be somewhat differentially affected; pragmatic skills may be better than syntactic and morphological skills; a diagnosis made on negative grounds (no other factor, such as mental retardation or neurologic deficits, explains the disorder); some believe that SLI suggests limited language skills with no pathology; treatment procedures are the same as those for Language Disorders in Children.

Specific Normal Voice Facilitating Techniques. A collection of voice therapy procedures used to promote normal voice productions; see Voice Disorders; Specific Normal Voice Facilitating Techniques.

Stimulus Generalization. Production of a newly learned response to stimuli not used in training; an important goal of intervention; to promote stimulus generalization.
- Use a variety of stimuli during treatment
- Use common stimuli
- Ask clients to bring objects, toys, books, and so forth from home to use as stimuli
- Train multiple exemplars
- Periodically Probe the production of target behaviors to assess their generalized productions

Stimulation Versus Treatment or Teaching. In language intervention, stimulation tends to be less directed, more naturalistic, without specific language targets, without a requirement that the child imitate modeled responses, and is often implemented by nonclinicians; treatment or teaching tends to be more clinician-directed, less naturalistic, with specific language structures as targets, with the requirement that the child imitate modeled responses, and often implemented by speech-language pathologists.

Stimulus Withdrawal. A group of procedures used to reduce incorrect responses during treatment; a reinforcer or a reinforcing state of affairs is removed as soon as an incorrect response is made; includes Time-Out and Response Cost.

Story Grammar.   The structure of narratives which may be treatment targets for children with language disorders; described under Language Disorders in Children; Treatment of Language Disorders: Specific Techniques or Programs.

Stridency.   A voice disorder characterized by an unpleasant, shrill, and metallic-sounding voice; caused by excessive pharyngeal constriction and an elevated larynx.
- Use the Chewing Method
- Model and contrast good vocal production with a strident production
- Lower the pitch; use Glottal Fry
- Teach relaxation
- Teach oral openness
- Use Yawn-Sigh method

Stridor.   A harsh and shrill (high-pitched) sound during breathing; often found in persons with laryngeal obstruction; laryngeal stridor is associated with various laryngeal pathologies including congenital laryngeal cyst, congenital laryngeal papilloma, congenital subglottic stenosis, and laryngocele; treatment is medical.

Stuttering.   A disorder of fluency characterized by excessive amounts of Dysfluencies, excessive durations of dysfluencies, and unusual amount of muscular effort in speaking; has varied definitions including an involuntary loss of speech motor control, part-word repetitions and sound prolongations, efforts to avoid stuttering, a social role conflict, and so forth; may be associated with avoidance of certain words and speaking situations; experience of negative emotions and expression of negative verbalizations about himself or herself and about listeners.

Stuttering, Treatment.   Stuttering has varied treatment procedures; only a few have been tested for their efficacy; some are questionable; some have uncontrolled clinical support; several are purely rational; most clinicians combine

S

certain effective components of treatment to create some-what personal programs; airflow management, gentle phon-atory onset, and rate reduction through prolonged syllables are common elements across diverse contemporary treat-ment programs; these programs are empirically supported with some experimental evidence.

1. A Contemporary, Comprehensive Treatment Procedure for Stuttering in Older Children and Adults

- The goal of treatment is to reduce the rate of dysfluen-cies in conversational speech to less than 1% in clinic speech samples and no more than 5% in everyday sit-uations by:
  - teaching the client to manage his or her speech-related airflow properly
  - teaching the client to initiate speech softly and gently
  - teaching the client to prolong syllable durations to reduce the speech rate
  - shaping normal prosodic features of speech and sta-bilizing fluency
  - strictly managing the behavioral contingency by giv-ing prompt positive and corrective feedback
  - shifting treatment to more naturalistic settings
  - training significant others to manage the skills in the natural environment to promote maintenance of flu-ency over time and across situations
  - following up the client periodically and giving booster therapy when needed
- Make a thorough assessment; determine the forms and the frequencies of stuttering in both conversational speech and oral reading in clinical and extraclinical sit-uations; consult the cited sources and the *PGASLP*
- Before you start treatment, take note of suggestions un-der *Measure dysfluency rates in all treatment sessions* and *Vary the treatment procedures to suit the individual client,* both found at the end of this main entry

Stuttering: A Comprehensive Treatment

- Define stuttering in a measurable way; note that measuring specific dysfluencies generally leads to better interobserver reliability
- Baserate stuttering in the clinic
  - take extended conversational speech samples
  - count all types of dysfluencies and the number of words spoken
  - calculate the percent dysfluency rate
  - continue to record brief conversational speech samples in the next two sessions during the first 5 minutes
  - take additional samples if the three-sample dysfluency rates are highly divergent
- Select the three target fluency skills that are incompatible with stuttering, commonly used, and known to be effective in establishing stutter-free speech: Airflow Management, Gentle Phonatory Onset, and Rate Reduction through syllable prolongation; all described later under Treatment of Stuttering: Specific Techniques or Programs.
- Counsel the client and the family about the treatment program
  - Give an overview of the treatment program and its rationale (essentially tell them that the method prevents stuttering and helps practice fluency skills)
  - point out its known effects and research data that support its use
  - point out its drawback, which is initially an unacceptable artificial-sounding fluency
  - point out its advantages: it teaches fluency skills that the client can fall back on at any time in the future
  - caution about the potential need for Booster Therapy in the future; tell them that brief periods of repeated booster treatment over a period of several years may be needed
  - impress on the client and the family that a relapse of stuttering does not mean the treatment has failed;

S

      with booster treatment, fluency can be regained and stabilized

- answer all questions the client, the family, or both may have about the treatment

• Begin teaching one target skill at a time; complete this skill component training in one session

• Teach airflow management first
  - model airflow management for the client
  - inhale a slightly deeper than usual amount of air through your nose
  - exhale a slight amount of air through your open mouth as soon as inhaling the air; make sure the air is not impounded in the lungs
  - ask the client to imitate your airflow modeling
  - reinforce correctly imitated responses promptly
  - if the client has difficulty doing both, model only a deeper than the usual inhalation; reinforce correct imitation; then model exhalation of a small amount of air; reinforce correct imitation
  - stop the client at the earliest sign of mismanaged airflow; point out the error (e.g., too deep an inhalation; impounding the air in the lungs; exhausting the air supply when asked exhale a small amount of air); model again for imitation; reinforce the imitated response
  - continue until the client can, on request and without modeling, inhale through the nose and exhale a slight amount of air through the mouth; give several successful trials

• Introduce the next skill—gentle phonatory onset
  - model gentle onset and contrast that with hard glottal attacks, especially the kind exhibited by the client; use short and simple words (e.g., *hi, how, bye, my*)
  - initiate syllables softly, gently, slowly, and in a relaxed manner

- ask the client to imitate only the just modeled gentle onset; reinforce correctly imitated soft onset productions
- continue until the client can, upon request and without modeling, initiate sounds softly while producing several words
- Combine airflow management and gentle phonatory onset
  - model both the component skills—airflow management and gentle phonatory onset—for the client to imitate; use the same words as before
  - ask the client to imitate your modeling of airflow management and gentle phonatory onset; reinforce correct productions
  - go back to single skill training if the client mismanages a component; concentrate on the mismanaged component; combine them again
  - continue until the client can, on request and without modeling, inhale and exhale slightly and initiate sounds softly while producing several words; reinforce such evoked (unimitated) productions
  - stop the client at the earliest sign of mismanaged airflow, abrupt or tensed onset of phonation, or stuttering (dysfluency); explain what went wrong, concentrate on the missed target if necessary, combine the skills again, and give additional practice
- Introduce the next skill—rate reduction through syllable prolongation
  - prefer the clinician-induced rate reduction; use Delayed Auditory Feedback if necessary (described later under Treatment of Stuttering: Specific Techniques or Programs); note that instructions and modeling and strict management of behavioral contingencies can be very effective in reducing the rate
  - model a slow speech through syllable prolongation; use the same words used until this stage; stretch the

syllable duration; reinforce correct imitation of slow, prolonged speech
- stop the client as soon as you hear the sign of increased rate of speech or the production of a dysfluency; explain the error, model again, and reinforce correct imitations
- continue until the client can, on request and without modeling, stretch syllables in all the words being practiced until now
- model stretched-out syllable durations with continuous phonation
- Combine all three skills of fluency—airflow management, gentle onset of phonation, and syllable prolongation—into an integrated skill
  - model inhalation and slight exhalation, gentle onset, and syllable prolongation using the same words practiced until this point
  - ask the client to imitate your modeling of all three target skills in words; reinforce correct imitations of airflow management, gentle phonatory onset, and syllable prolongations
  - monitor all three skills at this stage and stop the client for mismanaged targets or production of stuttering; pause briefly and continue
  - provide training in skills with single words initially modeled and later evoked by questions that lead to one-word responses (e.g., "What is your first name?" "What is your last name?" and several similar questions to evoke single word names of family members and friends; "What is the name of the city you live in?" "What is the name of your street?" and several similar questions)
  - continue until the client can, on request and without modeling, produce all three target behaviors and with stutter-free speech at the word level with 98 to 100% accuracy

452

- note that within the first one or two sessions, the client should be producing words (some clients can be moved to phrases even in the first session) with little or no stuttering; if this is not happening, perhaps the skills are not managed properly; make a careful analysis of errors and pay close attention to skill execution; be more prompt in reinforcing stutter-free speech and to stop and give corrective feedback at the earliest sign of a stutter
- Shift training to the phrase level as soon as possible
  - for the initial phrase training, form two-word phrases with the words already trained (e.g., the first and the last name of the client and his or her family members; name of the town and that of the city)
  - for subsequent training, form phrases with one trained and one untrained word
  - finally, form phrases with both untrained words
  - model the target phrases using all three skills in a smoothly integrated manner
  - make sure that you do not give a phonatory break between the two words; blend the two words; produce the two words as though they are a string of syllables with no break; stretch all the syllables; emphasize this aspect to the client
  - ask the client to imitate the phrase
  - reinforce correct imitations with good airflow, gentle onset, prolonged syllables, and continuous phonation throughout the utterance
  - stop the client at the earliest sign of a trouble (mismanaged airflow, hard glottal attacks, increased speech rate, or a stutter); explain the error and concentrate on the skills that broke down (e.g., the client failed to exhale before starting phonation; this would then be pointed out and practiced two or three times)
  - when the client has imitated several phrases with no stuttering and all skills efficiently exhibited, fade

S

modeling; ask questions that can be answered by two-word phrases (e.g., "What are your first and the last names?")

- promptly reinforce the completely stutter-free productions of phrases with inhalation and slight exhalation, gentle phonatory onset, and rate reduction through syllable prolongation
- stop the client for mismanagement of any of the targets and production of dysfluencies; make an error analysis, repeat the skill mismanaged, and continue the training

- Shift training to the sentence level
  - For the initial phase of sentence training, expand already trained phrases into sentences (e.g., "I live in Fresno" or "My name is Kopitron Stratofearopolis.")
  - model and have the client imitate sentences if necessary; target completely stutter-free productions with efficient use of the skills in a smooth and integrated manner with no phonatory breaks between words; continue to model until the client imitates several stutter-free sentences with smooth efficiency; use reinforcement and corrective feedback as before
  - fade modeling and ask questions the client will answer with complete sentences; monitor all target behaviors and fluency closely
  - stop the client promptly for mismanagement of any of the targets and production of dysfluencies; make an error analysis and concentrate on the particular skill break down
  - continue until the client speaks in sentences with stutter-free speech by using airflow management, gentle phonatory onset, and rare reduction through syllable prolongation
  - note that treatment at the spontaneous conversation speech level may have to be continued the longest; in fact, most clients should reach this stage soon in ther-

apy and stay on this stage long enough to maintain stutter-free speech with little or no modeling, thinned out contingency management with only an occasional reinforcement and corrective feedback

- during treatment at the conversational speech level, probe periodically; at the beginning of treatment sessions, conduct 5 minutes of probe; do not provide any modeling or positive or corrective feedback; ask the client to speak in his or her typical manner; the client will probably use the skills, but neither encourage nor discourage the client to do so; record these samples and calculate the percent dysfluency rate

- Shape normal prosody
  - begin shaping normal prosody when three successive probes show a dysfluency rate around 1% of the words spoken
  - instruct the client about normal prosodic features; tell the client that gradually increased rate and typical intonations are the key to normal-sounding speech
  - model a slightly higher speech rate and ask the client to imitate it
  - after a few imitated sentences at the new rate, withdraw modeling and engage the client in conversational speech maintained at the slightly increased speech rate
  - monitor the skills and dysfluent productions carefully; if dysfluencies appear as the rate is increased, ask the client to slow down to a rate that eliminates dysfluencies; after some practice at this slower level, ask the client to increase the rate again
  - reinforce the client for increased rate and maintained fluency; note that at this level, the primary criterion to deliver reinforcement is stutter-free speech that is moving in the direction of more natural speech; airflow and gentle onset are not emphasized, although they should be if fluency begins to break down

S

- ask the client to speak at progressively higher rate while maintaining stutter-free speech
- model pitch variations and let the client imitate and then talk spontaneously with increased intonational patterns
- model appropriate vocal intensity and let the client imitate and then talk with sufficient loudness; note that excessively monitored airflow and rate results in too soft speech
- make continuous judgments about speech naturalness and modify the speech to approximate normal prosodic features
- reinforce all appropriate productions
- stop the client for excessively slow rate and monotonous speech; pause and continue
- continue until the speech is judged both normally fluent and natural-sounding

- Implement a maintenance program
  - teach the client Self-Control (Self-Monitoring) skills by having him or her count dysfluencies, the production of target behaviors, increase in rate, abrupt phonatory onset, and breath holding; let the client chart these behaviors as you do in treatment sessions
  - ask the client to judge the appropriateness of airflow, gentle onset, rate reduction, and prosodic variations to encourage self-evaluation of skills
  - teach the client to stop talking and to pause briefly when he or she stutters or mismanages a target skill
  - hold informal treatment sessions in naturalistic settings; move treatment out of the treatment room, out of the clinic environment
  - monitor the skills and fluency in naturalistic settings by giving the client subtle signals: prompt a slightly slower rate by a hand gesture, prompt a gentler onset of voice by touching your own throat, and so on

S

- train the family members, teachers, friends, colleagues, and others in prompting and reinforcing the production of target skills and fluency
- train teachers and family members to provide opportunities to practice fluency skills
- train family members to hold informal treatment sessions at home

- Dismiss the client only when natural sounding fluency is established in natural settings and in conversational speech
- Urge the client and the family to contact you as soon as an increase in stuttering is noticed to schedule a follow-up assessment and booster therapy
- Give a follow-up schedule to bring the client back to the clinic periodically regardless of the outcome
- Take conversational speech samples during a follow-up assessment and offer booster treatment when dysfluency rates reach or exceed 5% of the words spoken
- Measure dysfluency rates in all treatment sessions
  - record at least a few minutes of speech sample in every treatment session, perhaps a 2-minute sample in the beginning (after the previously described probe measure) of treatment session, 2 minutes in the middle of the session, and 2 minutes at the end
  - calculate the number of words spoken and the number of dysfluencies to derive a percent dysfluency rate for the entire session
  - check your own reliability by periodically measuring the sample twice; make sure that you measure dysfluency rates with at least 90% reliability
- Vary the treatment procedures to suit the client
  - note that the procedures described are highly structured and the steps are specified somewhat rigidly
  - note that a beginning clinician might find it easier or efficient to follow a highly structured format where

S

decision points and decision criteria are specified; however, with some experience, clinicians begin to skip steps, move faster or slower, and even skip a particular target skill if that does not make a difference

- try if only a rate reduction would be sufficient for a given client; add airflow only if it enhances the rate of improvement (quickly eliminates certain kinds of dysfluencies)

- de-emphasize or stop explicitly monitoring a skill sooner or later if you did employ all the skills to begin with; probe to see if fluency is sustainable without an explicit monitoring of that skills

- use oral reading initially if that seems to give a better control on the fluency skills; some clients do better in oral reading where they do not have to focus on what to say

- start treatment at any level the client can handle the skills; some need not be started at the word level; phrases might work and, with a few clients, even short sentences may be the starting point

- if you did start at the word level, try moving to the short sentence level briefly to see if stutter-free speech can be sustained; if so continue at this level (thus skipping the phrase level)

- let the client's performance data dictate the sequence, speed, relative emphasis on skills, and the number of steps involved in treatment

2. *A Contemporary, Comprehensive Treatment Procedure for Stuttering in Very Young Children (2- to 5-Year-Olds)*

- Make a thorough assessment; determine the forms and the frequencies of stuttering in conversational speech in clinical and extraclinical situations; consult the cited sources and the *PGASLP*

- Baserate stuttering in the clinic

Stuttering Treatment for Young Children

- Use toys, objects, pictures, storybooks, and a loosely structured play situation to evoke and manage speech from the child
- Experiment informally with all three targets used with older children and adults: airflow management, gentle phonatory onset, and rate reduction through syllable prolongation; possibly, with very young children, only a slower rate may be effective in inducing stutter-free speech; if so, skip the others; most likely to be skipped is airflow management; the next most likely to be skipped is gentle phonatory onset; the younger the child, the more likely it is that you will use only slow speech
- Counsel the family about the treatment program, its known effects, its drawback (initially unacceptable, artificial fluency), and the potential need for booster therapy in the future; impress on them the need to regularly work with the child at home and the critical role they play in fluency maintenance
- Even if you use gentle phonatory onset and airflow management, emphasize slow normal speech; if you use all three, teach one target skill at a time; refer to the preceding program for steps involved in implementing the optional airflow management and gentle phonatory onset; model more frequently and use simple language with younger children
- Model rate reduction through syllable prolongation; use a rubber band to show stretching of syllables; use hand gestures to slow speech; use any other means the child will comprehend; model more frequently than you would for older children and adults; reduce your own rate; if selected, add rate reduction to airflow management and gentle phonatory onset; do not use DAF with very young children
  - begin at the word level

- model stretched-out syllable durations with continuous phonation
- Ask the child to imitate your modeling
- Reinforce correct imitations
- Stop the child for mismanaged targets or production of stuttering; pause briefly and continue
- Continue until the child can produce slow speech (or with the optional targets), upon request and without modeling, and with stutter-free speech at the word level with 98 to 100% accuracy
- Shift training to the phrase level
  - model often
  - fade modeling
  - promptly reinforce stutter-free production of phrases
  - stop the child for mismanagement of the target or targets and production of dysfluencies; pause briefly and continue
- Shift training to the sentence level
  - model frequently and have the child imitate sentences; target completely stutter-free productions
  - ask questions the child will answer with complete sentences; monitor target behavior or behaviors and fluency
  - stop the child for mismanagement of the target or targets and production of dysfluencies
  - continue until the child speaks in sentences with stutter-free speech
- Shape normal prosody
  - model a slightly higher speech rate and ask the child to imitate it
  - encourage the child to speak at progressively higher rates while maintaining stutter-free speech
  - model pitch variations and let the child imitate and then talk spontaneously with increased intonational patterns

- model appropriate vocal intensity and let the child imitate and then talk with sufficient loudness
- make continuous judgments about speech naturalness and modify the speech to approximate normal prosodic features
- reinforce all appropriate productions
- stop the child for excessively slow rate and monotonous speech; pause and continue
- continue until the speech is judged both normally fluent and natural-sounding
- Implement a maintenance program
  - teach the client to stop talking and to pause briefly when he or she stutters or mismanages the target skill or skills
  - hold informal treatment sessions in naturalistic settings
  - signal the client in a subtle manner to use the target skills
  - train family members, baby-sitters, preschool teachers, and day care workers in prompting and reinforcing slow, normal, and fluent speech in the child
  - train teachers and family members to provide opportunities to practice fluency skills
  - ask parents to participate in all treatment sessions you conduct
  - train family members to evoke a slow, normal rate of speech and to positively reinforce fluency
  - ask them to withhold random, noncontingent negative feedback to the child
  - teach them the skills of gently stopping the child when stuttering occurs and to pause and continue
  - teach parents to hold informal treatment sessions at home; ask them to submit tape-recorded sessions for your analysis and feedback to the parents
  - teach the parents to monitor fluency in a subtle and nonpunitive manner most of the time

S

- Dismiss the child only when natural-sounding fluency is established in natural settings and in conversational speech
- Counsel the family about the potential for relapse and the need for booster treatment
- Follow up and arrange for booster treatment

3. A Simplified, Minimal Therapy for Very Young Children (2- to 5-Year-Olds): An Exclusive Fluency Reinforcement Program

Treatment of stuttering in very young children can be simplified greatly; there is evidence that systematic positive reinforcement for fluency in very young children may be just as effective as any other procedure; in many cases fluency shaping that involves such skills as syllable prolongation and airflow management can be avoided; an advantage of an exclusive fluency reinforcement program (nothing else is used) is that the parents may be trained more easily to use the technique at home than perhaps any other method; another advantage is that the procedure does not negatively affect the prosodic features of speech; follow the steps outlined here to use a straightforward fluency reinforcement program; see the following entry to combine fluency reinforcement with direct stuttering reduction strategy.

- Make a thorough assessment of stuttering in the child; see the cited sources and the *PGASLP*
- Explain the method to the parents and recruit them to do treatment at home at least three times a week; each session should last 15 to 20 minutes
- Baserate dysfluencies for at least three consecutive sessions; offer treatment only if stuttering does not show systematic decline over baserate sessions
  - hold play-oriented conversational speech sessions and tape-record the sample
  - count all dysfluencies and the number of words spoken
  - calculate the percent dysfluency rates

S

- do not treat if the dysfluency rates show consistent decline over the three sessions; counsel the parents to return to clinic if the child shows an increase in the frequency of dysfluencies
- note that a few children may show such decline and recover without formal treatment

- Begin treatment in conversational speech mode only, although the child's utterances may be words, phrases, or short sentences
- Select stimulus materials the child likes; toys, arranged play situations, big, colorful picture, storybooks with attractive pictures, and so forth; consult the parents before selecting the materials; if practical, ask parents to bring the child's favorite toys and storybooks to the treatment sessions
- Ask the parents to observe the first few treatment sessions and then have them join you and the child
- Evoke speech from the child in a play-oriented format; use the toys, pictures, and other materials to stimulate speech
  - show a picture and ask the child such general questions as "What do you see here?" and "What is happening here?"
  - show a picture and ask such specific questions as "What is the boy doing here?" "What is the girl eating here?" "What is this Mommy doing?" "What is the kitty doing here?" and so forth
  - tell a short story about a picture and ask the child to retell it
  - ask the child to tell you a story
  - let the child engage in controlled play and ask questions about what he or she is doing
  - comment on what the child is doing to stimulate speech
  - role play such situations as cooking or shopping to stimulate speech from the child

S

- use hand puppets and carry on a conversation that is appropriate to the characters
- build simple blocks with the child and pretend difficulty on your part and ask questions about how to do it
- give slightly more difficult block designs to stimulate questions and requests for help
- show an array of toys placed on a high shelf and ask the child to describe them and request specific items
- use your imagination to provoke speech in the context of play and story telling but do not allow the child to get lost in play
- Manage a behavioral contingency as you evoke speech in the play-oriented treatment sessions
  - positively reinforce the child for all fluent productions, be they single word productions, phrases, or short or long sentences
  - use verbal praise as the main reinforcer ("That was nice speech"; "That was not bumpy! It was smooth"; "I like the way you talk.")
  - ignore all stutterings completely
  - if verbal praise is not effective, begin a token reinforcement program; give a token for every fluent production to begin with; use a fixed ratio schedule in which progressively more fluent responses are required to earn a token; exchange the token for a small gift of child's choice at the end of the session
  - train parents in reinforcing the child for fluent productions
  - ask the parents to hold informal treatment sessions at home
  - ask the parents to submit a tape-recorded sample of home treatment sessions
  - go over the tape and fine-tune the parents' skill in immediately and positively reinforcing fluent productions and to completely ignore stuttering

- measure stuttering as described in the previous section
- vary the treatment as found appropriate in light of treatment data
- dismiss the child from therapy when the child has sustained fluency at 95% or better in conversational speech produced in naturalistic settings over at least a 3- week period
- tell the parents to contact you if there is an increase in stuttering
- give them a follow-up schedule and conduct follow-up assessments
- if the dysfluency rate is below 5% during any assessment session, schedule booster treatment sessions

4. *Fluency Reinforcement Program Combined With Direct Stuttering Reduction Methods.* In treating children who stutter, the effects of positive reinforcement for fluency may be enhanced by adding an optional direct stuttering reduction program (nonexclusion time-out, called here pause-and-talk or response cost); to do this, take the following steps.

- Use all procedures described under the previous entry, An Exclusive Fluency Reinforcement Program
- Note that the fluency reinforcement program requires you to react only to fluent productions (with positive consequences) but nothing is done when the child exhibits a stutter; in this combined procedure, a direct stuttering reduction procedure is added to fluency reinforcement

Add Response Cost to Fluency Reinforcement. Response Cost is a procedure to reduce an undesirable response directly; this procedure includes giving the child a token for every fluent production and removing a token contingent on every stuttering; thus, the procedure is a combination of fluency reinforcement and reinforcement withdrawal (corrective feedback or operant punishment) contingent on stuttering; there is evidence that this is an effective procedure.

Stuttering: Combined Treatment

- Describe the procedure to the child and the parents; point out its effectiveness
- Baserate stuttering, select stimulus materials, and structure the treatment session as described under the previous entry on <u>An Exclusive Fluency Reinforcement Program</u>
- Use practically all procedures described in the previous entry; except that to reinforce fluency, adopt a token system; explain the procedure to the child and the parents
- Design a token system; select plastic tokens to be used as reinforcers; assemble a variety of back-up reinforcers; note that tokens themselves are not the true reinforcers—the back-ups are.
  - consult with parents and the child in selecting back-up reinforcers
  - select small toys, stickers, other inexpensive gift items such as pencils, balloons, and crayons
  - note that the most effective back-up reinforcers for many children might be activities, not gift items
  - arrange opportunities to engage in such activities as listening to a story that you read, drawing on the chalkboard, a play activity that the child selects, and listening to taped music
- Give the tokens to reinforce fluent productions
  - at the beginning of the session, ask the child to select one tangible reinforcer he or she will get at the end of the session in exchange for the tokens; make sure you offer only those choices that you have access to
  - evoke conversational speech (as described in the previous entry) and give the child a token for every fluent production; continue to use verbal praise as in the previous entry
  - make sure the child is able to accumulate enough tokens at the end of the session; if necessary, give

two tokens for every fluent production; this may be necessary if the child's stuttering rate is very high and opportunities for earning the tokens are somewhat limited

- at the end of the session, exchange the token for the selected reinforcer (e.g., a sticker or a pencil)
- alternatively, give back-up reinforcers throughout the session if that is feasible (e.g., after every 5 minutes of work or as soon as the child accumulates a certain number of tokens required to earn the back-up reinforcer, take a break for 1 or 2 minutes and allow the child to draw, listen to part of a story, listen to music, etc.); promptly terminate the activity and return the child to conversational speech and fluency monitoring

- Withdraw tokens to directly reduce stuttering while increasing fluency with reinforcement
  - explain this aspect of treatment to the child; inform him or her that you will be taking away a token for every instance of stuttering or bumpy speech
  - model a stutter and immediately remove a token from your own pile to demonstrate the procedure to the child
  - tell the child that his or her goal is to keep as many tokens as possible so as to earn a gift or an activity and not to lose the tokens to stuttering and thus lose the gift or the activity
  - watch for the earliest sign of a dysfluency or stutter (a lip puckering, an increased tension anywhere in the facial region, the beginnings of a sound prolongation or a sound repetition, twitching of the eyebrow)
  - as soon as a sign of stuttering or stuttering itself appears, take away a token the child has accumulated by producing fluent speech

S

- take the token back in a matter-of-fact manner; do not show unpleasant reactions
- Continue the procedure until fluency is stabilized in conversational speech in natural settings
  - measure stuttering in all sessions as describe in the previous entry
  - probe fluency and stuttering periodically as described in the previous entry
  - periodically probe the speech rate to make sure that the client is sustaining fluency without a rate change that affects prosodic features; available evidence suggests that the rate is not negatively affected and may even increase slightly when stutterings decrease
  - train parents to conduct home treatment sessions
  - monitor the home treatment sessions with taped samples and refine the parents' skills in administering the treatment
  - schedule follow-up and booster treatment sessions

Add Pause-and-Talk to Fluency Reinforcement. Pause-and-talk is a procedure to directly reduce an undesirable response; more often described as time-out; because of variations in time-out procedures and some common misapplications of them, a more descriptive pause-and-talk is preferred here; there is evidence that pause-and-talk is an effective procedure to reducing stuttering without affecting the natural prosodic features of speech; pause-and-talk can easily be combined with positive reinforcement for fluency.

- Describe the procedure to the child and point out its effectiveness
- Baserate stuttering, select stimulus materials, and structure the treatment session as described under An Exclusive Fluency Reinforcement Program
- Use all procedures described under An Exclusive Fluency Reinforcement Program in the previous en-

try; as described, reinforce fluent productions with verbal praise

- Add pause-and-talk to fluency reinforcement
  - continue to engage the client in conversational speech and to reinforce fluent productions with verbal praise
  - at the earliest sign of a stutter, say "Stop," turn your face away to avoid eye contact with the client, and freeze for 5 seconds; you may look at your watch to count 5 seconds
  - at the end of the pause (time-out) duration, look at the client to re-establish eye contact, smile, and say something that will let the client continue talking (e.g., "You can talk now"; "You were saying . . ."; "OK"; etc.); note that soon the client will begin talking again as soon as you re-establish your eye contact
  - make sure that the client completely ceases talking when you say "Stop"; the method is ineffective if the client continues to talk even though you have terminated eye contact and have turned away
- Continue the procedure until fluency is stabilized in conversational speech in natural settings
  - measure stuttering in all sessions as describe in the previous entry
  - probe fluency and stuttering periodically as described in the previous entry
  - periodically probe the speech rate to make sure that the client is sustaining fluency without a rate change that affects prosodic features; available evidence suggests that the rate is not negatively affected and may even increase slightly when stutterings decrease
  - train parents to conduct home treatment sessions
  - monitor the home treatment sessions with taped samples and refine the parents' skills in administering the treatment

S

> • schedule follow-up and booster treatment sessions

5. Direct Stuttering Reduction Procedures Combined With Fluency Shaping Techniques. A novel approach to treating stuttering in which fluency shaping techniques are combined with direct stuttering reduction methods; may be the most suitable for certain clients with whom pause-and-talk or response cost may not produce the maximal effects partly because of excessive frequency of stuttering; involves only a minimal use of fluency shaping (minimal syllable prolongation, only of the initial syllable of the first word of an utterance); thus it avoids the negative side-effects of fluency shaping (excessively slow and monotonous speech); although minimal prolongation may not be effective in itself, it may be effective when combined with pause-and-talk or response cost; experimental evidence is emerging in its favor; note that this technique may be used with adults or older children who stutter; this procedure may be unnecessary for very young children (3- to 5-year-olds) who may benefit the most from An Exclusive Fluency Reinforcement Program, described earlier under #3.

- Assess the client's stuttering thoroughly; determine the forms and frequency of dysfluencies in conversational speech in clinical and extraclinical situations; consult the cited sources and the *PGASLP*
- Select a combination of a *minimal syllable prolongation* (MSP) with *either* pause-and-talk (P-&-T) *or* response cost (RC); possibly, a child will react better to one combination (e.g., MSP plus RC) than to the other (e.g., MSP plus P-&-T); therefore, be prepared to experiment
- Describe the procedure to the client and the family; tell them you will be using a slight syllable prolongation with either RC or P-&-T and that you will be initially trying both the combinations to select the one that works best with the child

Stuttering: Combined Treatment

- Engage the child in conversation within a play-oriented, semistructured situation; see <u>An Exclusive Fluency Reinforcement Program</u> under #3 for details on structuring play-oriented treatment sessions with young children
- Apply the MSP plus P-&-T combination; begin with MSP (it does not matter what combination you try first; your preference for either RC or P-&-T may influence your initial selection)
  - model a slight prolongation of the initial syllable of the first word in an utterance; do *not* prolong all the syllables of all the words as it is done in the full-fledged fluency shaping technique
  - ask the child to imitate your production; make sure the child imitates a slight prolongation of the initial syllable of the first word only
  - reinforce the child for correct prolongation with verbal praise or with a token backed up with other reinforcers
  - simultaneously, every time the child stutters or you observe an earliest sign of a stutter, say "Stop," turn your face away from the client, freeze, look at your watch for 5 seconds
  - make sure the client ceases talking
  - re-establish the eye contact, smile, and indicate in some way that the client can now resume talking (e.g., say "You can talk now," "You were saying . . .," "OK"; etc.); note that after a few trials of this kind, most client will resume their speech as soon as you re-establish your eye contact and smile
  - after a few successful imitations of MSP, drop modeling and prompt the syllable prolongation by a hand signal; continue to apply P-&-T for all stutterings; client now is talking with MSP and pausing after each stuttering
  - continue this for two or three sessions to evaluate the effects of this combined procedure

S

- measure the exact frequency of all dysfluencies and the number of words spoken; calculate the percent dysfluency rate for all sessions so you can later compare the effect of this combination with that of the other
- do not try the other combination and continue with this combination only if the changes are impressive, consistent, and the client seems happy with the technique (smiling and cooperative in the sessions and eager to work with you) with no signs of stress or negative reactions to the procedure
- try the other combination if you do not find the results impressive (reductions in stuttering are minimal, the client does not seem to enjoy the session, is reluctant to work with you, the client is not punctual to the sessions, or even misses them)
- note that tokens, exchanged for backup reinforcers, may be used to reinforce fluent productions; but do not withdraw a token for dysfluent productions, as this would be response cost; in this MSP and P-&-T combination, consequate dysfluent productions only with P-&-T

- Try the MSP plus RC combination (this could very well be the first combination you try); note that RC involves reinforcing fluent productions with a token backed up by other reinforcers and removing a token for every dysfluent productions
- Assess the client's stuttering thoroughly; determine the forms and frequency of dysfluencies in conversational speech in clinical and extraclinical situations; consult the cited sources and the *PGASLP*
- Describe the procedure to the client and the family; tell them you will be using a slight syllable prolongation with RC (or P-&-T if you already have tried the RC combination); tell them that you will select the one that works best with the child

Stuttering: Combined Treatment

- Engage the child in conversation within a play-oriented, semistructured situation; see <u>An Exclusive Fluency Reinforcement Program</u> under #3 for details on structuring play-oriented treatment sessions with young children
- Apply the MSP plus RC combination; begin with MSP
  - model a slight prolongation of the initial syllable of the first word in an utterance; do *not* prolong all the syllables of all the words the way it is done in the full-fledged fluency shaping technique
  - ask the child to imitate your production; make sure the child imitates a slight prolongation of the initial syllable of the first word only
  - reinforce the child for correct prolongation resulting in stutter-free speech with a token the child will later exchange for a backup reinforcer
  - simultaneously, every time the child stutters or you observe an earliest sign of a stutter, withdraw a token from the child (this is the response cost aspect of the combination)
  - continue this MSP, token presentation for fluent productions, and token withdrawal for stuttering for two or three sessions to evaluate the effects of this combined procedure
  - if unsure of the effects, administer for another session or two
  - measure the exact frequency of all dysfluencies and the number of words spoken; calculate the percent dysfluency rate for all sessions so you can later compare the effect of this combination with that of the other
  - compare the rate of stuttering in treatment sessions involving MSP plus P-&-T that you have already tried and MSP plus RC
  - pick the combination that reduced stuttering faster compared to the other combination

S

473

- consider other factors that may be important in treatment technique selection: client's intense dislike of the technique, uncooperative behavior during treatment sessions in spite of good treatment effects, poor treatment attendance that may be attributable to a dislike of treatment, and strong parental objection in spite of positive effects and a good effort to convince them; in such cases, use an alternative, which may be the other combination as long it is effective (even if not to the same extent as the just applied procedure); note that the alternative my be a positive reinforcement of fluency, fluency shaping with syllable prolongation and airflow management, or any other techniques described in this section on <u>Stuttering</u>
- tell the client and the family about the combination (or other technique) you have picked; explain why you picked that combination by showing the data demonstrating greater or faster reduction in stuttering
- if selected (because of its more impressive effects compared with the other combination, client satisfaction with the technique as indexed by smiling and cooperativeness in the sessions and an eagerness to work with you with no signs of stress or negative reactions to the procedure), continue with the MSP plus RC combination until fluency is stabilized in the clinic and in natural settings
- if MSP plus RC is not selected, continue with the technique selected (may be the other combination or a different technique altogether)
- dismiss the client when fluency is sustained in the treatment setting as well as in the client's natural setting
- arrange for follow-ups and booster treatment sessions

Ahlander, E., & Hegde, M. N. (2000, April). *The relative effects of pause-and-talk and response cost.* Paper presented at the Treatment Efficacy Research Conference, Vanderbilt University, Nashville, TN.

Hegde, M. N. (1998). *Treatment procedures in communicative disorders* (3rd ed.). Austin, TX: Pro-Ed.

Shipley, K. G., & McAfee, J. (1998). *Assessment in speech-language pathology: A resource manual* (2nd ed.). San Diego: Singular Publishing Group.

Treatment of Stuttering: Specific Techniques or Programs

Airflow Management in Stuttering Treatment. Regulated airflow used in the treatment of stuttering; also called Regulated Breathing; a component in many stuttering treatment procedures; effective in inducing stutter-free speech; supported by clinical research; often combined with other treatment targets including Gentle Phonatory Onset and Prolonged Speech (described later in this section).

- Preferably, combine it with prolonged speech and gentle phonatory onset
- Model Regulated Breathing to produce stutter-free speech
  - take an inhalation through the nose, slightly deeper than the usual so it is easily observed
  - exhale a small amount of air through the mouth before initiating phonation
  - initiate phonation slowly, gently, and softly only *after* the start of exhalation
  - model the production of single words or phrases
  - prolong the vowels and reduce the rate
- Ask the client to imitate your modeled productions
- Reinforce the imitative productions
- Model frequently and stabilize regulated breathing of inhalation and slight prevoice exhalation
- Fade modeling and evoke regulated breathing and speech production

S

- Move through the sequence of words, phrases, and sentences as you add other components (soft and gentle phonatory onset, prolongation of vowels, and slow rate of speech)
- Fade the explicit management of airflow into a more natural use of airflow to sustain fluency in conversational speech in and out of the clinic
- Reinstate regulated breathing throughout the treatment when found necessary

Continuous Airflow. Maintaining airflow throughout an utterance; typically used in conjunction with such other treatment targets as exhalation, slight inhalation before phonation and rate reduction; helps induce stutter-free speech.

- Instruct the client to take enough air before beginning speech production
- Ask the client to exhale a slight amount of air before initiating phonation
- Ask the client to initiate phonation gently and softly
- Ask the client to maintain an even airflow throughout an utterance
- Model the technique
- Reinforce the client for correct production of the target behavior

Continuous Phonation. Maintaining phonation throughout an utterance; a stuttering treatment target; often combined with Gentle Phonatory Onset, Airflow Management, and Prolonged Speech (all described in this section).

- Instruct the client in maintaining phonation throughout an utterance
- Model continuous phonation in such a way as to blur the word boundaries
- Ask the client to imitate your modeling
- Reinforce correctly imitated productions

- Begin with shorter phrases and progress to longer sentences
- Combine it with other targets, including syllable prolongation, gentle phonatory onset, and airflow management

Counseling as Treatment for Stuttering. A collection of varied approaches to treating stuttering by giving information, advice, and strategies to deal with the problem; a range of techniques most of them psychologically oriented; recipients are parents of children who stutter and adults who stutter; often combined with direct methods of treating stuttering; efficacy of counseling when used exclusively with no direct work with stuttering by either the clinician or the parent is not established; when combined with direct work on stuttering, whether counseling had any effect is unclear.

Counseling Parents of Children Who Stutter. Using the psychological methods of counseling to indirectly treat stuttering in their children; an Indirect Stuttering Treatment method (described later in this section); the main approach is talking with the child's parents to change their feelings, attitudes, ideas, and expectations about stuttering and fluency; efficacy of this approach not established; often combined with Direct Stuttering Treatment (described later in this section).

- Be a sensitive, uncritical, accepting listener
- Find out what the parents wish to accomplish through counseling
- Let the parents explore their feelings, emotions, perceptions, and expectations relative to their child's stuttering
- Let the parents freely talk about their fears, possible feelings of guilt, and their overt reactions to stuttering in their child

- Let the parents talk about their strategies of dealing with stuttering in their child
- Help the parents find their own solutions by offering professional views and ideas they may not have known or considered
- Express approval of their positive feelings and helpful reactions toward their child
- Help them realize their child's strengths and limitations
- Reduce their negative thoughts and feelings, including potential feelings of guilt by reassuring them that they may not have created the problem
- Let the parents put their child's stuttering in perspective so that they do not exaggerate its negative effects
- Let the parents realize that no child is fluent all the time
- Explore actions the parents may have taken with positive effects on the child's fluency and encourage them to increase or strengthen them
- Explore actions the parents may have taken that have worsened the child's problems and encourage them to eliminate or reduce them
- Explore the parents' ideas about fluency and stuttering to encourage a more realistic view of them
- Discuss the kinds of communicative demands the parents make and ask them to reduce such demands
- Encourage the parents to create more positive speech experiences for the child by withholding criticism and accepting the child's stuttered attempts at communication

Counseling Persons Who Stutter. Using psychological methods of counseling to indirectly treat persons who stutter; an <u>Indirect Stuttering Treatment</u> (described later in this section); the main approach is talking with the client to change feelings, attitudes, and expectations; efficacy of this approach is not established; often combined with <u>Direct Stuttering Treatment</u> (described later in this section).

- Be a sensitive, uncritical, accepting listener
- Find out what the client wishes to accomplish through counseling
- Let the client explore his or her feelings, emotions, perceptions, and expectations relative to stuttering
- Let the client talk about the difficult speaking situations, listener reactions, and his or her own emotional reactions
- Help the client find his or her own solutions by offering professional views and ideas the client may be unaware of or may not have considered
- Discuss the client's strengths that he or she may not have realized
- Reduce negative thoughts and feelings by having the client concentrate on positive experiences, including positive speech experiences
- Let the client put stuttering in perspective so that he or she does not exaggerate its negative effects
- Let the client realize that no one is fluent all the time
- Explore actions the client takes that may exacerbate stuttering and encourage the client to eliminate or reduce them
- Explore actions and situations that enhance fluency and encourage the client to increase them or strengthen them
- Encourage the client to talk more positively about himself or herself

Delayed Auditory Feedback (DAF). Hearing one's own speech after a delay introduced by a mechanical device; most typical effect is to slow down the rate of speech; used in treating persons who stutter and those who clutter to slow their speech rate; reduces or eliminates stuttering, but induces unnatural sounding speech; a widely used stuttering treatment technique; a component in many programmed or comprehensive treatment approaches; useful in establishing <u>Stutter-Free Speech</u> (described later in this section) but needs additional procedures to make the speech sound natural and to make the fluency last over time and across situations.

- Assess the client thoroughly and establish baserates of stuttering and the speech rate
- Select a miniaturized, electronic feedback devise that the client can use in most situations
- Ask the client to wear the portable device (may use a desk-top unit with a loss in flexibility)
- Experiment with different delays to set a client-specific delay that induces stutter-free speech (most clients are stutter-free at 250 milliseconds of delay)
- Begin by asking the client to respond to questions that evoke two- or three-word phrases or short sentences
- Drop down to word level only if the client cannot maintain stutter-free speech at the phrase or short-sentence level
- Model slow, prolonged speech if necessary
- Use oral reading to stabilize a slow, prolonged production if necessary (some initially find oral reading under DAF easier than speaking)
- Establish stutter-free speech with the initial delay over a few sessions
- Increase the length of utterances gradually
- Move to more spontaneous conversational speech containing longer and more complex utterances
- Fade the DAF by initially decreasing the delay in gradual steps; reduce it in 50-millisecond intervals

or other intervals that still help maintain stutter-free speech
- Reduce the intensity of DAF
- Increase the rate of speech while still maintaining stutter-free speech; reinforce the client for speaking at progressively faster rates
- Eliminate the delay altogether, but let the client wear the unit
- Increase the rate further to move it closer to the pretreatment, judged normal, or natural sounding rate
- Shape the normal prosodic features including normal rhythm, intonation, intensity variations, emotional connotations, and so forth
- Conduct informal treatment sessions in varied nonclinical settings
- Train family members, teachers, and others to reinforce fluent, natural sounding speech in nonclinical settings
- Teach Self-Control (Self-Monitoring) skills (charting one's own stuttering, stopping soon after a stuttering or at the earliest sign of increased rate)
- Dismiss only after a natural sounding fluent speech is established
- Counsel the client about the possibility of relapse and the need for Booster Treatment
- Follow up and arrange for booster treatment (relapses are common; follow-up and booster treatment are critical in maintenance)

Direct Stuttering Reduction Strategy: Pause-and-Talk (Time-Out). A brief period of nonreinforcement during which the client stops talking and the clinician avoids eye contact with the client; the period is imposed at the earliest sign of an imminent stuttering or associated behaviors or immediately following those behaviors; duration typically does not exceed 10 seconds; effective in reducing stuttering; supported by

S

controlled experimental evidence; has the advantage of not inducing an artificial and unacceptable pattern of fluency; especially effective with children.

- Assess the client thoroughly and baserate stuttering, dysfluencies, as defined
- Use pictures, objects, storybooks, and toys to evoke continuous speech from young children,
- Use topic cards initially to promote extended monologues from adults
- Introduce natural conversation with both adults and children as soon as practical
- Instruct the client about the procedure: "I will be saying 'Stop' at the earliest sign of stuttering. I want you to stop talking immediately. I will also look away from you and count to five seconds. I will then look at you again. When I look at you, continue talking."
- Ask the child to state the rule and repeat the instructions if necessary
- At the earliest sign of stuttering, say "Stop," look away for 5 seconds, and then reestablish eye contact
- If the client does not begin talking immediately, prompt verbally or nonverbally (e.g., "You were telling me"; "Yes, continue"; a hand gesture to continue)
- Stop the client for every instance of stuttering or dysfluencies; be prompt, forceful, and unambiguous in your feedback
- Ensure that the client does stop talking when you say so
- Watch for undue emotional responses; they tend to disappear; however, if they persist, switch to another procedure
- Measure the frequency of stutterings or dysfluencies as you have defined them in each session or after the session through tape-recorded samples

- Begin with words and phrases and progress to controlled sentences and natural conversational speech
- Teach Self-Control (Self-Monitoring) skills in which the client measures and records his or her stutterings and learns to pause at the earliest sign of stuttering (self-imposed time-out)
- Train family members, teachers, siblings, friends, and others to give subtle signals for the client to stop when they observe stuttering in all situations
- Fade time-out and keep the client on social, verbal reinforcers for fluency
- Shift treatment to naturalistic settings; give unobtrusive feedback to the client in such settings
- Train parents or spouses to hold informal training sessions at home; let them use time-out initially for stuttering and only verbal praise for fluency later
- Have the client or the family members submit tape-recorded home conversational speech samples for your analysis of stuttering frequency
- Dismiss the client only when the rate of dysfluencies is below the set criterion (e.g., less than 3%)
- Counsel the client, the family members, or both about possible relapse of stuttering and the need for booster treatment; ask the client to contact you as soon as stuttering increases
- Follow up the client and arrange for booster treatment

Direct Stuttering Reduction Strategy: Response Cost.
Withdrawal of a positive reinforcer made contingent on stuttering; each stuttering costs the client a reinforcer he or she has access to; effective in reducing stuttering; supported by controlled experimental evidence; especially applicable with children; does not induce an artificial pattern of fluency that should be faded out.

- Assess the client thoroughly and establish baserates of stuttering or dysfluencies, as defined

Stuttering Treatment: Specific Programs

- Use pictures, objects, storybooks, and toys to evoke continuous speech from young children,
- Use topic cards initially to promote extended monologues from adults
- Introduce natural conversation with both adults and children as soon as practical
- Instruct the client about the procedure: " I will give you a token for every word (*later phrases and sentences*) you speak without stuttering. At the end of the session, you can exchange the tokens for this gift here. You should have at least five tokens (*or any such low number that ensures the gift for the child*) at the end of the session. The main thing is that I will take a token away from you every time you stutter. You should try to keep as many tokens as possible by speaking without stuttering."
- Ask the child to state the rule and repeat the instructions if necessary
- Reinforce initially for every fluently spoken word; progress to phrases, controlled sentences, and conversational speech
- Take a token away promptly and in a matter-of-fact manner immediately following a stuttering or at the earliest sign of it
- Watch for undue emotional responses at token loss; they tend to disappear; however, if they persist, switch to another procedure
- Measure the frequency of stutterings or dysfluencies as you have defined them in each session or after the session through tape-recorded samples
- Teach Self-Control (Self-Monitoring) skills in which the client measures and records his or her stutterings and learns to hand you a token at the earliest sign of stuttering (self-imposed response-cost)
- Fade response cost and keep the client on social, verbal reinforcers for fluency

- Train family members, teachers, siblings, friends, and others to give subtle signals for the client to stop when they observe stuttering in all situations
- Shift treatment to naturalistic settings; give unobtrusive feedback to the client in such settings
- Train parents or spouses to hold informal training sessions; let them initially use your token system; later let them fade the tokens and use only verbal praise
- Have the client or the family members submit tape-recorded home conversational speech samples for your analysis of stuttering frequency
- Dismiss the client only when the rate of dysfluencies is below the set criterion (e.g., less than 3%)
- Counsel the client, family members, or both about possible relapse of stuttering and the need for booster treatment; ask the client to contact you as soon as there is an increase in stuttering
- Follow up the client and arrange for booster treatment

Direct Stuttering Treatment. Methods in which the clinician concentrates on reducing stuttering in the client as against trying to indirectly reduce it through counseling and other methods; in behavioral treatment, includes Direct Stuttering Reduction Strategy: Pause-and-Talk (Time-Out) and Direct Stuttering Reduction Strategy: Response Cost (described earlier in this section); a contingency is imposed on stuttering itself, contrasted with counseling parents of stuttering children or stuttering adults.

Fluency Reinforcement Techniques. Techniques of stuttering treatment in which durations of fluency or fluent utterances of varied lengths are positively reinforced; may be used exclusively, in which case, there is no contingency on rate reduction, airflow management, or other targets; may be more effective with younger children than with older children or adults; when not effective, other targets added.

- Assess the child's stuttering
- Baserate the child's stuttering frequency in the clinic
- Arrange a loosely structured treatment setting in which toys, objects, picture books, and storybooks serve as stimuli
- Evoke controlled conversational speech in a relaxed, play-oriented manner
- Select a duration-based (e.g., fluent speech sustained for 20 seconds) or topographically based (e.g., a word, phrase, or a sentence) fluency responses for reinforcement
- Describe and model fluent utterances for the child; describe and model dysfluent utterances as well
- Describe the contingency in simple terms (e.g., "I will give you a token for easy speech.")
- Evoke controlled, limited utterances; use modeling
- Reinforce promptly and generously for fluent utterances or durations
- Ignore stuttering
- Increase the length of utterances or duration of utterances in gradual steps
- Train at the level of conversational speech
- Shift training to nonclinical settings
- Train parents in similar techniques and ask them to conduct home treatment sessions
- Counsel parents about the possibility of relapse and the need for booster treatment
- Follow up and arrange for booster treatment

Fluency Shaping Techniques. A collection of somewhat varied treatment procedures for stuttering with an emphasis on teaching skills of fluency; contrasted with the Fluent Stuttering (described in this section) approach of Van Riper; the goal is natural-sounding normal fluency in everyday situations sustained over time; children are more likely to achieve this goal than adults; most adult stutterers may realize only controlled (monitored) fluency; include <u>Fluency Reinforcement Techniques</u>, <u>Delayed Auditory Feedback</u>, <u>Regulated Breathing</u> or <u>Airflow Management</u>, <u>Gentle Phonatory Onset</u>, <u>Rate Reduction</u>, and <u>Prolonged Speech</u> (all described in this section); little or no attention paid to feelings and attitudes; emphasis on programmed instruction and objective data collection; to use a comprehensive fluency shaping procedure that includes airflow management, gentle phonatory onset, and syllable prolongation, see at the beginning of the main entry <u>Stuttering,</u> and follow the procedures described under 1. A Contemporary, Comprehensive Treatment Procedure for Stuttering in Older Children and Adults.

Fluent Stuttering: Van Riper's Approach. An extensive, early, and influential treatment program for stuttering; also described as stuttering modification therapy; goal is to teach less abnormal, socially more acceptable stuttering, not necessarily normal fluency; contrasted with <u>Fluency Shaping Techniques</u> (described in this section); includes counseling and psychotherapy to change feelings and attitudes.

• Teach stuttering identification
  • teach the client to identify his or her stuttering and all associated problems including negative feelings, avoidance, word fears, and easy and difficult stutterings, with discussion, demonstration, reading, modeling, and so forth
  • teach the stutterer to identify his or her stuttering and associated problems in everyday speaking situations
• Desensitize to toughen the client to his or her stuttering
  • encourage the stutterer to be open and honest with his or her stuttering
  • ask the stutterer to freeze stuttering; teach the client to continue stuttering until told to stop

S

- ask the client to face different audiences and stutter voluntarily to learn that most people do not react negatively, and if some do, he or she can tolerate it
- Modify stuttering by teaching more fluent, easier, and less abnormal stuttering
  - ask the client to face all feared and avoided words and begin to use them
  - teach cancellation by asking the client to pause after a stuttered word and say the word again with easy and more relaxed stuttering (soft articulatory contacts and slower rate); do not ask the client to say the word fluently; ask the client to use cancellation outside the clinic
  - teach pull-outs by asking the client to change stuttering in its midcourse; let the client pull himself or herself out by slowing down and using soft articulatory contacts; let the client use them outside the clinic
  - teach preparatory sets by asking the client to use the techniques of modifying stuttering (easy, relaxed stuttering) as he or she anticipates difficulty on a word
- Stabilize the treatment gains
  - teach the client to continue to assign himself or herself speech tasks that help stabilize the use of cancellations, pull-outs, and preparatory sets
  - ask the client to constantly practice the stuttering modification skills on difficult words
  - reduce the frequency of client contacts
  - continue to seek out difficult and previously avoided speaking situations
  - reintegrate the stutterer's self-concept to include the role of a speaker who speaks mostly fluently but stutters on occasion

Van Riper, C. (1973). *The treatment of stuttering.* Englewood Cliffs, NJ: Prentice-Hall.

Gentle Phonatory Onset. Soft, easy, slow, and relaxed initiation of sounds as against harsh, abrupt, and tensed, initiation; a target behavior in the treatment of stuttering; often combined with such other target behaviors as Airflow Management, Prolonged Speech, or Rate Reduction (described in this section).

- Combine it with prolonged speech, airflow management, or both because gentle onset alone is not a sufficient treatment target
- Instruct the client on the need for gentle phonatory onset; contrast it with its opposite; point out the relationship between abrupt onset and stuttering
- Demonstrate (model) gentle and tensed/abrupt onset and show how speech may be dysfluent with the latter
- Ask the client to initiate sound softly, gently, with a relaxed posture
- Model soft and easy initiation of some vowels
- Ask the client to imitate and reinforce correct imitative productions
- Model soft articulatory contacts for consonants and relaxed production in general
- Reinforce imitative productions of soft articulatory contacts and relaxed speech production
- Model a few single-syllable words (e.g., *I, bye, Hi*) with soft and slow onset and ask the client to imitate
- Reinforce correct imitative productions of single-syllable words
- Ask the client to produce selected simple words and phrases with gentle onset (evoked, not modeled)
- Add airflow management, prolonged speech, or both to gentle onset

S

- Continue treatment with the two or three targets; move through the sequence of words, phrases, controlled sentences, and conversational speech

Gradual Increase in Length and Complexity of Utterances (GILCU). One of two highly structured and programmed operant treatment approaches of the <u>Monterey Fluency Program</u> (described later in this section); developed and researched by B. Ryan and B. Van Kirk; involves reinforcing fluent speech starting with single-word productions and ending with conversational speech; the length and complexity of utterances are increased gradually in the intermediate steps; supported by clinical evidence.

Indirect Stuttering Treatment. Methods in which the clinician tries to manage stuttering in the client without concentrating on reducing stuttering directly; includes <u>Counseling as Treatment for Stuttering</u> (described earlier in this section); there is no direct work on reducing stuttering.

Integration of Stuttering Modification and Fluency Shaping. A dual approach that uses both the <u>Stuttering Modification</u> and <u>Fluency Shaping Techniques</u> (both described in this section); a procedure of treatment developed by T. Peters and B. Guitar; the dual approach is more forcefully applied to advanced stutterers than to beginning stutterers; uses a variety of handouts (e.g., understanding stuttering, how to be open about stuttering, and how to use feared words) during treatment sessions.

- Let the client understand his or her stuttering
  - be warm and friendly; describe the treatment program to the client
  - ask the client to read a brief description of stuttering, what it is, and how it develops; use the authors' handout "Understanding Your Stuttering"; answer all questions; share and reinforce the client's insights

S

- catalog all aspects of the client's stuttering to give a good understanding of the problem; model stuttering, use videotapes or mirrors to demonstrate stuttering
- Reduce negative feelings and attitudes and eliminate avoidance behaviors
  - encourage the client to discuss his or her stuttering openly with family, friends, and acquaintances; use the authors' handout "Discussing Stuttering Openly" in the treatment session
  - ask the client to create a hierarchy of feared and avoided words and situations; encourage the client to use feared words and enter previously avoided speaking situations freely and frequently; use the authors' handout "Using Feared Words and Entering Feared Situations"
  - teach the client the technique of *freezing or holding onto the moment of stuttering*; use the authors' handout; when the client stutters, ask to continue (to repeat, prolong) until you signal to stop; teach the client to be calm while doing this
  - teach the client Voluntary Stuttering; use the authors' handout "Using Voluntary Stuttering"; explain the rationale for it; model brief, easy repetitions or prolongations for the client to imitate; take the client to naturalistic settings where the client will stutter voluntarily
- Teach fluency enhancing skills and modify the moments of stuttering
  - teach Rate Reduction in Treating Stuttering induced by DAF, Gentle Phonatory Onset (both described in this section) and Soft Articulatory Contacts; use the authors' handout, "Using Fluency Enhancing Behaviors"; fade DAF in gradual steps
  - stabilize fluency enhancing skills in conversational speech without DAF

S

- initiate activities to generalize fluency to situations outside the clinic and with an audience other than the clinician
- teach easy stuttering; teach cancellation, pull-outs, and preparatory sets described under Fluent Stuttering: Van Riper' Approach (described in this section); teach the stutterer to integrate fluency enhancing skills with stuttering modification.
- initiate activities to generalize stuttering modification skills to situations outside the clinic and with other audiences
- Help maintain improvement
  - help the stutterer become his or her own clinician; use the authors' handout "Becoming Your Own Clinician"; help the client learn to design assignments to reduce fear and avoidance (e.g., voluntary stuttering in a difficult situation); encourage the client to work on stuttering and fluency everyday
  - establish long-term fluency goals; use the authors' handout; help the client set the goal of spontaneous (unmonitored) fluency whenever possible; controlled (monitored) fluency when it is important to be fluent; and controlled stuttering (mild, stuttering with which the stutterer is comfortable) when it is acceptable

Peters, T. J., & Guitar, B. (1991). *Stuttering: An integrated approach to its nature and treatment.* Baltimore, MD: Williams & Wilkins.

Lidcombe Program. An early intervention program for preschool children who stutter; administered mostly be parents; involves the behavioral methods of positive reinforcement for fluency and corrective feedback for stuttering; parents and their stuttering children visit the clinic once a week to get training in 1-hour sessions; includes systematic methods to obtain at-home and in-the-clinic measures of stuttering throughout the treatment phases; problem solving and maintenance procedures are included; developed and researched by Onslow, Packman, and associates; published clinical trial data are available.

- Measure stuttering
  - engage the child in conversation for about 10 minutes and count the syllables stuttered and syllables spoken fluently
  - obtain percent syllables stuttered (%SS) before the onset of treatment
    continue to collect %SS throughout the treatment phase
- Train parents to rate their child's stuttering severity
  - train them to use a 10-point scale (1 = No stuttering; 10 = extremely severe stuttering)
  - assess agreement between your measures and the parents' ratings by rating the clinic-measured %SS together with the parent
- Train parents to record 5- to 10-minute speech samples at home and count the number of stutterings and the duration of the child's speaking time
  - obtain such samples from time to time throughout the treatment phase
  - calculate stutters per minute of speaking time from these recordings (SMST)
- Train parents to deliver treatment in 5- to 10-minute sessions held at home one or two times a day, preferably when the child is better able to cooperate (such as in the mornings and early afternoons); conduct parent training during the first weeks of clinic visits
  - set the goal of effortless, stutter-free speech for the child

S

- train the parent to engage the child in structured play with storybooks, picture books, selected toys, and so forth
- train them to tell the child that "We will be playing a game and let's see if you can say a lot words smoothly. I will say 'Great talking' when I hear smooth talking."
- train parents to evoke single words with the help of flash cards with a child whose stuttering is very severe; train parents to use more play-oriented conversational speech with a child whose stuttering is mild
- train parents to decrease the treatment structure as the child becomes more fluent
- train parents to praise the child for stutter-free speech with such verbal statements as "Good talking!" "Your speech sounds great!" or "Your words are smooth!" and so forth; train them to deliver such praise promptly, consistently, and with enthusiasm and sincerity; train them to supplement praise with such tangible reinforcers as stickers or tokens

- Train parents to react in one of several ways when their child stutters in structured treatment sessions at home:
  - ignore stuttering
  - say something like "That was a bumpy word" and continue conversation
  - model a fluent production of the stuttered word and continue conversation
  - say "A bumpy word occurred" and ask the child to repeat the word correctly or fluently
  - ask the child to repeat the stuttered word fluently and, if successful, ask the child to do that one or two more times; reinforce fluent productions

- watch for signs of distress in the child and postpone the use of correction if the child reacts emotionally to it; reintroduce correction gradually and after the child experienced success with reinforcement for stutter-free speech
- deliver significantly fewer corrections than praise in all sessions
- Train parents to deliver treatment on-line
  - train parents to monitor speech in everyday speaking situations (e.g., the parents correct a child's stuttering while shopping or on a playground)
  - initiate this step when the parent can measure and correct stuttering reliably and stuttering has begun to decrease as a result of treatment sessions conducted at home
- Train parents to teach their child self-monitoring skills by
  - periodically asking the child whether a production was smooth or bumpy to encourage self-evaluation
  - praising the child for self-correction of stuttered production
- Initiate a maintenance program when the child's daily SR at home is 2.0 or lower and the clinic %SS is 1 or less for 3 consecutive weeks
  - decrease the frequency of clinic visits gradually, building such decreases as rewards for maintaining fluency at home
  - schedule maintenance clinic visits at 2 weeks, 2 weeks, 4 weeks, 4 weeks, 8 weeks, 8 weeks, 16 weeks, and 32 weeks
  - assess stuttering when they visit the clinic
  - advance the child to the next visit if the child maintains an SR average of 2.0 and SMST 1.0 or less

S

- discuss reasons for increase in stuttering should this happen and design a strategy for the parent to implement it; set a returning date
- continue monitoring as scheduled
- train parents to gradually reduce on-line monitoring while maintaining fluent speech

Lincoln, M., & Harrison, E. (1999). The Lidcombe program. In M. Onslow & A. Packman (Eds.), *The handbook of early stuttering intervention* (pp. 103–117). San Diego: Singular Publishing Group.

Metronome-Paced Speech. Speech that is regulated by the beats of a metronome; a form of treatment used for stuttering and cluttering; syllables or word initiations may be regulated; may be used to slow down or accelerate the rate of speech; documented immediate effects of reduced or eliminated stuttering, but timed, rhythmic, and unnatural sounding speech; research needed to document long-term effects; possibility of client adaptation to the beats (no more effective); De-layed Auditory Feedback (DAF) (described earlier in this section), with its similar effects, is preferred over metronome speech in the treatment of stuttering.

- Assess the client and baserate stuttering
- Select a miniaturized, battery-operated, electronic metronome the client can wear like a hearing aid
- Find the client-specific beat rate that reduces or eliminates stuttering
- Have the client time the production of syllables with the beats in the early stages of treatment
- Have the client time the production of words with the beats in the later stages
- Have the client time the production of phrases and sentences as fluency increases and stabilizes
- Increase the rate of beats or vice versa, depending on the starting point

- Ask the client to initially wear the unit in all situations
- Fade the metronome beats by reducing its intensity in gradual steps
- Ask the client to wear the unit with the power turned off
- Ask the client to remove the unit
- Continue conversational therapy without the unit to stabilize fluency
- Conduct informal treatment sessions in varied non-clinical settings
- Counsel the client about the possibility of relapse and the need for Booster Treatment
- Follow up and arrange for booster treatment

Monterey Fluency Program (MFP). A programmed operant approach to establish, transfer, and maintain fluency in persons who stutter; uses one of two specific methods: Delayed Auditory Feedback (DAF) and Gradual Increase in Length and Complexity of Utterances (GILCU); DAF is often used with older or more severe stutterers and GILCU is more frequently used with younger and less severe stutterers; contains establishment, transfer, and maintenance phases; supported by clinical evidence; developed and researched by B. Ryan and B. Van Kirk.

MFP Delayed Auditory Feedback Method

- Give an overview of the program to the client, the parents, or both; describe the role the parents or other family members will play in fluency maintenance at home
- Give a criterion test consisting of 5 minutes of reading, monologue, and conversation to baserate stuttering; measure stuttering in terms of stuttered words per minute (SW/M)
- Implement the fluency establishment program

S

- teach the client to identify and measure his or her stuttering with 75% or better accuracy
- begin by reading with the child in a slow, prolonged, and fluent manner; reinforce verbally and with tokens and require a 0 SW/M in this and the subsequent steps
- instruct the child to read with a 250-millisecond (msec) DAF
- reinforce verbally and with tokens for fluent speech and say, "Stop, use your slow, prolonged speech" when the client stutters
- decrease the DAF to 200, 150, 100, 50, and 0 msec in successive steps
- at each step of the decreasing DAF, require a 0 SW/M (100% fluency) during a 5-minute oral reading
- switch to monologue with 250- msec DAF when the client meets the 5-minute 0 SW/M criterion in oral reading with no DAF
- decrease DAF in steps similar to those for oral reading
- switch to conversational speech with 250-msec DAF when the client meets the performance criterion (0 SW/M in 5 minutes of monologue with no DAF)
- repeat the steps to progressively decrease the DAF to zero and have the client meet the performance criterion
- Implement the fluency transfer program
  - vary the physical setting; have the client read for 1 minute and converse for 3 minutes with you in each of five physical settings; verbally reinforce for fluency and say "Stop, speak fluently" when stuttering occurs
  - vary the audience; bring in one person (e.g., the child's classmate), then two persons, and finally

S

three persons; each time, let the child converse with 0 SW/M

- ask parents to join you in treatment sessions; train them to conduct home reading, monologue, and conversational practice sessions
- ask parents to conduct practice sessions at home; have the client read, engage in monologue, or conversation at home with increasing audience size as the corresponding steps are completed in the clinic
- ask the parents to require fluent speech all the time at home and let them reinforce the child
- transfer training to classroom; initially, let the child read and converse with you in the classroom
- eventually, have the child give an oral presentation to the class
- have the child make telephone calls and require a 3-minute fluent conversation on the phone
- have the child speak to strangers and require 3-minutes of fluent speech
- instruct the child to speak fluently at all the time and in all situations

- Implement the fluency maintenance program
  - follow up the child for 22 months; schedule follow-up sessions 2 weeks, 1 month, 3 months, 6 months, and 12 months
  - give the criterion test at each visit (5 minutes of oral reading, monologue, and conversation with 0.5 SW/M or less)
  - if there is regression, recycle through selected steps of the treatment program
  - dismiss the child after 22 months of maintained fluency

MFP Gradual Increase in Length and Complexity of Utterances (GILCU)

- Give an overview of the program to the client, the parents, or both; describe the role the parents or

other family members will play in fluency maintenance at home
- Give a criterion test consisting of 5 minutes of reading, monologue, and conversation to baserate stuttering; measure stuttering in terms of stuttered
words per minute (SW/M)
- Implement the fluency establishment program
  - teach the client to identify and measure his or her
    stuttering with 75% or better accuracy
  - instruct the client to "read fluently"; have the cli-
    ent read one word fluently; reinforce with verbal
    praise for fluent production; say "Stop, read flu-
    ently" when stuttering occurs; obtain 10 consecu-
    tive fluently read words
  - gradually increase the length of orally read re-
    sponses; steps include 2, 3, 4, 5, and 6 fluent
    words; 1, 2, 3, and 4 fluent sentences; fluency for
    30 seconds and 1, 1.5, 2, 2.5, 3, 4, and 5 minutes
  - instruct the client to "speak fluently"; ask the cli-
    ent to engage in monologue (first step with a non-
    reader); use pictures and topic ideas and other
    necessary stimulus procedures with the same
    gradually escalating steps
  - engage the child in conversation; use the same
    gradually escalating steps
  - reinforce fluent productions with verbal praise and
    tokens
  - say "Stop, read fluently" or "Stop, speak fluently"
    when the client stutters
  - model the target response when the client persists
    with stuttering
  - require 100% fluency (0 SW/M) at each step
  - give a criterion test at the end of the establishment
    phase (5 minutes of reading, monologue, and con-
    versation with 0 SW/M)
- Implement the fluency transfer program

S

- use the procedure outlined earlier under *MFP Delayed Auditory Feedback Method*; skip or modify steps to suit the client (e.g., skip telephone training for a young child; select appropriate extraclinical settings for an adult)
- Implement the fluency maintenance program
  - use the procedures outlined earlier under *MFP Delayed Auditory Feedback Method*

Ryan, B., & Van Kirk, B. (1971). *Monterey fluency program.* Palo Alto, CA: Monterey Learning Systems.

Prolonged Speech. Speech produced with extended duration of speech sounds, especially vowels, and particularly those in the initial position of words; a target behavior in stuttering treatment; not a treatment procedure but the effect of treatment; induces <u>Stutter-Free Speech</u>; results in fluency that sounds unnatural and socially unacceptable; useful in establishing stutter-free speech; often combined with such additional targets as <u>Natural Sounding Fluency, Airflow Management,</u> and <u>Gentle Phonatory Onset</u>; a common component in many contemporary stuttering treatment programs; supported by clinical evidence, some experimentally controlled; procedurally, either DAF-induced or clinician-induced.

Prolonged Speech, DAF-Induced. Speech that is produced by prolonging speech sounds, especially the vowels, and particularly in the word-initial positions; prolongation of sounds forced by the <u>Delayed Auditory Feedback (DAF)</u>; induces stutter-free speech that sounds fluent but unnatural and socially unacceptable; a target behavior in many stuttering treatment programs; often combined with such other targets as <u>Airflow Management, Gentle Phonatory Onset, Normal Prosody</u> and <u>Natural-Sounding Fluency</u>; supported by clinical evidence, some experimentally controlled; clinical procedures under <u>Delayed Auditory Feedback.</u>

S

Prolonged Speech, Clinician-Induced. Speech that is produced by prolonging speech sounds, especially the vowels, and particularly in the word-initial positions; prolongation of sounds taught by clinicians without mechanical help; Instructions, Modeling, and Differential Reinforcement are the most effective techniques to induce it; supported by clinical evidence, some experimentally controlled; induces stutter-free speech that sounds fluent but unnatural and socially unacceptable; a target behavior in many stuttering treatment programs; often combined with such other targets as Airflow Management, Gentle Phonatory Onset, Normal Prosody, or Natural-Sounding Fluency.

- Assess the client and baserate the stuttering rate and speech rate
- Instruct the client in producing prolonged speech and describe its need, effects, and justification
- Ask the client to prolong the vowels, especially those at the beginning of words, phrases, and grammatical clauses
- Ask the client to reduce the rate of speech throughout the utterance
- Model the prolonged speech and overall reduced speech rate
- Model words, phrases, and sentences to give the client an idea, but ask the client to imitate only what he or she can (perhaps only words); model frequently
- Reduce your own rate of speech and talk in a noticeably prolonged manner
- Reinforce the client's prolonged speech promptly and lavishly
- Tell the client to "stop" (discontinue talking) at the earliest sign of increased rate, shortened vowels, or stuttering

- Repeat modeling, especially in the early stages of treatment whenever the client fails to maintain the target behaviors or produces stuttering
- Establish stutter-free (prolonged) speech at the topographic levels of words, phrases, sentences, and spontaneous conversational speech
- Use such performance criteria as 98 or 100% fluency at each topographic level, observed for a period of time or for a certain number of responses
- Increase the length of utterance as the client meets a particular performance criterion
- Decrease the extent of prolongation gradually as the client becomes more fluent
- Ask the client to increase the rate of speech and reinforce fluency at progressively increased speech rates
- Model normal prosodic features and ask the client to imitate
- Let the client slowly and gradually return to normal rate, rhythm, and prosody while maintaining fluency
- Train family members to signal the client to speak slowly and to reinforce fluent speech in daily situations
- Train the client in Self-Control (Self-Monitoring) skills by having him or her count stutterings
- Train the client to stop and slow down every time the rate increases or stuttering returns
- Conduct informal treatment sessions in varied nonclinical settings
- Counsel the client, the family, or both about the possibility of relapse and the need for booster treatment
- Follow up and arrange for booster treatment

Rate Reduction in Treating Stuttering. A speech rate slower than normal or below a client-specific baserate;

a typical target to reduce stuttering; a component of many treatment programs; similar to prolonged speech; supported by clinical evidence; may use Delayed Auditory Feedback to induce rate reduction; appropriate with very young children especially when the DAF is omitted.

* Establish the baserate of speech rate, measured in terms of syllables per minute or words per minute
* Instruct the client in rate reduction and describe its desirable effects
* Reassure the client that a more acceptable rate is the final target of treatment
* Reduce the rate by prolonging the vowels, not by increasing pause durations between words, phrases, and sentences
* Experiment with slower rates that reduce stuttering to near zero
* Model the effective rate selected for the client
* Ask the client to imitate the slower rate in producing multisyllable words and phrases by extending the duration of syllables (not pauses)
* Use delayed auditory feedback if instructions and modeling are not effective
* Shape slower rate in multisyllable words, phrases, sentences, and conversational speech to induce Stutter-Free Speech
* Fade the excessively slow rate of speech while the client maintains stutter-free conversational speech and moves toward more Natural Sounding Fluency
* Shape the normal or near-normal rate along with Normal Prosody
* Teach Self-Control (Self-Monitoring) of rate control that the client can use when needed in everyday situations

Regulated Breathing. A direct stuttering reduction method in which the client is asked to modify breathing patterns along with the use of such other strategies as thought formulation and relaxation; some clinical evidence supports its use but the effective component of the eclectic program is not clear; developed and researched by N. Azrin and his associates; only the components inhalation and slight exhalation before initiating phonation have been incorporated into several current treatment programs; more effective with older children and adults than with very young children.

* Ask the client to formulate thoughts before speaking
* Instruct the client to inhale and exhale a small amount of air before talking; model the target behaviors
* Ask the client to continue to exhale a little even after the last sound is produced
* Instruct the client to pause at natural speech junctures and formulate thoughts again
* Ask the client to stop soon after a stuttering occurs and relax, especially the chest muscles
* Ask the client to seek out previously avoided speaking situations
* Ask the client to practice the new method of speaking daily
* Train and ask the client to measure and record his or her stutterings in natural settings
* Train a family member in the procedure and let the person help the stutterer at home
* Maintain phone contact with the client to follow up

Azrin, N. H., & Nunn, R. G. (1974). A rapid method of eliminating stuttering by a regulated breathing approach. *Behavior Research & Therapy, 12,* 279–286.

Replacing Stuttering with Normal Speech. A method of stuttering treatment based primarily on Delayed Auditory Feedback (DAF); includes Continuous Airflow throughout utterances and psychotherapeutic discussions; developed and researched by W. Perkins and his associates, including R. Curlee.

- Establish fluent speech
  - set the DAF at 250 msec to generate about 30 words per minute (wpm) and stutter-free speech
  - use reading or conversation, whichever is easier for the client
  - use clinician-induced prolongation if a DAF unit is not available
- Establish normal breath flow
  - begin this in the second session if not toward the end of first session
  - limit the phrase length to three to eight syllables
  - teach the client to maintain airflow continuously throughout an utterance; ask the client to blend words in a smooth, continuous manner
  - teach a soft, breathy voice
  - teach gentle initiation of the initial syllable of phrases
- Establish normal prosody
  - teach normal intonation, stress pattern
  - have the client prolong stressed syllables longer and produce them louder
  - have the client produce unstressed syllables with light contacts and with less prolongation
- Shift responsibility for taking all subsequent steps to the stutterer
  - impress on the client that all subsequent steps are his or her own responsibility
  - ask the client to tape-record a treatment step taken and make decisions about the degree of control, the ability to slow down when the rate accelerates, and the need to move back to an earlier step
  - ask the client to move at a comfortable speech rate
- Establish slow-normal speech in conversation

- begin with oral reading if fluency skills have not been practiced in conversation
- progress to slow-normal conversational speech with 250-msec DAF
- eliminate avoidance behaviors
- Incorporate psychotherapeutic discussion
  - respond affirmatively to client's positive statements about himself or herself regarding the speech experiences
- Establish normal speech rate
  - reduce DAF to 200 msec and increase speech rate to 45–60 wps
  - reduce DAF to 150 msec and increase speech rate to 90–120 wps
  - reduce DAF further in 50-msec intervals until a normal 150–wpm rate is achieved
  - reduce the volume of DAF
  - stabilize a "home base" rate to which the client can return when stuttering increases
- Establish normal speech without DAF
  - turn the DAF unit off
  - remove one earphone at a time
  - remove the DAF headset
- Establish a clear voice
  - if voice sounds breathy or soft, reinforce a clear, louder voice
  - ask the client to use the most effective fluency skills in everyday situations (not necessarily all those taught in the program)
- Use strategies for generalizing normal speech
  - teach the client to rate his or her fluency, rate, breath flow, prosody, and self-confidence
  - if the rating is below expected, ask the client to return to relevant shaping procedures
  - teach the client to rehearse a slow rate and breath management when he or she anticipates stuttering

S

- change the therapy room and add one and then more listeners to treatment sessions
- ask the client to face speaking situations from the least difficult to the most difficult and try to maintain normal fluency (e.g., talking on the telephone, ordering in a restaurant, talking to strangers)
- reduce the frequency of treatment sessions
- facilitate living pattern changes by encouraging the stutterer to participate in enjoyable speech activities previously not tried; ask family members to accept the newly learned normal fluency in the client

Perkins, W. H. (1973). Replacement of stuttering with normal speech: II. Clinical procedures. *Journal of Speech and Hearing Disorders, 38,* 295–303.

Shadowing. A stuttering and cluttering treatment technique in which the client, without seeing the text, repeats (shadows) everything the clinician reads from a book; the client stays a few words behind the clinician; typical effect is to reduce the frequency of stuttering; popular in the 1960s and 1970s, especially in Europe; some clinician evidence suggests its effect in reducing stuttering; no research on maintenance of fluency.

- Assess the client and baserate the stuttering frequency
- Select a reading material that is suitable to the client
- Instruct the client to say everything that you read
- Give practice by reading a few sentences at a time, stopping, and reinstructing, if necessary
- Do not show the text to the client
- Read normally; do not change the rate, rhythm, or phrasing
- Tape-record the client's shadowing to measure the frequency of stuttering during treatment sessions

Stutter-Free Speech. Speech of a person who stutters that contains no or few stutterings; often not the same as normally fluent speech because it may not sound natural when achieved by the use of Delayed Auditory Feedback, Rate Reduction, or Prolonged Speech induced by clinicians, and by Metronome-Paced Speech; a result of initial stages of such treatment methods; needs additional procedures to make the speech sound naturally fluent and make it last over time and across situations.

Stutter-Free Speech: A Stuttering Treatment Program. A method of stuttering treatment developed and researched by G. Shames and C. Florance; uses Delayed Auditory Feedback (DAF) to induce slow, stutter-free speech; uses operant procedures to shape natural-sounding fluency.

- Teach volitional control over speech (slower rate and continuous phonation)
  - reduce the speech rate through DAF (initial delay of 250 msec)
  - train the client to produce 30 minutes of stutter-free conversational speech at progressively reduced delays of 200, 150, 100, and 50 msec to increase the speech rate
  - teach the client to stretch each word into the following word to produce continuous phonation
- Teach Self-Control (Self-Monitoring) and self-reinforcement
  - teach the client to self-monitor fluent and stuttered speech so that he or she deliberately produces an acceptable rate and continuous phonation
  - teach the client to evaluate his or her fluent and stuttered productions
  - teach the client to self-reinforce by talking without monitoring after a period of deliberately monitored speech
- Implement transfer and generalization procedures

S

- develop a contract with the client that specifies speaking situations in which he or she will use the newly acquired fluency
- ask the client to use stutter-free speech in a few situations initially and all day subsequently
- let the client control the number and types of situations to which to transfer
- let the client self-reinforce with unmonitored (but fluent) speech
- Replace monitored speech with unmonitored speech
  - ask the client to gradually decrease the duration for which he or she monitors fluency
  - ask the client to use unmonitored but fluent speech all the time or use monitored speech only on special occasions
- Follow up the client
  - Follow up the client for 5 years

Shames, G. H., & Florence, C. L. (1980). *Stutter-free speech.* Columbus, OH: Charles E. Merrill.

Stuttering Modification. A collection of approaches to treating stuttering in which the emphasis is on changing the form of stuttering so that it is less severe and more socially and personally acceptable; the goal is not normal fluency, but less abnormality; approach exemplified by Fluent Stuttering approach of Van Riper (described earlier in this section); includes attempts to change attitudes and feelings; treatment sessions loosely structured; little emphasis on measurement of behaviors; contrasted with Fluency Shaping Techniques (described earlier in this section).

Stuttering Prevention: A Clinical Method. An early treatment program for children who stutter; developed by W. Starkweather and his associates; based on the Demands and Capacities Model (DCM) of fluency and stuttering; goal is to reduce demands made on the child's fluency and increase fluency capacities.

Stuttering Treatment: Specific Programs

- Assess the child's capacity for fluency and the demands the child faces
- Counsel the parents
  - educate the parents about stuttering, the treatment program, and prognosis; give an optimistic outlook on improvement with treatment
  - change attitudes of parents by discussing their negative feelings and possible guilt
  - change behaviors of parents; ask them to speak at a slower rate; ask them to use shorter, simpler sentences while speaking to the child; let them know that negative reactions and punishment can worsen stuttering; encourage polite turn taking in conversation; ask them to arrange a special talking time with the child; ask parents to demand speech less often; teach parents the direct treatment techniques
- Modify directly the child's stuttering and fluency
  - reduce the tension and struggle behaviors associated with dysfluency
  - initially, model behaviors (slower rate, less struggled word and phrase repetitions) without necessarily requiring the child to imitate them
  - later, ask the child to imitate slower rate by syllable prolongation
  - implement such fluency enhancing strategies as no interruption and no demands for verbal performance (silent periods are fine)
  - control play activities so that they are appropriate for the child's cognitive level and allows for conversation
- Include direct intervention strategies and fluency shaping procedures as found necessary
  - use gentle phonatory onset and light articulatory contacts
  - time-out contingent on struggle behaviors
  - self-correcting

S

- Promote a level of language use that is normal for the child's age and gender
  - model a level of language use that is appropriate for the child
  - change parent's language as specified earlier
- Dismiss the child only when both the parents' and the child's behaviors have changed

Starkweather, W., Gottwald, S. R., & Halfond, M. (1990). *Stuttering prevention: A clinical method.* Englewood Cliffs, NJ: Prentice-Hall.

Stuttering, Voluntary. A technique of stuttering modification in which the client is asked to stutter deliberately; the goal is to reduce the fear and embarrassment associated with it and to eliminate avoidance of stuttering; part of Van Riper's Fluent Stuttering approach.

Subcortical Aphasia. Aphasia presumably due to damage to subcortical structures, especially to basal ganglia and surrounding areas; somewhat controversial; to produce aphasia, subcortical damage must be extensive; some experts suspect that subcortical aphasia involves cortical damage as well; characterized by generally fluent speech, intact repetition, and articulation problems.

Submucous Cleft. Unexposed cleft of the hard palate, soft palate, or both because of normal mucosal covering; speech in some cases may be hypernasal.

Substitution Processes. A group of phonological processes in which one class of sounds is substituted for another; in phonological treatment, the target is to eliminate such processes; major substitution processes include:

- *Deaffrication:* substitution of a fricative for an affricate (e.g., a /t/, /s/, or a /k/ for /tʃ/; a /d/ or a /z/ for /dʒ/)
- *Denasalization:* substitution of an oral consonant for a nasal consonant (e.g., /d/ for /n/)
- *Gliding:* substitution of a glide for a liquid (e.g., /w/ for /r/)
- *Stopping:* substitution of a stop for a fricative or an affricate (e.g., /p/ for /f/; /p/ for /v/, /t/ for /s/)

Super-Supraglottic Swallow

- *Velar Fronting:* substitution of an alveolar for a velar (e.g., /t/ for /k/, /d/ for /g/, /n/ for /ŋ/)

Super-Supraglottic Swallow. A swallowing maneuver that helps close the airway entrance before and during the swallow; it helps close the false vocal folds by tilting the arytenoid cartilage anteriorly to the base of the epiglottis before and during the swallow; arytenoids are tilted when the breath is held and the patient bears down; to implement this maneuver, ask the patient to:
- inhale and hold the breath tightly by bearing down
- swallow while holding the breath and bearing down

Supraglottic Swallow Maneuver. A procedure to reduce or control aspiration while modifying swallowing behavior during the oral phase of the swallow; teaches the client to voluntarily protect the airway.
- Ask the patient to inhale and hold the breath
- Place food in the mouth
- Ask the patient to tilt the head back and swallow
- Teach the patient to cough after each swallow to clear any residual food from the pharynx

Swallow Reflex. A series of reflexive actions needed to complete the swallow act; includes the reflexive elevation of the soft palate, closure of the airway, peristalsis (constriction of the pharyngeal constrictors), relaxation of the cricopharyngeal muscle to passage of food into the esophagus; often delayed in patients with dysphagia; may be triggered by stimulating the base of the anterior faucial arch.

Syndrome. A constellation of signs and symptoms that are associated with a morbid process.

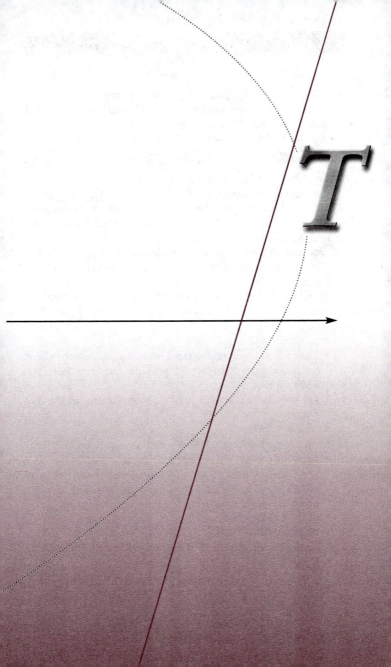

Teflon™ or Collagen Injection. A medical treatment procedure for clients with paralyzed vocal folds; injected into the middle third of the fold, the two materials increase the bulk and the chances of abduction.

Terminal Response. The final response targeted in Shaping.

Time-Out (TO). Time-out from positive reinforcement; also described as pause-and-talk as used in Stuttering treatment and in reducing a variety of undesirable behaviors; direct response reduction procedure in which one of the following three contingencies is placed on a behavior to be reduced: (1) a brief period of no reinforcement (nonexclusion TO); (2) exclusion of the person from the stream of activity (exclusion TO), but not from the current environment; or (3) removal of the person from the current environment and placing the person in an isolated place for a brief period (Isolation TO).

Exclusion TO
- Contingent on an undesirable response, exclude the client from the current stream of activities, but not from the environment
- Let the client resume the activity at the end of the TO duration

Isolation TO
- Contingent on an undesirable response, remove the client from the current environment
- Place the client in a specially designed situation for a certain duration
- Bring the client back to the normal environment at the end of the TO duration

Nonexclusion TO
- Begin TO as soon as the client produces an undesirable response
- During TO, do not interact with client
- Ask the client not to respond for the specified duration
- At the end of the TO duration, resume interaction

T

Tokens

Tokens. Conditioned generalized reinforcers; objects that are earned during treatment and exchanged later for back-up reinforcers.
* Always have back-up reinforcers the child can exchange the tokens for
* Let the child choose a back-up reinforcer in the beginning of each session
* Let the child understand the ratio of tokens to a back-up reinforcer
* Set a low ratio in the beginning and gradually raise the number of tokens needed to receive the back-up reinforcer

Tongue Thrust. A deviant swallow in which the tongue is pushed forward against the central incisors.

Topic Initiation. A pragmatic language skill to initiate conversation on a topic; a frequent language intervention target; procedures described under Language Disorders in Children; Treatment of Language Disorders: Specific Techniques or Programs.

Topic Maintenance. A pragmatic language skill to maintain conversation for socially acceptable time periods; a frequent language intervention target; procedures described under Language Disorders in Children; Treatment of Language Disorders: Specific Techniques or Programs.

Topographic Sequence of Treatment. Sequencing treatment based on response complexity; most clients learn better if the target skills are simplified in the initial stages of therapy.
* Begin treatment with simpler topographic levels (words, phrases) and increase the topographic complexity in gradual steps (sentences, conversational speech)
* In treating articulation disorders, begin teaching a phoneme at the word or syllable level; as the client becomes proficient in producing the sound at this level, shift training to the phrase level; finally provide training in conversational speech

- In language therapy, teach grammatic morpheme in words or phrases (e.g., cups or two cups); as the client becomes proficient in producing the morpheme at this level, shift training to sentences and conversational speech
- In fluency therapy, train such skills as gentle onset, prolonged speech, and airflow management initially in words and phrases and subsequently in sentences and conversational speech
- In voice therapy, use single vowel productions (e.g., /a/) and words to improve voice quality; subsequently, shift training to sentences and conversational speech

Topography. Description of natural and physical properties of an object or event; topographic aspects of skills refer to their physical form or shape including how complex they are, and how they appear, sound, and feel.

Total Communication. The simultaneous use of multiple modes of expression to enhance communication; includes speech, gestures, informal and formal (e.g., American Sign Language and AMER-IND) signs, and facial expressions.

Tracheoesophageal Fistulization/Puncture (TEF/ TEP). A surgical procedure that helps laryngectomy patients to produce laryngeal speech with the help of a voice prosthesis; the tracheal wall is punctured to create a small tunnel into the esophagus; the puncture acts as a shunt to allow air into the esophagus through a Voice Prosthesis inserted into the opening; air goes up through the P-E Segment and results in the production of sound.

Andrews, M. L. (1995). *Manual of voice treatment: Pediatrics to geriatrics.* San Diego: Singular Publishing Group.

Casper, J. K., & Colton, R. H. (1993). *Clinical manual for laryngectomy and head and neck cancer rehabilitation.* San Diego: Singular Publishing Group.

Traditional Orthography. Written natural language; a normal form of communication; a method of nonvocal communication for the speechless; used in teaching <u>Augmentative Communication Gestural-Assisted (Aided)</u>.

Training Broad. An approach to treating articulation disorders in which several sounds are treated simultaneously; practice, limited on any one sound, is given over a broad range of sounds; contrasted with <u>Training Deep</u>.

Training Criterion. A rule that specifies when an exemplar or a target skill has met a specified performance level; a 90% correct response rate is an often accepted training criterion.
- Specify a training criterion in measurable terms (e.g., 9 out of 10 correct responses)
- Continue training until that criterion is met
- Probe when the training criterion is met
- If the probe criterion (90% correct in untrained contexts) is not met, resume training

Training Deep. An approach to treating articulation disorders in which one or a few sounds are trained intensively; other sounds are selected for training only when the child has mastered the initial targets; contrasted with <u>Training Broad</u>.

Training Sessions in Natural Environments. Part of extraclinical training strategy used to promote maintenance.
- Initially, hold training in varied settings in and around the clinic
- Next, hold informal training sessions in nonclinical settings
- Train parents to hold training sessions at home
- Take the client to such natural setting as shopping centers and restaurants
- Let the training in natural settings be less conspicuous, involving mostly conversational speech
- Prompt the target responses in a subtle manner
- Deliver reinforcers and corrective feedback in a subtle manner

T

Transcortical Motor Aphasia. A type of nonfluent aphasia characterized by agrammatic, paraphasic, and telegraphic speech; differential diagnosis is made on the basis of intact repetition skills; lesion or lesions, often sparing the Broca's area, are found deep in the frontal lobe or above or below Broca's area. See Aphasia; Treatment of Aphasia: Specific Types.

Transcortical Sensory Aphasia. A type of fluent aphasia that is similar to Wernicke's aphasia; the lesion or lesions, often sparing Wernicke's area, are found in the temporoparietal regions; characterized by fluent speech, poor auditory comprehension, impaired naming, paraphasic speech, and echolalia.

Traumatic Brain Injury (TBI) in Adults. An injury to the brain; may be Penetrating (Open-Head) Injury or Nonpenetrating (Closed-Head) Injury; major symptoms include restlessness, irritation, disorientation to time and place, disorganized and inconsistent responses; impaired memory, attention, reasoning, drawing, naming, and repetition; also known as craniocerebral trauma; immediate concern is medical; long-term concern is rehabilitation.

Treatment of Traumatic Brain Injury: General Principles

- Plan for long-term treatment and rehabilitation, especially in the case of more severe injury
- Use direct behavioral treatment procedures, as they are known to be effective; these include simplifying the tasks with shaping procedure, measurable, practical skill targeting instead of indirect underlying process training; and immediate positive reinforcement for skill management
- Schedule different kinds of therapeutic activities at different stages of recovery from TBI (acute, postacute, outpatient, and long-term)
- Work with the family and medical and rehabilitation staff from the beginning; make sure that the family members

understand the effects of TBI and the initial, limited goals for functional communication

- Serve as member of rehabilitation teams that include different professionals
- Plan on communication training gaining momentum as the patient recovers from the initial effects of TBI
- Consider physical rehabilitation as an important aspect of treatment
- Select client-specific functional treatment goals that help improve immediate communication, orientation to the environment, memory for events and persons, and those that help reduce confusion
- Revise treatment targets as the patient's condition improves (or deteriorates); select goals that are appropriate and practical for the physical condition of the client
- Let the client's family members participate in treatment target selection; have them rate the importance of potential communication skills and skill hierarchies
- Emphasize communication effectiveness instead of grammatical accuracy; accept gestures, words, phrases, or grammatically incorrect expressions if they are effectively communicate
- Integrate such cognitive skills as orientation, memory, and attention into communication training instead of concentrating on them in an isolated manner (e.g., reinforce increasingly longer durations of attention while training such communication skills as maintaining eye contact or topic maintenance) instead of paying attention to printed dots or squares
- Include behavioral self-management exercises in your treatment program
- Select treatment activities that are real-life activities (e.g., in improving memory skills, use pictures of family members instead of irrelevant pictures or geometric shapes)
- Begin with simple activities and move through a sequence of more complex activities

T

TBI: Treatment Procedures

- Hold brief and frequent treatment sessions in the initial stages of rehabilitation
- Increase the duration of sessions as the client's general physical condition improves; hold longer sessions less frequently
- Consider teaching compensatory strategies whenever necessary
- Structure treatment sessions to eliminate distraction, especially in the initial stages of recovery; loosen the structure gradually to better resemble everyday living conditions
- Carefully sequence treatment tasks
- Work closely with the members of the interdisciplinary team so that an integrated plan of rehabilitation is implemented
- Note the similarities in treatment goals and procedures for patients with TBI and those with Right Hemisphere Syndrome
- Note that there is little research on ethnocultural variables that affect treatment; consequently, consider general guidelines given under Ethnocultural Variables in Treatment

Traumatic Brain Injury: Treatment Procedures
Treatment During the Initial Stage
- Simplify activities and routines
- Decrease variability in activities and stimulation; let the patient experience only a few structured activities to begin with
- Induce consistency in staff care and stimuli
- Improve the client's orientation and attention to surroundings
  - arrange familiar cues by pasting familiar pictures, posters, and objects
  - play favorite music
  - post written signs and lists about the daily routines; train the patient to consult the signs and lists; ask the patient to read them aloud; ask the patient to describe scheduled activities and their timings

- ask questions about time, place, and people (e.g., "Where are you now?" "What time is it?" "Who am I?" "Who is she?") and prompt correct responses
- frequently model any response you expect from the client; reinforce correct imitative responses
- increase the patient's attention to the surroundings and communication patterns by drawing the patient's attention to surrounding events, persons including health care workers; by encouraging the patient to talk about surroundings and persons and giving corrective feedback and positive reinforcement
- simplify all demands so that the client experiences successes
- use tangible reinforcers as the patients with TBI may not initially respond to verbal praise (use such tangible reinforcers as sweets, music, touching, massage)
- keep the treatment sessions brief
- prompt and assist the client to engage in self-care activities (dressing, eating)
- gradually reduce the amount of physical help offered
- have the client participate in group treatment sessions as soon as it is practical
- place behavioral contingencies on appropriate behaviors
- shape desired targets
- Pair gestures with verbal explanations
- Use auditory stimulation as the chief method of input
- Do not overstimulate
- Use brightly colored objects and pictures in treatment
- Start with strong cues and fade later
- Use graphs and charts to show the patient relationships between objects
- Relate the information to experiences that have occurred in the patient's life
- Teach the patient to respond with yes or no

T

TBI: Treatment Procedures

- Introduce familiar sounds from the patient's home (e.g., dog bark)
- Use familiar odors to reorient patient to previously identifiable smells
- Gain the patient's attention before talking to him or her (e.g., "Listen, carefully, now"; "I want to say something to you."); educate the clinical staff to do the same
- Give introduction to new topic (e.g., "I am now going to tell you about . . ."); do not introduce topics abruptly
- Assess comprehension of spoken speech frequently by asking the patient to restate what was just said or summarize the main points of discussion; prompt correct responses to minimize errors
- Reinforce nonverbal communication or signs of attention (e.g., eye contact, smiling, nodding); still, assess comprehension to make sure the patient understands
- Withhold attention from irrelevant, inappropriate, and tangential responses; without responding, ask a simple question that might evoke a more relevant response; reinforce it; use <u>Time-Out</u> to decrease more serious undesirable behaviors
- Reduce complexity and rate of speech if necessary
- Use statements instead of questions when initially communicating with the patient
- Prompt, gesture, and use verbal instructions to help the patient comprehend
- Allow the patient time to listen to instructions
- Use sentence completion tasks for patients with initiation or inhibition difficulties
- Place contingencies on appropriate behaviors

Treatment During the Intermediate Stage

- Continue to place contingencies on target behaviors
- Establish more complex routines
- Teach the patient to request information (e.g., requesting information about time, space, or persons)

TBI: Treatment Procedures

- Continue to provide additional stimuli as needed (written instructions, alarms, posters, verbal reminders of activities and appointments)
- Repeat treatment trials
- Improve selective attention and comprehension by asking the patient to:
  - match pictures to sentences
  - follow spoken instructions
  - retell a message to another person
  - answer simple questions
- Work closely with health care workers; teach them to
  - recognize the client's problems
  - respond promptly to positive changes in communication skills
  - provide additional stimuli as needed
- Work with family members; teach them to
  - prompt the client when there is hesitation
  - model appropriate behaviors
  - reinforce the behaviors naturally and sustain those behaviors
- Increase awareness of deficits
  - use simple explanations to describe the problem to the patient
  - give contingent feedback on problem behaviors
  - use group therapy to allow the patient to see that others have similar problems
- Continue group treatment to have peer modeling, monitoring, and self-awareness of problems
- Begin to diminish special stimuli and reminders as performance improves toward the end of the intermediate stage
- Begin to teach <u>Self-Control (Self-Monitoring)</u> skills
- Begin to teach compensatory skills

Treatment During the Late Stage
- Train more complex activities that enhance independence

T

TBI: Treatment Procedures

- Teach narrative skills in graded steps (e.g., initially tell a brief and simple story and ask the client to retell it; prompt correct responses; subsequently, tell progressively more complex stories the patient will retell; reduce the frequency of your prompts)
- Ask the patient to describe daily activities and complex skills (e.g., ask the patient to describe how he or she would fix a sandwich, make a grocery list, pay utility bills; prompt correct responses in correct sequence of steps; reinforce)
- Integrate such pragmatic skills as topic maintenance and topic initiation into narrative skill teaching (e.g., promote topic maintenance; prompt the patient to "Say more," "Give details," "What happened next?" "What about this?" or "What about that?"; prompt the client to initiate conversation on new topics; fade the prompts)
- Integrate work-related words, phrases, and sentences if the patient is expected to return to work; make this activity client-specific
- Further diminish special stimuli (posters, verbal reminders, written instructions) that control behaviors
- Continue to use shaping, modeling, prompting, and manual guidance to enhance correct responses and to reduce the probability of errors
- Treat Motor Speech Disorders
- Teach Self-Control (Self-Monitoring) skills; teach the client to
  - keep possessions in specific places
  - count his or her own errors in treatment
  - self-correct errors
  - use self-cueing strategies (pausing after an error)
- Teach compensatory strategies if necessary, by teaching patients to:
  - break down tasks into smaller, more manageable components; teach the patients to write down steps

526

involved in performing an action (e.g., steps in preparing a breakfast)
- request information relative to time, date, and so forth
- request others to modify their speech (e.g., teach the client to request others to speak slowly or to repeat)
- rehearse important information (e.g., teach the client to self-talk about how to perform such activities as fixing lunch or changing light bulbs)
- write down instructions, appointments, important information, and so forth
- ask for written instructions from people
- use active instead of passive cues (an alarm instead of a reminder in a diary that may not be consulted)
- use electronic devices (digital watches that display time, day, and date; auditorily signal appointments); use data bank watches that store messages and appointments; use electronic pill boxes that remind the patient to take medications; use microcassette recorders to record lectures, instructions, and discourse they can listen to later; use hand-held electronic spell checkers; use notebook computers for more complex information management
- limit distractions or modify environment by finding quiet places to study or rearrange work environments
- keep possessions at specific and constant places to improve access
- cue himself or herself to activities, names, paces, and appointments
- Teach organizational strategies by teaching the patient to:
  - separate relevant from irrelevant material
  - summarize, highlight, and take notes
  - self-monitor
- Ask patients to copy symbols, letters, and words that commonly occur in their surroundings (e.g., signs that read, "No drinking, smoking, and eating")

T

TBI: Treatment Procedures

- Develop a core vocabulary that the patient is likely to use every day
- Teach the patient to recognize letters, syllables, words, phrases, and sentences
- Hold group treatment sessions; note, however, there is no strong empirical evidence to support this, although it is a common practice; structure these group interactions to:
  - promote pragmatic communication skills (discourse, topic maintenance, and topic initiation)
  - increase general socialization
  - increase socially appropriate verbalization
  - self-evaluation of strengths and limitations
- Promote community reentry; note that rehabilitation should end with successful community reentry in which steps are taken to ensure a smooth transition from the rehabilitation setting to home, school, work, and the larger social situations
  - prepare the patient for reentry; in the final stages of treatment, emphasize self-help skills and independent living skills; stimulate the patient's interest in academic, social, occupational, and household activities
  - educate family members, teachers, and supervisors about the current status of the patient; let them appreciate the patient's strengths and limitations; let them understand the patient's compensatory strategies and the continued support needed
  - modify the communication styles of family members and significant others to suit the remaining and perhaps permanent deficits (e.g., teach them to speak slowly, repeat often, and speak in simpler sentences)
  - modify the number and nature of demands people make (e.g., the teacher may give reduced amount of work or simplified work; work supervisor may have to give extra time to complete a task)

T

- teach family members and others to recognize reasons for oppositional behaviors (e.g., oppositional behaviors may diminish if the demands are modified or tasks are simplified)

Beukelman, D. R., & Yorkston, K. M. (1991). *Communication disorders following traumatic brain injury: Management of cognitive, language, and motor impairments.* Austin, TX: Pro-Ed.

Bilger, E. D. (Ed.). (1990). *Traumatic brain injury.* Austin, TX: Pro-Ed.

Hegde, M. N. (1998). *A coursebook on aphasia and other neurogenic language disorders* (2nd ed.). San Diego: Singular Publishing Group.

Brookshire, R. H. (1997). *An introduction to neurogenic communication disorders* (5th ed.). St. Louis, MO: Mosby Year Book.

Ylvisaker, M. (1985). *Head injury rehabilitation: Children and adolescents.* Austin, TX: Pro-Ed.

Traumatic Brain Injury (TBI) in Children. Cerebral injury due to external force; may be <u>Penetrating (Open-Head) Injury</u> or <u>Nonpenetrating (Closed-Head) Injury</u>; communicative disorders are a common consequence of TBI; treatment procedures described under <u>Traumatic Brain Injury, Treatment</u> and many described under <u>Language Disorders in Children</u> are generally applicable with the following special considerations:

- Assess residual language and communication difficulties
- Design a treatment program that will address the residual deficits
- Consider the child's social and family communication needs
- Work closely with educators and teach skills that help academic achievement:
  - discuss the child's needs with other school professionals including teachers, educational psychologists, reading specialists, and others
  - develop a treatment plan that addresses the concerns of educators

T

- target functional communication skills necessary for classroom adjustment
- target specific academic terms for language intervention
- integrate reading and writing into your treatment tasks
- Work with the teacher to help her with classroom communication and general behavior; suggest to the teacher that she should
  - simplify the academic tasks for the child
  - shape difficult tasks
  - use simpler language spoken in slower rate
  - limit distractions in the classroom
  - keep the classroom situation organized with little variation
  - use gestures and signs along with verbal expressions
  - repeat instructions, give written instructions
  - ask the child to repeat her instructions
  - make sure that the child takes adequate notes
  - encourage the child to request help and promptly reinforce such attempts
  - accept any mode of expression initially but should expect more refined verbal communication eventually
- Keep the teacher and other educators serving the child informed of your treatment targets, general procedures, and outcome
- Ask other professionals to reinforce the skills you have taught
- Work closely with family members; train them to support the child's communicative attempts by positive reinforcement
- Develop a home treatment program and train parents in its implementation
- Select relevant recommendations from "Promote community reentry" under Treatment During the Late Stage (previous entry)

Bilger, E. D. (Ed.). (1990). *Traumatic brain injury.* Austin, TX: Pro-Ed.

Mira, M. P., Tucker, B. F., & Tyler, J. S. (1992). *Traumatic brain injury in children and adolescents.* Austin, TX: Pro-Ed.

T

Ylvisaker, M. (1985). *Head injury rehabilitation: Children and adolescents.* Austin, TX: Pro-Ed.

Treatment. Application of a variable that can induce changes; use of any effective procedure in teaching new communicative skills; behaviorally, management of contingent relations between antecedents, responses, and consequences; conceptually, a rearrangement of communicative relationships between a speaker and his or her listener.

Treatment of Communicative Disorders: General Procedures That Apply Across Disorders. Common procedures used in treating most if not all disorders of communication; modified to suit the individual client, his or her specific problems, the specific target behaviors, and in light of the performance data.
- Assess the client
  - determine the diagnosis
  - describe the strengths and limitations of the client
  - describe the client's current level of communicative performance
- Evaluate the client's family constellation
  - describe the family support and resources
  - describe the social, educational, or occupational demands made on the client
- Select functional, client-specific target behaviors
  - select behaviors that, when treated, will have the greatest effects on the client's communication in social situations
  - select both short- and long-term targets
  - define the dismissal criterion
- Establish the pretreatment measures or baselines of target behaviors
  - select stimuli for evoking the target behaviors
  - repeat the measures to establish reliability
  - use the Baseline Evoked Trials and Baseline Modeled Trials

- take an extended conversational speech sample
- obtain home sample if possible
- Design a flexible therapeutic environment
  - use the degree of control and structure that is necessary
  - gradually, loosen the structure to make the treatment environment more like the client's everyday environment
- Write a treatment program; specify
  - the target behaviors
  - treatment procedures
  - reinforcing or feedback procedures
  - Criteria for Making Clinical Decisions (moving from one level of treatment to another)
  - Probe procedure
  - maintenance procedure
  - follow-up
  - booster treatment
- Implement the treatment program
  - use objects, pictures, demonstrated actions, and so forth to evoke the target behaviors
  - give instructions, demonstrations, explanations
  - model the target responses
  - prompt the target responses
  - use manual guidance to assist the client in producing the target responses
  - shape the responses
  - fade the special stimuli including pictures, objects, modeling, prompts, and manual guidance
  - give prompt, positive feedback to the client; use natural reinforcers; if you used tangible reinforcers, fade them; decrease the amount of feedback given
  - give prompt, corrective feedback to the client; say "No" or "Wrong"; use other procedures as found appropriate (time-out, response cost)
  - start treatment at a simpler level; however, if the client can perform at a higher level, do not use the lower level
  - probe for generalized production as often as necessary

T

- shift treatment, in progressive steps, to more complex levels as the client meets the probe criterion
- always train the target behaviors in conversational speech with natural consequences
- Implement the maintenance program
  - train family members, teachers, friends, and professional caregivers in supporting the client's communicative behaviors
  - teach them to evoke the target behaviors and reinforce the client naturally
  - shift training to nonclinical settings
  - invite other persons to treatment sessions
  - have family members conduct informal treatment sessions at home
  - have teachers focus on the target skills you teach and integrate those skills in the classroom work
  - teach the client to self-monitor his or her errors and target behaviors
  - teach the client to count his or her relevant behaviors
  - teach the client to self-correct mistakes
  - teach the client to cue himself or herself
  - teach the client to pause soon after an error response is produced
  - dismiss the client when responses are reliably produced in natural settings
- Follow up the client
  - set up a schedule for follow-up
  - follow up a client for a duration necessary to show maintenance
  - take a conversational speech sample during follow-up sessions
  - measure the production of relevant communicative skills
  - recommend booster treatment if the skills have deteriorated
- Arrange for booster treatment
  - give the same or better treatment

- probe the response rates
- schedule the next follow-up if necessary

Hegde, M. N. (1998). *Treatment procedures in communicative disorders* (3rd ed.). Austin, TX: Pro-Ed.

Treatment of Communicative Disorders: A General Sequence that Applies Across Disorders. Stepwise progression of treatment used in treating disorders of communication; the sequence may be based on response topography, response modes, multiple targets, training and maintenance, and response consequences.

- Sequence and simplify the target behaviors topographically
  - syllables or words
  - phrases
  - sentences that are imitated or otherwise controlled
  - sentences that are more spontaneously produced
  - sentences that are fully spontaneously produced
  - conversational speech
  - begin treatment at the simplest level that is necessary for the client; do not routinely start training at the syllable or word level; experiment to see if the client can manage at a higher level
- Sequence the response modes
  - begin treatment with imitation as the initial response mode if necessary
  - move to evoked responses
- Sequence the multiple targets
  - teach the most useful behaviors earlier than the less useful ones
  - teach the simpler behaviors earlier than the more complex behaviors
  - teach first behaviors that are building blocks for other behaviors
  - when one target behavior reaches the probe criterion, select another behavior or shift training to more complex level on the behavior under training
- Sequence training and maintenance strategies

- initially establish the behavior under structured clinical situations
- loosen the structure gradually and make treatment conditions more similar to natural conditions
- shift treatment to more natural conditions in and around the clinic
- shift training to natural conditions away from the clinic
- shift training to home situations, but do this as soon as possible (do not wait until the last stage of training)
- Sequence response consequences or feedback variations
  - give more frequent and consistent feedback in the beginning
  - reduce the amount of feedback as the learning stabilizes
  - give tangible reinforcers if necessary and only in the beginning
  - shift to social and more natural reinforcers
  - train others to give natural feedback in naturalistic settings

Hegde, M. N. (1998). *Treatment procedures in communicative disorders* (3rd ed.). Austin, TX: Pro-Ed.

Treatment of Communicative Disorders: Procedural Modifications.   Changes made in treatment procedures because of their ineffectiveness or less than optimum effectiveness; modifications may be made in antecedents, responses, and consequences; treatment procedures, not principles, are modified; based on performance data.

- Modification of antecedents
  - change stimuli that are ineffective in evoking the target responses
  - shift from pictures to objects
  - shift from line drawings to photographs
  - shift from abstract to concrete stimuli
  - shift from pictorial representation to enacted stimuli
  - discard clinical stimuli in favor of stimuli from the client's home
  - model if evoking is not effective

- prompt if evoking is not effective
- provide manual guidance (physical assistance to execute a response) if the evoking techniques are not effective
- give instructions and repeat them
- ask effective, common questions to evoke the responses
- rephrase ineffective questions
- Modification of responses
  - simplify the response if a more complex topographic feature is ineffective (too difficult)
  - if the target is not produced in sentences, shift downward in progressive steps
  - abandon training on a behavior that is too difficult for the client in favor of one that is easier; use the baseline data for guidance
  - abandon training on a behavior that is not imitated in favor of the one that is
  - return to abandoned behaviors at later date; shape them in small steps
- Modification of consequences
  - use the operational definition of consequences; events should increase behaviors to be called reinforcers; decrease to be called punishers or corrective
  - change consequating events that do not increase behaviors
  - change consequating events that do not decrease behaviors
  - use primary reinforcers if social consequences do not reinforce
  - shift back to social reinforcers after the behaviors are established
  - use tokens backed up by a variety of reinforcers if other forms fail
  - use biofeedback if other forms fail

Hegde, M. N. (1998). *Treatment procedures in communicative disorders* (3rd ed.). Austin, TX: Pro-Ed.

Treatment Evaluation. Testing the immediate effects and long-term efficacy of treatment procedures by controlled experimental analysis; an important criterion in treatment selection; see Treatment Selection Criteria; treatment evaluation involves:

- Group or single-subject experimental designs
- Comparison of treatment versus no treatment to show that treatment is better than no treatment
- Ruling-out of extraneous variables to show that it was the treatment, and not some other factor (e.g., maturation, teacher's work, parents' actions), responsible for the documented effects
- Replication by the experimenter and others to show that the technique is effective (or not effective) when applied in different settings, by different clinicians, and in treating different clients

Hegde, M. N. (1994). *Clinical research in communicative disorders: Principles and strategies* (2nd ed.). Austin, TX: Pro-Ed.

Treatment Evoked Trials. Structured and temporally separated opportunities for the client to produce a target response in the absence of clinician's modeling; useful in establishing target behaviors, especially with clients who perform better under a highly structured treatment session.

- Place stimulus item in front of client or demonstrate an action
- Ask the relevant predetermined question
- Wait a few seconds for client to respond
- If the response is correct, reinforce the client
- If the response is incorrect, give corrective feedback
- Record the response on the recording sheet
- Remove stimulus item
- Wait 2–3 seconds to signify the end of the trial
- Begin the next trial
- Calculate the percent correct response rate

Treatment Modeled Trials. Structured and temporally separated opportunities for the client to produce a target response when the clinician models the response for the client to imitate.

Treatment Selection Criteria

- Place a stimulus item in front of the client or demonstrate an action
- Ask the predetermined question
- Immediately model the correct response
- If the response is correct, reinforce the client
- If the response is incorrect, give corrective feedback
- Wait a few seconds for client to respond
- Record the response on the recording sheet
- Remove the stimulus item
- Wait 2–3 seconds to signify the end of the trial
- Calculate the percent correct response rate

Treatment Selection Criteria.   General guidelines on selecting treatment procedures; select procedures according to the following criteria.

General Comments About Treatment Selection.
Note that:

- Many treatment procedures in communicative disorders have not been experimentally tested to show that treatment is better than no treatment
- It is the ethical responsibility of clinicians to use techniques that have been shown to be effective in controlled experimental research
- It is necessary for clinicians to have a general knowledge of treatment research designs without which they cannot evaluate treatment procedures offered to them
- Many specialists vigorously advocate and offer "new and revolutionary" treatments in the absence of controlled experimental data
- Rejection of treatment procedures based solely on opinions, speculation, questionable theories, bandwagon, popularity, also is a clinician's ethical responsibility
- Technique that appears logical, appealing, likeable, and so forth may not necessarily be effective
- Widespread use of a technique is not an assurance of its effectiveness

- Certain unpopular techniques (e.g., time-out and response cost in the treatment of stuttering) are known to be effective, as shown by controlled research
- Speech-language pathology is not immune to faddish trends in treatment
- Getting on a bandwagon quickly is not the best sign of staying current in the discipline
- Some of the techniques you have been using with enthusiasm for years may never have been tested and may in fact be useless

Evaluating the Levels of Evidence to Select or Reject Treatment Procedures. Note that the criteria are hierarchically arranged based on the levels of evidence; a higher criterion is more stringent, more difficult to meet, although more preferable than a lower criterion; a treatment technique is accepted or rejected based on the level of evidence on which it is advocated:

- **Level 1. Expert Advocacy.** Some techniques are simply advocated by experts; no evidence of any kind is offered; may sound logical, appealing, and the advocate may be influential or well-known; reject all such procedures
- **Level 2. Unreplicated, uncontrolled case studies.** Some techniques may have been clinically tried with a few clients and a case study published; the study has not been repeated (replicated); no control groups or controlled conditions were used; clients have improved under treatment; no assurance that treatment was effective because extraneous variables have not been ruled out; because at least improvement with the technique was documented, you may select this type of treatment and use it with caution
- **Level 3. Replicated, uncontrolled case studies.** A technique has been applied more than once and multiple case studies have been published; no control groups

T

or controlled conditions yet; clients have improved under treatment; such a technique may be used, although no one can claim that the treatment is effective

- **Level 4. Unreplicated, controlled experimental studies.** The technique has been experimentally evaluated with a control group or a single-subject experimental design with control conditions; treatment was shown to be effective by ruling out extraneous variables; but the generality and applicability of the technique is unknown because it has not been applied in different settings by different clinicians (replication); clinician can use a technique that has been experimentally verified; not just improvement, but effectiveness is claimed for the technique

- **Level 5. Replicated, controlled experimental studies.** A technique has been shown to be effective in experimental research and then shown to have generality by repeating its application in different settings, by different clinicians, in treating a variety of clients; therefore, this technique is the most desirable; this is the kind of technique the clinician would want to select

Hegde, M. N. (1994). *Clinical research in communicative disorders: Principles and strategies* (2nd ed.). Austin, TX: Pro-Ed.

Treatment Targets. Skills or behaviors that are taught to clients during treatment.

- Select treatment targets after a thorough assessment
- Select functional targets that are useful to the client
- Select targets that are linguistically and culturally appropriate to the client
- Select skills that can make an immediate and socially significant difference in the communicative skills of the client
- Select behaviors that serve as building blocks for more complex functional skills

Treatment or Teaching Versus Stimulation. See <u>Stimulation Versus Treatment or Teaching</u>.

Treatment Variables.   Technical operations performed by the clinician to create, increase, or decrease behaviors; these include:
- Antecedents or stimuli used in treatment, including modeling, instructions, demonstrations, manual guidance, pictures, objects, recreated events, storytelling (by the clinician), topics of conversation, and so forth
- Consequences or feedback the clinician gives, including verbal praise, tokens, tangible reinforcers, opportunities to indulge in various activities, privileges offered by parents, and so forth

Tremor.   A pattern of shaking, defined as an involuntary rhythmical movement of small amplitude.

Trials.   Measurable sequentially repeatable opportunities to produce a response; may be more or less structured; include Baseline Evoked Trials, Baseline Modeled Trials, Treatment Evoked Trials, and Treatment Modeled Trials.

Hegde, M. N. (1998). *Treatment procedures in communicative disorders* (3rd ed.). Austin, TX: Pro-Ed.

T

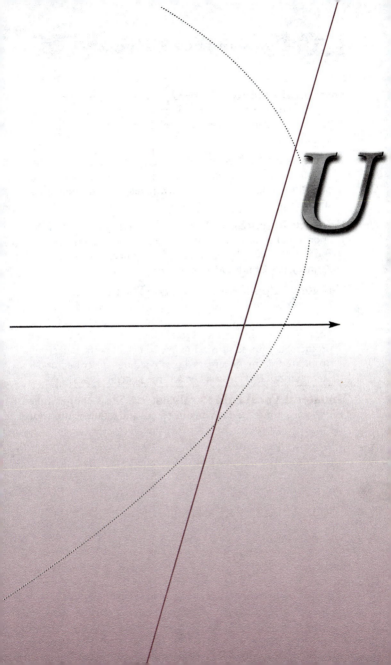

Unconditioned Reinforcers.   Reinforcers whose effects do not depend on past learning or conditioning (e.g., food items); the same as Primary Reinforcers; see Conditioned Reinforcers.

Unconditioned Response.   A response given to unconditioned stimulus; typically a response without a conditioning or learning history (e.g., salivary response to food in the mouth); see Conditioned Response.

Unconditioned Stimulus.   A stimulus that elicits a response without the benefit of conditioning or learning (e.g., food in the mouth that automatically elicits a salivary response); see Conditioned Stimulus.

Unilateral Upper Motor Neuron Dysarthria.   A type of motor speech disorder; its neuropathology is damage to the upper motor neurons that supply cranial and spinal nerves involved in speech production; the dominant speech problem is imprecise production of consonants; select appropriate treatment targets and procedures described under Treatment of Dysarthria; Dysarthria: Specific Types.

Unilateral Vocal Fold Paralysis.   Paralysis of one of the two vocal folds; leads to breathy voice and reduced intensity.

U

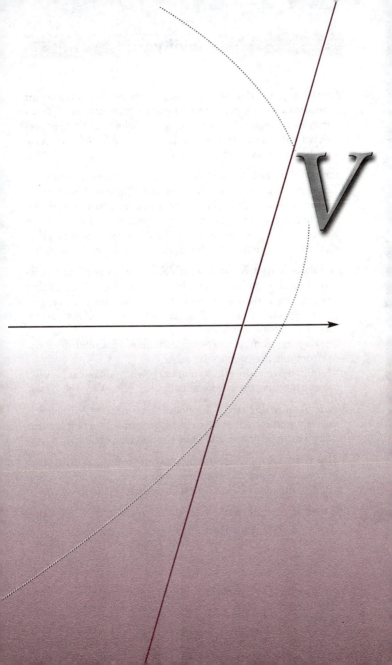

V

Validity. The degree to which a measuring instrument measures what it purports to measure; treatment procedures may have Logical Validity, Empirical Validity, or both; procedures that have empirical validity are preferable to those with only logical validity.

Variable Interval Schedule (VI). An intermittent reinforcement schedule in which the time duration between reinforcers is varied around an average; not as applicable as the Fixed Interval or Variable Ratio Schedules in the treatment of communicative disorders; difficult to use in routine clinical work; efficient with electronic programming equipment.

Variable Ratio Schedule (VR). An intermittent reinforcement schedule in which the number of responses needed to earn a reinforcer is varied around an average; more effective in generating response rates that last; useful in a maintenance strategy.
- Vary the number of responses required for reinforcement from one occasion to the other
- Initially, reinforce on a smaller ratio schedule (e.g., a VR_4) and increase the ratio gradually (e.g., VR_6, VR_8, VR_{12}, etc.)

Velar Assimilation. A phonological process in which a velar sound is used in place of a nonvelar sound (e.g., /g/ for /d/); see Articulation and Phonological Disorders.

Velar Fronting. A phonological process in which velar sounds are replaced by nonvelar sounds (e.g., /t/ for /k/); see Articulation and Phonological Disorders.

Velopharyngeal Insufficiency. Also known as velopharyngeal incompetence, a clinical condition in which the velopharyngeal mechanism cannot adequately close the velopharyngeal port, resulting in hypernasal speech; see Cleft Palate.

Ventricular Dysphonia. A voice disorder resulting from the use of the ventricular (false) vocal folds for phonation;

- Select facial, neck, and head muscles for relaxation training; ask the client to relax one set of muscles and tense them to appreciate the difference
- Manipulate head positions to induce relaxation
- Ask the client to imagine speaking situations that induce greater tension and immediately let the client relax the speech muscles
- Use relaxing head movements (positions) if necessary
- Use other appropriate voice therapy techniques in combination with relaxation
- Stabilize a relaxed speaking posture and improved voice quality

Respiration Training. Teaching clients to manage inhalation–exhalation cycles optimally for the purpose of phonation and sustained vocalization; recommended for clients with functional voice disorders who do not seem to use their breath stream properly in voice production.

- Explain the relation between breathing and speaking and between airflow and vocal fold vibrations
- Teach the client to inhale more quickly, more deeply than usual but exhale more slowly and in a controlled manner; to extend exhalation, ask the client to count to 5 slowly and then to 10 slowly
- Ask the client to prolong vowels to teach controlled and prolonged exhalation that would better support speech; in progressive steps, teach the client to prolong a vowel for about 20 seconds
- Teach the client to inhale quickly between utterances
- Teach good posture, which promotes normal airflow management

Tongue Position Modification. Manipulating tongue position in the oral cavity to affect changes in voice quality and resonance; tongue typically positioned too far back results in cul-de-sac resonance; tongue typically carried too far forward creates "thin voice" giving the baby talk effect.

- Teach clients to carry tongue in its neutral position
- Modify the excessively backward tongue position
- Modify the excessively forward tongue position
- Instruct, model, demonstrate, and reinforce correct tongue positions

Vocal Rest. A voice therapy technique that requires little or no talking, typically for 4–7 days; vocal rest may be complete or partial.

- Recommend mandatory vocal rest for clients who have undergone any form of laryngeal surgery; this helps promote normal healing of the surgical wounds
- Recommend vocal rest as initial treatment for clients who have such types of laryngeal lesions as vocal fold hemorrhage and mucosal tear to let the healing process begin
- Recommend partial (modified) vocal rest for clients who have a severe cold (and resulting laryngeal inflammation), vocal nodules, and vocal fold edema; note that partial vocal rest means talking only when absolutely essential and with appropriate vocal habits
- Instruct the client either to totally avoid or markedly reduce
  - speaking
  - shouting or screaming
  - singing or humming
  - whispering
  - coughing or throat clearing
  - laughing or crying
  - lifting or pushing heavy objects
- Have a family member monitor these activities
- Teach the client to keep a record of such activities
- Teach the client to self-monitor

Warble Tone Approach. A voice treatment method in which the vocal pitch is constantly and continually shifted up and down to move the client out of the habitual monotonous pitch and thus to establish a pitch that is more appropriate to the client; recommended for clients with hoarse, strained, breathy, or rough voice regardless of its origin.

- Using a visual feedback device (such as the Visi-Pitch), model a tone that is varied up and down in pitch and ask the client to imitate what you model
- Ask the client to produce the vowel /i/, constantly varying the pitch (loudness should also vary with it); when the most desirable tone is heard, ask the client to extend it
- Begin fading the warble tone after a few successful trials; ask the client to reduce the warble portion of the tone and extend the steady, desirable portion of the tone; give several trials
- Withdraw the warble completely and have the client practice the desirable steady tone
- Introduce phrases with vowel-initial sounds in the first word of the phrase (e.g., *even now, easy day*), and ask the client to produce them with the new steady, desirable voice
- Use more complex utterances and sentences to stabilize the new voice

Whisper-Phonation Method. A voice therapy technique that uses <u>Prephonation Airflow</u> to reduce <u>Hard Glottal Attack;</u> the client is required to whisper sustained vowel productions; gentle phonation is introduced as the vowel is being sustained.

- Ask the client to whisper monosyllabic words that have vowel initiates
- Teach the client to whisper the initial vowel very gently

- Introduce gentle phonation as the end of the vowel is prolonged
- Gradually increase the loudness of the whisper until phonation is introduced
- Teach the client to blend the whisper into a soft phonation
- Reinforce speaking in a relaxed, breathy voice

Yawn-Sigh Method. A voice therapy technique for clients with hypervocal function; uses the relaxing effects of the inspiratory yawn followed by an expiratory sigh and phonation.

- Instruct and demonstrate the relaxing effects of prolonged inspiration involved in a yawn and the relaxed phonation that results with a sigh
- Ask the client to yawn and then exhale slowly while phonating lightly
- Ask the client to say words that start with /h/ after each yawn
- Teach the client to produce a gentle, voiced sigh while exhaling
- Teach the client to produce an easy, prolonged, open-mouthed exhalation after each yawn
- Ask the client to skip the yawn and teach the client to inhale normally and exhale a prolonged sigh with the open mouth
- Ask the patient to say "hah" after beginning each sigh
- Ask the patient to say additional words all beginning with the glottal /h/
- Ask the patient to blend in an easy, relaxed, phonation during the middle of a sigh
- Fade the sigh and move on to words, phrases, and sentences

Andrews, M. L. (1999). *Manual of voice treatment: Pediatrics through geriatrics* (2nd ed.). San Diego: Singular Publishing Group.

Boone, D. R., & McFarlane, S. C. (2000). *The voice and voice therapy* (6th ed.). Boston: Allyn & Bacon.

Case, J. L. (1996). *Clinical management of voice disorders.* Austin, TX: Pro-Ed.

Deem, J. F., & Miller, L. (2000). *Manual of voice therapy* (2nd ed.). Austin, TX: Pro-Ed.

Voice Prosthesis.   A small (1.8 to 3.6 cm) silicone device that has a valve at the back end and an opening at the front end; inserted into the tracheoesophageal puncture in patients who have undergone laryngectomy; allows air into the esophagus, which vibrates; the sound is shaped into speech; see <u>Laryngectomy.</u>

Voluntary Stuttering.   A treatment target in fluent stuttering approach of Van Riper; for procedures see <u>Stuttering, Treatment; Treatment of Stuttering: Specific Techniques or Programs.</u>

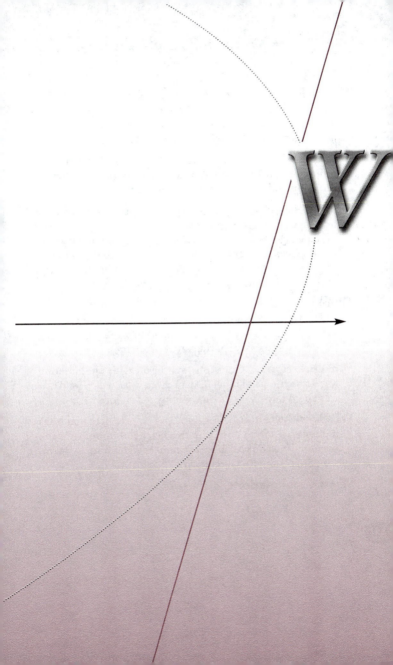

Wernicke's Aphasia. A type of aphasia caused by lesions in Wernicke's area; characterized by fluent but meaningless speech, with impaired comprehension of speech; see Aphasia; Treatment of Aphasia: Specific Types.

Wernicke's Area. The posterior portion of the superior temporal gyrus in the left hemisphere responsible for formulation and comprehension of language.

Whole Language Approach. An approach to teaching language and literacy that requires the teaching of all aspects of language (speaking, reading, writing) simultaneously; lacking in experimental support and now highly questioned; see Language Disorders in Children; Treatment of Language Disorders: Specific Techniques or Programs.

Whole Word Accuracy (WWA). A criterion measure used in multiple-phoneme approach of articulation treatment; the entire word is judged for accuracy (as against judging the accuracy of only the target phoneme).

Wh-Questions. Questions that begin with wh-; interrogative statements that begin with *what, when, where,* and *who*; treatment targets for language impaired children.

Wireless Systems. Assistive Listening Devices that transmit messages from a speaker to a listener without wire connections; include FM auditory trainers and infrared systems; see under Aural Rehabilitation.

Word Combinations. The same as Phrases.

Hegde's
PocketGuide to
Treatment in
Speech-Language Pathology